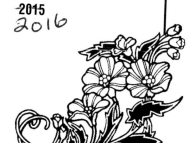

WILLIAM B. FARRAR MEMORIAL COLLECTION

In Memory Of

BLANCHE A. FARRAR, HIS MOTHER and

HENRY B. FARRAR, HIS FATHER

~~2015~~
2016

© DEMCO, INC. 1990 PRINTED IN U.S.A.

IT HAPPENED TO ME

Series Editor: Arlene Hirschfelder

Books in the It Happened to Me series are designed for inquisitive teens digging for answers about certain illnesses, social issues, or lifestyle interests. Whether you are deep into your teen years or just entering them, these books are gold mines of up-to-date information, riveting teen views, and great visuals to help you figure out stuff. Besides special boxes highlighting singular facts, each book is enhanced with the latest reading lists, websites, and an index. Perfect for browsing, there are loads of expert information by acclaimed writers to help parents, guardians, and librarians understand teen illness, tough situations, and lifestyle choices.

1. *Epilepsy: The Ultimate Teen Guide,* by Kathlyn Gay and Sean McGarrahan, 2002.
2. *Stress Relief: The Ultimate Teen Guide,* by Mark Powell, 2002.
3. *Learning Disabilities: The Ultimate Teen Guide,* by Penny Hutchins Paquette and Cheryl Gerson Tuttle, 2003.
4. *Making Sexual Decisions: The Ultimate Teen Guide,* by L. Kris Gowen, 2003.
5. *Asthma: The Ultimate Teen Guide,* by Penny Hutchins Paquette, 2003.
6. *Cultural Diversity—Conflicts and Challenges: The Ultimate Teen Guide,* by Kathlyn Gay, 2003.
7. *Diabetes: The Ultimate Teen Guide,* by Katherine J. Moran, 2004.
8. *When Will I Stop Hurting? Teens, Loss, and Grief: The Ultimate Teen Guide to Dealing with Grief,* by Ed Myers, 2004.
9. *Volunteering: The Ultimate Teen Guide,* by Kathlyn Gay, 2004.
10. *Organ Transplants—A Survival Guide for the Entire Family: The Ultimate Teen Guide,* by Tina P. Schwartz, 2005.
11. *Medications: The Ultimate Teen Guide,* by Cheryl Gerson Tuttle, 2005.
12. *Image and Identity—Becoming the Person You Are: The Ultimate Teen Guide,* by L. Kris Gowen and Molly C. McKenna, 2005.
13. *Apprenticeship: The Ultimate Teen Guide,* by Penny Hutchins Paquette, 2005.
14. *Cystic Fibrosis: The Ultimate Teen Guide,* by Melanie Ann Apel, 2006.
15. *Religion and Spirituality in America: The Ultimate Teen Guide,* by Kathlyn Gay, 2006.
16. *Gender Identity: The Ultimate Teen Guide,* by Cynthia L. Winfield, 2007.

EATING DISORDERS

THE ULTIMATE TEEN GUIDE

JESSICA R. GREENE

IT HAPPENED TO ME, NO. 39

ROWMAN & LITTLEFIELD
Lanham • Boulder • New York • London

Published by Rowman & Littlefield
4501 Forbes Boulevard, Suite 200, Lanham, Maryland 20706
www.rowman.com

10 Thornbury Road, Plymouth PL6 7PP, United Kingdom

British Library Cataloguing in Publication Information Available

Library of Congress Cataloging-in-Publication Data

Greene, Jessica R., 1964– author.
  Eating disorders : the ultimate teen guide / Jessica R. Greene.
    pages cm. — (It happened to me ; no. 39)
  Includes bibliographical references and index.
  ISBN 978-0-8108-8773-2 (cloth : alk. paper) — ISBN 978-0-8108-8774-9 (ebook) 1. Eating disorders in adolescence—Popular works. 2. Teenagers—Life skill guides. I. Title.
  RJ506.E18G74 2014
  616.85'2600835—dc 3   2014005390

∞™ The paper used in this publication meets the minimum requirements of American National Standard for Information Sciences—Permanence of Paper for Printed Library Materials, ANSI/NISO Z39.48-1992. Printed in the United States of America

Contents

Acknowledgments

I'm extraordinarily grateful to everyone whose efforts made the creation of this book possible, these individuals in particular:

Dr. Timothy Brewerton, Carolyn Costin, Dr. Michael P. Levine (the great triumvirate of ED specialists), Lynn S. Grefe, Dr. Kimberly Dennis, Dr. Joel Jahraus, and Kourtney Gordon took time from their professional lives to contribute their expertise.

Harriet Brown, Dr. Cynthia Bulik, Kjerstin Gruys, and Ryan K. Sallans are incredibly generous.

Darryl Roberts and Christopher Hines are as awesome as the work they do.

Carolyn Jennings rocks as a writer, cheerleader, and friend.

Mark Taris gave me the confidence to complete the odyssey, granted me leave, and then welcomed me back.

Anya Chrystal at EDC; Diana Kalogridis, Maggi Flaherty, Yasemin Merwede, and Claire Mysko at NEDA; Aimee-Leigh Lerett at Hal Leonard Corporation; Ilse Jung at the Museum of Art History–Vienna; and Chris Wild at Retronaut helped make the pages come to life.

Every writer should be blessed with wonderful readers to critique and proofread work in progress. Thank you, Kelly Miller, Chris Coad Taylor, Lisa Vogt, and Larry Judd. Joni Fisher gave her time in the early stages of the manuscript. Carmen Cool came to my rescue in the eleventh hour.

Arlene Hirschfelder, Christen Karniski, Stephen Ryan, Jessica McCleary, and Debra Kass-Orenstein are the nuts and bolts of this project.

Last, but never least, thanks to Chris and Libby, who keep my light on.

Permissions

Chapter 3

"Perfect"
Lyrics by Alanis Morissette
Music by Alanis Morissette and Glen Ballard
Copyright © 1995 SONGS OF UNIVERSAL, INC., VANHURST PLACE, UNIVERSAL MUSIC CORP. and AEROSTATION CORPORATION

Chapter 5

Chapter 7

Chapter 8

Prologue: Eating Disorder Issues and Attitudes

What's Eating You?

When was the last time you heard someone say, "How many calories are in that?" Or "I hate the way my stomach sticks out." Or "If I could just lose ten pounds, my life would be perfect." We hear statements like these all the time. They echo across America, showing our preoccupation with eating choices, body appearance, and self-control. Usually, our choices about food—what, when, and how much to eat—and criticisms about how we look are momentary concerns. They are only a few of our many daily decisions and debates that leave little lasting impression. We hear them so often, and think such similar thoughts ourselves, we rarely recognize that the underlying emotions are not so healthy.

Teens everywhere consider issues surrounding healthy eating, fitness, and personal image as they evaluate what kind of life to lead and what kind of person to be. Parents, peers, food advertisers, health educators, and pop culture icons shower you with conflicting messages about what to like, what to buy, and how to improve yourself. You want to please your friends and your parents and still be comfortable with your choices. The information is overwhelming, filled with assumptions and half-truths. Processing it all is complicated. On top of this, for some teens, the feelings about self-image become obsessive, and behaviors concerning eating and exercise can go wildly out of control. I know what that's like because it happened to me. At the age of seventeen, I was diagnosed with an eating disorder. Recovery took years, as the eating disorder morphed from anorexia to binge eating to what I called "bulimia around the edges." As any sufferer will tell you, although our attention appears to be focused on controlling how we eat and the size and shape of our bodies, we are troubled by our emotions and are seeking to feel whole and valued in an imperfect world. The issues and attitudes take time and effort to repair in order to become healthy again.

This book focuses on issues and attitudes that most concern you about eating behaviors. It shows the road signs that lead to full-blown eating disorders, and determines who is most susceptible to developing one. It suggests why they happen, what it's like to have one, and how widespread they are. It also examines the issue of companion disorders—mental illness, substance abuse, and compulsive

Anorexic, Anorectic, Anoretic

Which is it?

We typically use the word *anorexic* to name someone with the illness of *anorexia nervosa* ("Eve's an anorexic"), or to describe the look and behaviors of someone showing signs of the disease ("Adam is anorexic"). In fact, the proper use of *anorexic* is as an adjective, so only the latter sentence is technically correct.

Anorectic (also *anoretic*) is the regular medical noun for a person diagnosed with anorexia, as in "Anorectics struggle with making food choices and determining how much to eat." It's also the term for something that depresses appetite (an appetite suppressant, or *anorexigenic*).

This book makes the distinction between the uses of these words. Whether it's wise to refer to anyone with a psychological illness by the name of the disorder (e.g., anorexic/anorectic, bulimic, binge eater, etc.) is a question we'll consider toward the end of chapter 3.

behavior that co-occur with disordered eating. You'll discover that true eating disorders are behavioral adaptations, similar in many respects to alcohol or drug dependency, carrying most of the same risk factors and requiring intervention and specialty therapy in order to recover. The book guides you through the historical legacy of disordered eating (Hey, it's always been with us!) and uncovers societal and cultural views on food choice, eating habits, and body consciousness. It even explains the consequences of long-term malnutrition, food abuse, and obesity (which may not be rising to the epidemic proportions previously predicted). Lastly, it investigates the kind of help that's available and takes a look at the process of recovery from those on the front lines of the battle to regain good health.

Here you'll find some of the latest research in behavioral health and statistics about America's "food-aholism," and explore feelings about eating and body image from teens around the world. Besides straightforward, frank discussion of

Here's an Extra Scoop

Eating disorders are misdirected strategies for coping with emotional issues, dressed up as an obsession with food, appetite, and body image.

> ## America's Diet Obsession
>
> Food advertisers spend millions on advertising, luring us to consume everything from peanut butter to pizza. Americans indulge, then spend *billions* of dollars per year on weight loss products and diet programs—around $60.5 billion in 2013, according to the market research firm Marketdata.[a]

what researchers have learned since the 1980s, you'll notice quick facts, quizzes, opposing viewpoints, case reports, celebrity profiles, topics for discussion with friends and family, and lots of quotes from health experts, family members, and teens speaking out about their experiences. Key terms appear in italics and are defined in the glossary, should you like further clarification.

Statements made by some of the sufferers may seem controversial, but they are only expressing true thoughts and feelings. For those who have never experienced an addiction, the mind-set of someone with an eating disorder may seem strange. Even doctors and therapists have difficulty understanding the complexities and often make inappropriate assumptions and remarks. What you'll discover here should help you become wiser about the nature of both disordered eating and true eating disorders, and should give you insight on what you can do to protect your health or the health of someone you care about.

America is obsessed with food and image. Many health advocates believe that the emphasis on food consumption, dieting, and fitness has reached a crescendo, pushing the buttons of those most vulnerable to eating disorders and turning all disordered eating into a public health crisis. Carolyn Costin, founder and director of Monte Nido® Treatment Centers and Affiliates, said it best: "In our current cultural climate, instead of asking, 'Why do so many people develop eating disorders?' one wonders, 'How is it that anyone, especially a female, does *not* develop one?'"[1]

Special Note from the Author

This book is intended as a thoughtful discussion on the subject of eating problems that arise in the teenage and early adult years. It is meant to add to your knowledge and understanding of the eating disorder spectrum, deepen your compassion, and stimulate conversation with others. It is not a diagnostic tool or proponent of any treatment method, or intended to glamorize the illness.

Everyone who struggles with eating issues experiences illness through an individual set of circumstances. Thus the road into and out of an eating disorder is unique to the person who has one. If you're feeling any serious distress or

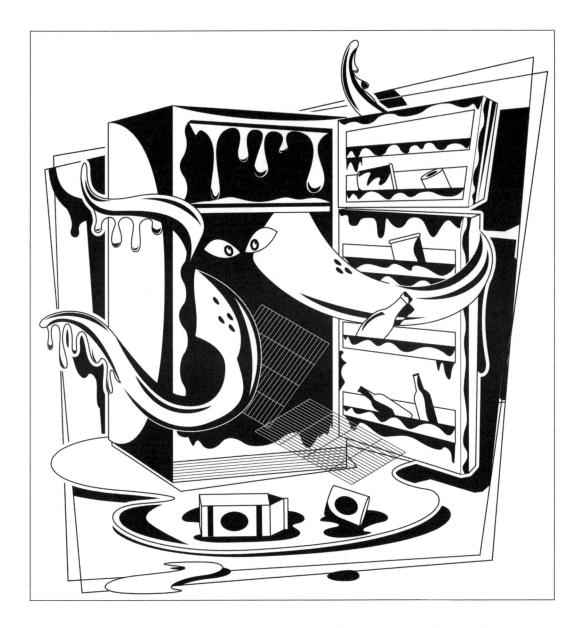

consequences from obsessive thoughts and activity around food and eating, I hope you'll seek the advice of a trustworthy professional in the field of psychological health. If you're a family member or concerned friend, I hope this text will prompt you to get the support you need to help your loved one.

I've drawn on many people's experiences in examining the current issues and attitudes, and have incorporated assertions from experts, as well as testimony from sufferers and those who love them. They have great insight that is important to highlight. The voice of Ruth is me. I'm recovered from my eating disorder—you'll learn part of the story in chapter 1.

EATING TO EXTREMES: MENTAL DISORDER OR LIFESTYLE CHOICE?

How do we define eating disorders? How do you know if you have one? How common are they? Are they really a sickness or a matter of personal preference? Explore attitudes about food, weight, and disordered eating from experts and teen contributors.

Food is central to our lives. No matter where you go, everyone you meet has an opinion about it. On any given day, you can find a seemingly endless array of cooking shows, blog posts, and web videos that tell us how to fix the tastiest recipes and how good food makes us feel. On other days, a host of experts give us the latest tips for staying fit and healthy. Eat low fat, low salt, no added sugar. Count carbs, count *calories*, get washboard abs. The conflicting information drives us all nuts. And every day, images of magazine models, celebrity actors, and sports stars relay to us what our bodies are supposed to look like. Haven't you got enough to worry about?

We must eat to live. Not only must a body satisfy nutritional needs for good health and caloric needs for energy, but food and eating are part of human culture. Food also feeds our emotional experience. The feelings we have about eating influence our everyday choices about what, when, and how much to eat, and whether we enjoy it. These feelings can cut into the natural and normal desires for food. Many who have experienced an eating disorder describe it as a voice inside their head, very real and very strong. It might insist they deserve to eat only a grilled chicken leg, a tablespoon of rice, and three peas for dinner, or it might say it's all right to pig out after a bad day at school. That's what it's like to have an eating disorder. I know this, because it happened to me.

Eating Disorder or Just Alternative Eating?

Have you ever skipped meals because you're trying to lose weight? Do you reward yourself with a favorite food when you do something good, or eat to feel better when you're feeling sad? Do you ever feel guilty for eating "fattening" foods, or judge your body size and shape against what you see in pictures or videos? You're not alone. We're a nation of funky eaters with disordered patterns of thinking about food and body weight. Being light and willowy, if you're female, or muscled and taut, if you're male, can become entrenched in our minds as the way to feel better about who we are. Thanks to society's emphasis on the value of a perfect physique, marketers' desire to sell food products, and our own cultural eating experiences, we're encouraged to build intense relationships with what we put in our mouths. Just about everyone makes a connection between food and emotion—as we'll see in chapter 2, human brain evolution has encouraged this development. Problems with eating can arise when you link how you feel about yourself to what you think about food and body size. Given various biological and environmental influences, you may be vulnerable to developing an eating disorder.

Having an *eating disorder* (ED) shows a preoccupation with self-image and self-control. This intense focus interferes with your physical and psychological health through an increasing obsession with eating and body weight. People can exhibit a wide variety of alternative eating characteristics, so there's a good deal of debate about the underlying causes and how best to define and categorize symptoms. Health professionals must have a standard method for making a proper diagnosis so patients can be treated appropriately. Although physicians have been treating people with "wasting disease" and atypical eating behaviors since the late nineteenth century, the psychiatric profession did not consider eating problems as a mental disorder until 1980. Since then, the American Psychiatric Association (APA) has continually refined the criteria for diagnosing *anorexia nervosa*, *bulimia nervosa*, *binge eating disorder*, and other forms that recognize abnormal and unhealthy eating behaviors. The *DSM-5* (*Diagnostic and Statistical Manual of Mental Disorders*, fifth edition) is the latest edition of the official textbook that clinicians use to determine who has an ED and who doesn't. Although many millions of people exhibit poor eating habits, such as skipping meals, or spend a lot of time at the gym or playing sports or even say they are "addicted" to food, it's often impossible to know from casual observation whether their body size or behaviors indicate a specifically classified ED.

Unusual eating behavior has been a part of human culture and religious practices since the beginning of recorded history. Until recently, however, public stigma of people with weird food choices and extreme eating patterns has inhibited research funding and has limited options for treatment. Clinicians and families alike have suspected teenagers—particularly girls and young women—

What Is the *DSM*?

Published by the APA, the *DSM* (*Diagnostic and Statistical Manual of Mental Disorders*) is used by mental health professionals to classify the signs and symptoms of psychological disturbances in patients needing treatment. All established mental disorders are numerically coded and defined using specific criteria—descriptions of physical and behavioral features, plus details pertaining to age, culture, and family environment. Besides clinicians and medical researchers, drug regulators, legislators, and health insurance and pharmaceutical company officials also consult the book when determining new policies. Assigned work groups evaluate the new information and propose changes to the text to improve the volume's validity and reliability as research studies uncover more details about mental illnesses.

The new edition, the *DSM-5*, published in May 2013, has reorganized and reinterpreted the section relevant to eating disorders as a result of documented observations and field studies made since the mid-1990s. The chapter lists eight categories of Feeding and Eating Disorders:

1. Pica
2. Rumination Disorder
3. Avoidant/Restrictive Food Intake Disorder (ARFID)
4. Anorexia Nervosa (AN)
5. Bulimia Nervosa (BN)
6. Binge Eating Disorder (BED)
7. Other Specified Feeding or Eating Disorder (OSFED)
8. Unspecified Feeding or Eating Disorder (UFED)

OSFED and UFED have reclassified the former EDNOS (Eating Disorders Not Otherwise Specified) distinction. OSFED recognizes variants of the main disorders, such as *purging disorder* and *night eating syndrome*, and forms of anorexia, bulimia, and binge eating that don't meet the threshold of the main definitions.

UFED is a catch-all term for everything else. Together, they are referred to as EDNEC (*Feeding and*) *Eating Disorders Not Elsewhere Classified.*

Dr. Timothy Walsh, chair of the committee that proposed the changes to the old *DSM-IV*, has said the new diagnostic criteria more closely identify the symptoms doctors and therapists see in their practices. He insists the research has shown that binge eating disorder is an actual pathology, and not idiosyncratic eating habits by people tempted with cheesecake or barbecued ribs. "[Binge eating] disorder is really a phenomenon of frequently eating an abnormal amount combined with feelings of shame, guilt, or disgust. The behavior is recurrent, and it feels wrong. It's that combination of factors that distinguish it from the overeating that we all occasionally do."[a]

of starving themselves on purpose for attention, or of lacking willpower when presented with overly tempting food items. Although these misconceptions and other myths still exist, increased public awareness and extensive research in a wide variety of clinical studies and surveys are changing that attitude. Results of a Zogby America poll taken in 2002 showed that nearly half of all Americans personally know someone with an eating disorder.[1] The National Eating Disorders Association (NEDA) reports that over 80 percent of Americans believe that eating disorders are serious illnesses that require treatment and, like any other physical illness, should receive insurance coverage.[2]

Many mental health professionals recognize EDs as one of many types of disordered activity that is symptomatic of *addiction.* In fact, scientists who study addiction medicine believe much compulsive behavior is severe enough to qualify as behavioral addiction. This includes disordered patterns of eating that fall into EDNEC, the category of unspecified eating conditions.

How Can You Tell Whether You or Someone You Know Has a True Eating Disorder, or Merely Quirky Eating Habits?

Good question! It can be confusing. Eating disorders arise gradually and take their toll on individuals in unique ways. Sometimes strange eating habits lead to eating disorders, sometimes not. Mental health is a spectrum; you can't tell what is happening inside someone's head, or predict how deeply one will progress into mental disorder. And, like many with addictive behaviors, sufferers can become well practiced in hiding abnormal signs from public view. The most important signs to note are those that significantly impact the quality of life. Answer the following questions with *always*, *sometimes*, or *never*.

Are you, or someone you know,

- obsessed with food amounts, food choices, and eating rituals
- highly self-critical, especially of body size and shape
- afraid of becoming fat or of losing control of your hunger
- binging on foods to feel better
- purging food through vomiting, use of laxatives or diuretics, or expending calories through continual exercise
- isolating from family and friends, either to eat in secret or to avoid eating altogether
- constantly thinking how to change your weight to become a better person or more like the images of people around you

The more often you answer "always," the more likely it is you have, or are on the way to developing, an eating disorder.

There are places online to learn what to watch for when identifying the potential for, or presence of, an eating disorder. Eating disorder associations and information referral centers in the United States and Canada are usually reliable sources. Treatment centers for eating disorders often have questionnaires that help evaluate signs and symptoms and determine if you should speak to a physician or mental health professional. Check out the self-evaluation quiz offered by the Klarman Center at McLean Hospital in Belmont, Massachusetts (see "More Food for Thought" at the end of the chapter).

Keep in mind, holiday overeating and occasional fasting are not classifiable mental illnesses. Neither is *disordered eating*—habits such as eating only once per day (or constant grazing), eating only a few types of foods, or maintaining strict food rituals. Disordered eating, though, is a gateway to a full-blown eating disorder. Borderline eating disorder activity patterns not only put you at risk for a host of behavioral disorders, but also make you more vulnerable to troublesome health problems. Severely deviant eating practices and abuse of food can lead to

Here's an Extra Scoop

Disordered eating—a term first identified in 1992 by the Women's Task Force of the American College of Sports Medicine[b]—is a serious health issue. It refers to a range of unhealthy eating practices that over time can damage body organs, lead to bone loss, and even cause early death.

serious illnesses such as heart disease and diabetes mellitus (type 2 diabetes), but even moderate food craziness leads to *malnutrition* that'll negatively impact your health in years to come.

Think of it like this—not everyone who boozes becomes an alcoholic. Not everyone who smokes or does drugs becomes a hard-core addict. But substance abuse takes its toll on a body, nevertheless, and the same is true for someone whose diet is continually out of whack. Whether or not a food abuser is categorically eating disordered, there's a good chance she'll eventually suffer ailments related to

Ruth's Remembrance

At the age of seventeen years, two months, eighteen days, I was practically a walking skeleton. I had huge eyes, hollow cheeks, and butt cheeks that failed to touch. I could feel the bones in my feet when I ran, and the skin over my arms had shrunk so much around the remaining sticks, the long veins stood out. Normally active, healthy, and never overweight as a child, I'd begun putting on extra pounds in high school. Since the age of thirteen, I'd tried to diet—mildly, haphazardly, never seriously, and without real success. This changed after I turned sixteen and moved with my family to spend a year in Europe. The regimen exploded into an obsession of calorie counting and distance running, and I steadily shed almost a third of my original body weight. Convinced I had cancer, my mom brought me to our pediatrician within days of arriving home. He diagnosed me with anorexia nervosa and directed me to the only in-patient hospital program in the state that was equipped for treating self-starved teenagers in the 1980s. "Put her to bed," he told my parents. "Don't let her move, and pray that she lives through the weekend."

I spent eight weeks in the hospital ward, sharing daily conversation, group therapy, and quiet meals with other anoretic girls who ranged in age from twelve to twenty. I was afraid of gaining weight and that I wouldn't be able to stop eating, but I didn't want a feeding tube, so I went with the program. I figured I could lose weight again after I got out, because I knew how to do it. I just needed to be pulled back from the brink of death. I left the hospital having regained half the weight I'd lost. I meant to finish high school, leave for college, and be independent, which I did, even though I continued to struggle with eating and exercise issues for years afterward.[c]

nutritional deficits and imbalances. Amy, twenty-three, of Boston, lived in this wilderness of disordered eating. "I eat the same thing every day: yogurt. I love the way it tastes. It's the perfect food," she said. She carefully spooned fat-free, plain yogurt into her mouth. By the end of the meal, she had downed a pound of yogurt. For lunch. Nothing else. This meal resembled almost all of what Amy had been eating for months. Yogurt, yogurt, and more yogurt. "Occasionally, I'll eat a bagel or drink some coffee," she admitted.[3]

The American College of Sports Medicine characterizes disordered eating as continual restrictive dieting or binging and purging for the purposes of weight control, although not at a frequency or intensity that would be considered a psychological disturbance. This behavior is widespread, and many of us know it well. "At the age of twenty-five, I can honestly say that the majority of the young women I know have either full-blown eating disorders or screwed-up attitudes toward food and fitness," wrote blogger and author Courtney Martin in 2007. "This is the daily reality of the women in my immediate circle of friends. Even those who I thought might be safe from the powerful distraction of the scale turn out to be affected once I start asking."[4]

Ruth's story on page 6 is my own, so I am one of the lucky ones. I had dipped into a deadly psychological disease and needed help to recover. Eating disorders have the highest mortality rate of all mental illnesses. The APA reported in 1993[5] that 5–10 percent of those with anorexia nervosa die within ten years of being diagnosed, 18–20 percent are dead within twenty years.[6] That's one or two out of every ten. Less than one half of people with any type of ED report ever being cured. Victims die young as a result of medical complications and from outright suicide. Studies of eating disorder outcomes have estimated that anorexia and bulimia cause early death from twelve to eighteen times the normal death rate of anyone else in the sufferer's age group. Some specialists suspect the mortality rate may be highest for those whose eating conditions are classified as OSFED or UFED. For those who have suffered from an ED a very long time, chronic malnutrition leads to organ failure, even when the body is not deathly thin.

So, How Common Are EDs, Really?

That depends on whom you ask. Estimating the prevalence of mental health disorders is not easy. *Prevalence* tells us how many people (or proportion of people) in a population are afflicted by a disease. Health statistics in the United States are based on independent research studies and surveys of people who come forward to take them. Some of these studies are funded by the government, some by private health foundations. Studies of mental health disorders rarely agree and there is no central reporting agency to track and interpret the data. There is plenty of inconsistency across the many thousands of eating disorder–related reports.

All findings have their special limiting factors, such as a small sample size and participant recidivism (dropout rate). Even the criteria used to define the eating disorders being investigated can be biased. Certain studies examine only one race or nationality. Some pertain only to one type of disorder; others combine two or three, or don't discriminate between any of them. Surveys are normally based on self-reports, leaving it up to the respondents to define their own symptoms. Many who would surely be clinically diagnosed with some form of ED are never evaluated, either because they don't believe they have a problem, or because they fear the stigma of having a mental disorder.

Determining the *incidence*—how many new cases are diagnosed per year—among young people under the age of twenty-five, might be slightly more accurate than for the entire U.S. population. Large, regular health surveys are done concerning youth, and minors are more likely than adults to be brought in for treatment by a worried family member. Respected studies since the mid-1990s are painting a clearer picture of the extent of the problem, even though most mental health experts believe that statistics about eating disorders are still vastly underreported and underestimated, especially for males and other subcultures, such as children under ten and those in midlife and older.

Here are some highlights of recently gathered statistics.

How Many

- A 2011 U.S. data analysis estimated 20 million females and 10 million males (approximately 10 percent of the nation's population) may be clinically diagnosed with anorexia, bulimia, binge eating, or an uncategorized type of ED at some time in their life.[7] This is a huge increase over previous estimates from the 1990s which assumed anywhere from 5 to 11 million (1.5–3.5 percent) suffered, or would suffer, from an eating disorder. It's probable these older, smaller figures didn't accurately account for the greater range of age, both genders, and all forms of EDs covered in the newer report.
- NEDA estimates close to a half million teens (including 10 percent of all female teenagers!) struggle with key symptoms of eating disorders.[8]
- Worldwide, it's been estimated that eating disorders affect approximately 70 million people.[9] Data reviews indicate rates of eating problems have been increasing in countries around the world since the 1950s.

The Effects

- Ninety-five percent of all eating disorder cases affect youth between the ages of twelve and twenty-five,[10] according to the Center for Mental

Health Services at the Substance Abuse and Mental Health Services Administration.

- Males are affected in 10 percent of all cases of anorexia, up to 25 percent of bulimia diagnoses, and make up nearly half (40–45 percent) of those who binge.[11]
- Ten percent of all people diagnosed with eating disorders in the United States claim their trouble began before age eleven.[12] A survey in Great Britain found thousands of girls are developing eating disorders by the time they are in primary school. Fifty-three percent stated their problems with food began by age ten.[13]
- Similar rates of eating disorders occur to all ethnic groups in the United States. Bulimia is more common among Latinos and African Americans than in non-Hispanic whites, who suffer a slightly higher rate of anorexia.[14] Binge eating, as a symptom, is quite common in adolescents around the world.
- A 2009 follow-up of almost 2,000 ED patients found people diagnosed with anorexia, bulimia, or an unspecified ED were almost equally likely to die in the eight to twenty-five years following the initial assessment.[15] Suicide rates were highest for those with bulimia.

The High School and College Set

- In face-to-face interviews of 10,123 teenagers in 2009, 273 (around 3 percent) admitted to suffering from an ED. Girls reported them twice as often as boys and were more likely to get them in late adolescence.[16] The 2011 Youth Risk Behavior Surveillance, a national survey of over 15,000 high school students, indicated that 46 percent were actively trying to lose weight, continuing an upward trend since 1991.[17]
- According to research reported in 2005, over one-half of teenage girls and nearly one-third of teenage boys have used unhealthy weight control behaviors such as skipping meals, fasting, smoking cigarettes, vomiting, and taking laxatives.[18]
- Since 2001, prevalence estimates of current eating disorders among college students have ranged from 8 to 17 percent.[19] According to NEDA's Collegiate Survey Projects, eating disorder rates have risen since the 1980s—10–20 percent of women and 4–10 percent of men.[20]
- Eighty-six percent of young adults with eating disorders revealed on a Ten-Year Study from the National Association of Anorexia Nervosa and Associated Disorders (ANAD) that their illness began by age twenty; 43 percent reported onset between age sixteen and twenty.[21] One-fifth of

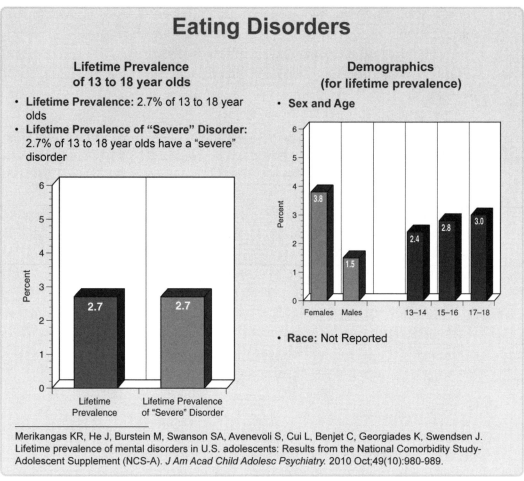

Eating Disorders

Lifetime Prevalence of 13 to 18 year olds

- **Lifetime Prevalence:** 2.7% of 13 to 18 year olds
- **Lifetime Prevalence of "Severe" Disorder:** 2.7% of 13 to 18 year olds have a "severe" disorder

Demographics (for lifetime prevalence)

- **Sex and Age**
- **Race:** Not Reported

Merikangas KR, He J, Burstein M, Swanson SA, Avenevoli S, Cui L, Benjet C, Georgiades K, Swendsen J. Lifetime prevalence of mental disorders in U.S. adolescents: Results from the National Comorbidity Study-Adolescent Supplement (NCS-A). *J Am Acad Child Adolesc Psychiatry.* 2010 Oct;49(10):980-989.

Courtesy of the National Institute of Mental Health, National Institutes of Health, U.S. Department of Health and Human Services, 2011.

2,822 college students sought mental health treatment for ED symptoms, but less than 10 percent had been officially diagnosed.[22]

Note the date of the report when acquiring facts and statistics. Data that was accurate for people, especially for children, tweens, and teens, might not be as applicable twenty years later. Researchers at the National Institute of Mental Health (NIMH) who conducted the National Comorbidity Survey Replication (NCS-R)—the largest survey of specific types of EDs prevalent in both women and men—pointed out that many respondents were reluctant to admit to symptoms during a structured interview. The authors believed the results were almost certainly underestimates. The report led NIMH to completely rewrite the information guide on eating disorders that it makes available to the general public, editing out all references to the numbers of those affected. In 2009, another research team replicated the NCS-R study to assess the prevalence of EDs in over 10,000 young people under age nineteen.

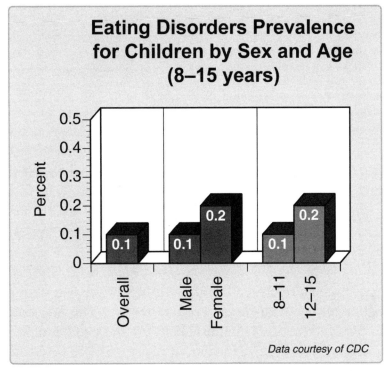

Courtesy of the National Institute of Mental Health, National Institutes of Health, U.S. Department of Health and Human Services,
2011.

Let's see how doctors and therapists are defining the symptoms of the best
known types of EDs: anorexia, bulimia, binge eating, and EDNEC (formerly,
EDNOS).

The Pursuit of Thin—Anorexia

Anorexia nervosa, literally, "nervous loss of appetite," is self-*starvation* leading
to significantly low body weight. Weight loss may occur quickly, or so slowly that
family and friends barely detect what is happening until the sufferer is profoundly
affected by the *psychopathology* of starvation. When children and tweens develop
the illness, it's possible that no actual loss occurs at all. Because they grow so
quickly, they simply never attain a normal body weight for their age and height.
Dramatic weight loss and low body weight are signs of other physical illnesses, so
doctors must use additional criteria to establish a firm eating disorder diagnosis.
The *DSM-5* notes that in addition to restricting food intake, sufferers intensely
fear gaining weight, or persistently avoid it, not recognizing the seriousness of
their health condition.[23] Although most anoretics don't realize how thin they've
become, some do. The classic, characteristic anorexic temperament involves lack
of self-regard, perfectionism, and rigid, highly structured routines.

Anoretics expend more energy than they consume. Some skip meals, even fasting for days at a time. Others eat regularly but limit calories to just a few hundred per day. Most all of them restrict themselves to "safe" foods, traditional diet food they can feel comfortable eating. Many rid themselves of calories through *purge* techniques. Forced vomiting and use of laxatives or diuretics are common means of purging, and many anoretics also burn calories in obsessive exercise. *Bulimirexia* unofficially refers to anorexia sufferers who use any method, or combination of methods, to control the consequences of having eaten. "Many people think anoretics are on starvation diets all the time, but that wasn't the case with me," says Ruth. "I ate breakfast, lunch, dinner, and snacks. But I was running and walking everywhere, so I got in a calorie deficit every week. I lost the weight I wanted to lose, but couldn't stop. The disease completely erases an accurate perception of how much you should be eating."[24]

Previous editions of the *DSM* defined anorexia characteristics as the "refusal to maintain" a "minimally normal" body weight and the loss of three consecutive menstrual cycles,[25] but this is no longer the case. The first criterion of the *DSM-5* states that food (energy) requirements are not being met, resulting in "a significantly low, body weight." No amount of weight loss is specified; it's only described as "a weight that is less than minimally normal, or for children and adolescents, less than that minimally expected."[26] The text provides numerical guidelines to help clinicians judge weight that is too low for a given patient. The new manual also allows that anorexia might not always be associated with *amenorrhea*. A few women continue to menstruate and young girls may not have reached puberty. Males can fall victim to anorexia as well and, of course, never have a menstrual cycle to lose. As more cases are evaluated, the APA revises the criteria for clinical diagnoses.

Over the course of time, malnutrition—the lack of sufficient calories and nutrients—leads to long-term health problems:

- Hair loss
- Brittle nails that break and peel
- Dry, yellowing skin
- Low body temperature (less than 98.6F)
- Lanugo—a fine, soft hair that covers the body
- Lethargy, sluggishness, or feeling tired all the time
- Muscle weakness and deterioration
- Thinning bones (*osteopenia/osteoporosis*)
- Tooth loss
- Brain cell damage
- Heart muscle wasting
- Mild anemia

- Swollen joints
- Constipation
- Insomnia
- Infertility
- Multi-organ failure
- Coma and death

The body has mechanisms to protect itself from the pain of starvation, so the lack of appetite that some anoretics claim to experience is real. The hormone *leptin* is primarily produced in fat cells. When we lose body fat, either intentionally as on a diet or unintentionally as with certain illnesses or drug reactions, shrinking fat cells release leptin into the bloodstream, which helps us to feel less hungry. This is an important adaptation for humans (and all animals) in times of famine when food is hard to get and we need to live off our energy stores. Dieters who follow a balanced eating plan where they consume dietary fat while reducing overall calories, and who stay moderately active, are less likely to feel hunger pangs. Leptin levels do appear to fluctuate with amount of body fat (lower with less, higher with more), but at least one study showed anorexic subjects had unusually high amounts of leptin circulating in their blood.[27]

For such anoretics who eat regularly, lose weight slowly, and are less restrictive with their food choices, losing weight can actually feel good. This sense may continue even as a dieter's weight slips below normal and is probably not due to leptin in particular, but because of complex changes in the way hunger is perceived. Researchers in Australia attempted to examine this "dieter's high." In 2007, Andrew Brown and his team noted that the early stages of low-carb dieting produces *ketones* as the body breaks down fat faster than its carbohydrate (glycogen) stores. The structure of one of these ketones, β-hydroxybutyrate (BHB), is almost identical to another produced by the brain, γ-hydroxybutyrate (GHB; γ is the Greek letter gamma), which has been recognized for its *analgesic* effects.[28] GHB is also synthesized as a club drug and is abused for its ability to lift the user's mood. It's possible that BHB has similar effects on brain chemistry. Moodiness is a common tendency during puberty as changes in hormonal activity take place. Manipulating their diet and adjusting their energy expenditure is one way some teenagers find relief.

The feeling of well-being from weight loss may be short-lived, and it's true the dieter's high doesn't happen to everyone. It might be impossible for people who periodically fast or eat and drink so little and irregularly that their bodies don't get enough energy for basic functions. Anoretics who are especially restrictive with their calories, perhaps averaging below 1,000 calories per day, develop elaborate rituals—pushing food around the plate, taking tiny bites, chewing for a set number of rounds, even spitting out food ("chew and spit"). These sufferers

Club Drug: GHB

GHB is a naturally occurring brain chemical that results from the break-down of the neurotransmitter gamma-aminobutyric acid, a central nervous system depressant. The Food and Drug Administration approved its synthesized form, *Xyrem*, in 2002—under severe use restrictions—to treat the sleep disorder, narcolepsy.[d] The street form of GHB is made into a clear liquid, white powder, tablet, or capsule by combining gamma-butyrolactone and sodium hydroxide or potassium hydroxide, substances more commonly used as floor stripping solvents and drain cleaners. Distributed as a sedative on the club scene, it's reportedly been used in date rape cases. Bodybuilders also seek out GHB for its anabolic effects, aiding protein synthesis and reducing fat to help build muscle.

High doses of GHB can lead to coma and death, and continual use can be addictive. Short-term symptoms of withdrawal include insomnia, anxiety, tremors, and sweating. Long-term use leads to hallucinations, slurred speech, headaches, and amnesia.

admit to feeling hungry but override the urge to eat because of their intense fear of gaining weight and the resounding guilt they feel after eating. Some anoretics believe that they don't deserve to satisfy hunger pangs. They respond to them by some form of distraction, such as extended exercise, drinking a lot of water, chewing sugarless gum, and using appetite suppressants. Sometimes sufferers even name their conflicting urges to eat and not eat and make deals about the size of the portions they allow themselves, how long they wait to eat, or how much exercise they engage in before eating. The rigid attention that anoretics have to pay to their daily activities increasingly isolates them from everything they formerly enjoyed.

Fear of Fat—Bulimia

British psychiatrist Gerald Russell first described bulimia nervosa, "hunger of an ox," in 1979. Until then, binge eating and purge techniques were just other abnormal eating behaviors, not uncommon in anorexia. Dr. Russell proposed that the routine of binging and purging could be categorized as a type of ED of its own because the majority of patients he was treating were not underweight, and did not so severely restrict day-to-day food intake as in classic anorexia. Even though significantly concerned with body image, his patients seemed not to share the same distorted thought processes that make anorexia so distinctive. They could accurately assess their body size, which for most of them was within normal range, but they were quite dissatisfied, obsessed with weight control, and had symptoms of depression. In 1987, the APA identified bulimia nervosa as a bona-fide type of eating disorder in the *DSM*.

The cycle of binging and purging is shameful to almost everyone with bulimia, who might see themselves as failed dieters. It's different from the binging and purging of those with anorexia, who are driven to binge from constant hunger and then purge frantically to regain self-control. Classic bulimics treat food more like a drug, and purging as a form of stress relief. The activity begins by consuming massive amounts of food, followed by a purge to relieve the physical and psychological effects of overeating. To be diagnosed with bulimia, the *DSM-5* specifies that a binge-purge cycle take place at least once per week, for three months.[29] People with bulimia can be any size, although rarely significantly underweight. (It's possible for someone with bulimic symptoms to be underweight, just as it's possible for someone with anorexic symptoms to be overweight. According to the *DSM*, however, being significantly underweight is a key diagnostic feature of anorexia nervosa. The key diagnostic feature of bulimia nervosa is the recurring cycle of binging and purging.)

Often, bulimics meticulously plan a binge session. They gather groceries—usually comfort food, high in mouth feel—and wait until they can consume it in secret. Fast food meals, whole pizzas, boxes of doughnuts, packages of cookies, and cartons of ice cream disappear within an hour or so. The feeling of relief that bulimics get from the purge can drive them multiple times a day to consume thousands of calories in a single sitting and then regurgitate them. "Most of my binges lasted for ten or thirteen hours," said Jordana, twenty-four, from Orlando, Florida. "It was always at night. . . . I would eat for forty-five minutes and then throw up for forty-five minutes, eat for forty-five minutes and go throw up. But it was never enough. I had to keep eating. I've done it for twenty-four hours nonstop."[30]

Chronic dieting, especially crash dieting, is common in many with bulimia. The diet need not be conscious, it might be from any lack of sufficient food. Nutrient cravings develop out of dietary imbalances. The same study that found heightened leptin levels in anoretics, conversely found lowered levels in bulimics, which at least partly explains the feeling of ravenous hunger that drives the binging.[31] They may, in fact, have previously been diagnosed with anorexia. It's been reported that roughly one-third of those with bulimia or bulimic patterns have

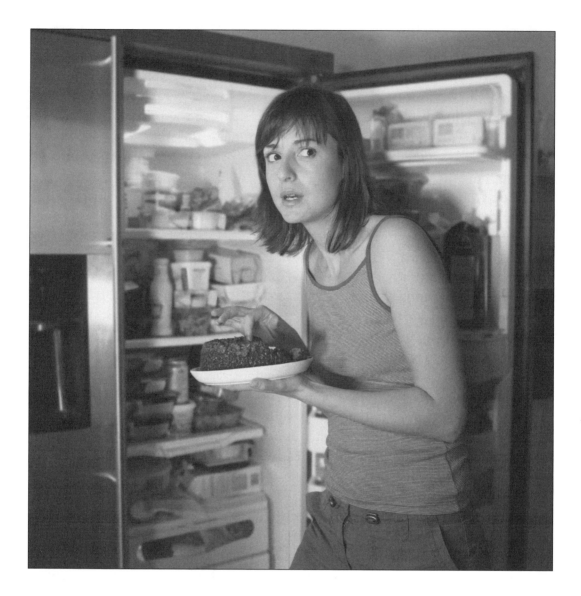

an anorexic history.[32] It's not unusual to become entrenched with eating disorders that float in and out and between classically defined *DSM* criteria.

Rather than tell-tale signs of malnutrition, bulimia, in its early stages, is characterized by other physical and behavioral symptoms:

- Chronic sore throat
- "Chipmunk cheeks" (swollen salivary glands)
- Eczema
- Red eyes from broken blood vessels; rosacea
- Bruised or callused knuckles—*however*, some bulimics become so efficient at purging, they need nothing to stimulate the gag reflex!
- Unexplained disappearances or immediate bathroom use after eating
- Overeating and undereating

- Constipation/diarrhea
- Weight fluctuation
- Irregular menstrual cycles
- Fatigue/lethargy
- Irritability
- Depressed mood

Over time, malnutrition develops. Symptoms can worsen and even become life threatening:

- Tooth enamel erosion and cavities from stomach acid
- Advanced gum disease (periodontitis)
- Inflamed or torn esophagus and stomach lining
- Gastrointestinal problems, such as acid reflux disorder
- Intestinal irritation from laxative abuse
- Anemia
- Severe dehydration
- Heart palpitations
- Electrolyte imbalance—fluctuating levels of sodium, calcium, potassium, and other minerals, which affect the heart and other organs

Bulimia can go undetected for long periods. Dramatic weight fluctuation is not necessarily evident, and many other signs and symptoms can be explained away as something else. Bulimics also disguise their disorder through other health concerns. Teen diabetics, for instance, must take *insulin* to keep their blood sugar level under control. The regimen provides a way to manipulate or skip an insulin dose as a means of weight control. This prevents the body from absorbing calories, forces it to excrete the circulating sugars in urine, and initiates the breakdown of fat and muscle for energy. The condition has an unofficial label, *diabulimia*, and has dangerous health consequences. Complications from diabetes—blindness, kidney failure, and neuropathy leading to loss of fingers, toes, or even limbs—occur much earlier in the diabetic's lifetime than they ordinarily would. Up to a third of adolescent girls with insulin-dependent diabetes

Here's an Extra Scoop

Although it's true bulimics are secretive about their behavior, not all of it is necessarily a completely solitary activity. Some college campuses have become known for dorm or sorority binge-purge parties where girls get together to chow down their "forbidden" foods and then go spew.

mellitus (type 1 diabetes) have eating disturbances that cause them to poorly control their insulin levels.[33]

Food Addiction—Binge Eating Disorder

Newly reclassified as a type of ED with its own distinct *pathology*, binge eating disorder (BED) can be described as bulimia without the puking, fasting, laxatives, or excessive exercise. Unlike the other eating conditions, almost as many males suffer from it as females. For every nine women who *binge* eat, about seven men do, too.

As with bulimia, binge eaters eat beyond the point that they know is rational, suffering significant physical and emotional discomfort afterward. Unlike bulimics, however, who admit to feeling excited as they anticipate and plan their binges, binge eaters often dread eating episodes. They feel helpless in the face of their uncontrollable urge to eat. Although binge eaters may be "closet" eaters, many are less likely than bulimics to eat in secret, especially when they are known to friends and family as big eaters. They're almost always overweight, have poor self-image, are distressed about their body size, and are ashamed about their lack of self-control. Many have a history of cyclic, or "yo-yo," dieting,[34] a key *risk factor* for developing any ED. They might eat rapidly or slowly, stretching their eating sessions out over several hours. Some binge eaters eat continually and confess to binges lasting days, or even a week or more. They are, it seems, addicted to food.

"Eating is something everybody does," says Josh, twenty-two, "and yet I do it to where it makes my life completely miserable. People say, 'Why can't you just not eat it? Why can't you just put it down?' I don't know how to."[35] Josh is morbidly obese—360 pounds over his ideal weight. Research suggests that from one-fifth to one-third of people who are obese may be diagnosed with BED[36]—or at least a *subthreshold* version.

The new *DSM-5* presents the symptoms for BED as follows: first, binges must occur again and again, with a sense of being out of control, averaging once per week for three months. Second, three or more of the following five indicators apply:[37]

1. Eating much more rapidly than normal
2. Eating until feeling uncomfortably full
3. Eating large amounts of food despite not feeling physically hungry
4. Eating alone because of feeling embarrassed by how much food is eaten
5. Feeling disgusted, depressed, or very guilty after overeating

In contrast to anorexia and bulimia, the APA has noted that binge eating disorder appears to arise in early adulthood. There are few statistics on the existence of BED in children, tweens, and teens, as prevalence and incidence studies tend to recruit older subjects seeking help to lose weight. Some specialists believe the disorder is not rare in adolescents. It's been suspected that a significant portion of obese youngsters suffer from BED. Considering the growing rate of *obesity* among young people, it won't be surprising to discover more cases of BED beginning at younger ages. Approximately 12.5 million children and adolescents (almost 17 percent of those ages two to nineteen) are obese. That's triple the prevalence since 1980, according to the 2009–2010 National Health and Nutrition Examination Survey.[38]

Individuals with BED are at a risk for developing health complications that are associated with obesity. As their weight climbs from "overweight" into the categories of "obese" and "morbidly obese,"[39] these risks tend to increase:

- Asthma
- Alcohol abuse—for those who drink
- Insulin resistance
- Heart trouble (cardiomyopathy)
- Circulatory problems (of lymph and other body fluids)
- Gall stones
- "Fatty" liver
- High blood pressure (hypertension)
- High cholesterol
- Joint deterioration
- Sleep apnea

Over time, these health abnormalities can morph into serious life-threatening diseases: diabetes mellitus (type 2 diabetes), cardiovascular (heart) disease, hypertension (high blood pressure) leading to stroke, certain cancers, and alcohol dependence (alcoholism). Psychological health is a serious problem for binge eaters, too. Like others with EDs, they also suffer from *mood disorders* at a greater rate than the rest of the population, especially

- depression
- chronic fatigue
- anxiety
- phobias
- panic attacks

Binge eating disorder is just beginning to be taken seriously. Dr. James Hudson, director of the Psychiatric Epidemiology Research Program at McLean Hospital and a professor of psychiatry at Harvard, headed a team of researchers

Sleep Apnea: The Silent Killer

Sleep apnea, a condition where the trachea is obstructed so that an individual fails to breathe regularly while asleep, is highly correlated with obesity. It has a host of dangerous consequences, the worst of which is sudden death. An eighteen-year study by the Wisconsin Sleep Cohort found that adult subjects, ages thirty to sixty, with this sleep disorder were two to three times more likely to die compared to those who did not have the disorder.[e] Forty-two percent of those deaths in people with severe sleep apnea were attributed to heart disease and stroke. A follow-up study by an Australian research team corroborated the findings. Thirty-three percent of study subjects with moderate to severe sleep apnea died during a fourteen-year period, compared to only 7.7 percent of those without sleep apnea. Terry Young, PhD, a professor at the University of Wisconsin, Madison who led the American study, is worried that the rise in obesity rates will also result in a rise in sleep apnea for both adults and youngsters. "People who think they have sleep apnea due to being told they snore and stop breathing should seek evaluation," she said. "People with mild sleep apnea should be cautious about progression of their sleep apnea due to weight gain."[f]

who coordinated the study of the prevalence of different types of eating disorders for the National Comorbidity Survey. He says most physicians aren't aware of the problem. "Doctors have a reasonable degree of awareness about anorexia and bulimia, but they're not tuned into binge eating. It's just not as well known."[40] From his sample of over 9,000 males and females, he found 2.8 percent of the general population over age eighteen suffers from BED. The numbers break down to one in thirty-five individuals—5.25 million women and 3 million men.[41] The rates are far higher than for bulimia (1 percent) or anorexia (0.6 percent). The study projected that 4.5 percent of Americans develop some binge eating behavior at some point in their lives. "Binge eating disorder represents a major public health problem," Hudson said. "We [doctors] need to be asking [patients] about it." Now that the APA agrees, more BED sufferers will be directed to get help.

Some therapists who treat eating disorders believe that binge (or *compulsive*) eating comes about for one of two reasons: either in response to calorie restric-

EATING TO EXTREMES **21**

> ### Eating to Feel . . . Nothing
>
> Perhaps even more consistently than any of the other ED types, binge and compulsive eaters are aware that they are using food to cope with emotions. Many of them speak of "filling the void" or "stuffing the feelings" when describing their inclination to begin an eating episode. "I don't eat normally," said Jennifer, twenty-three, of New Jersey. "I can eat an entire box of cereal at one sitting." While in high school, Jennifer sold candy as a fund-raiser and would eat the candy instead of selling it. "I tried to sell the ones I didn't like, but I thought about it and felt, well, it's chocolate and wafers. They can't be that bad. And they weren't," she said. "Food kills all my feelings. I stuff myself until I feel nothing."[g]
>
> Rickywayne, thirty-five, of Mont Belvieu, Texas, knows his eating is tied to his emotions. Always a compulsive eater, his binging deepened after his mother passed away. He turned to food even more to cope with depression. "I eat when I'm happy, I eat when I'm sad. Regardless of how I feel, I'm gonna eat. I'm a food addict. There's no off-switch to my brain with food. I just can't stop it."[h]

tion, or, as Jennifer stated (above), because of desire to calm one's feelings, a need to "numb out." The first, *deprivation-sensitive BED*, follows periods of extreme dieting and can lead to the yo-yo cycle that so many dieters recognize. In fact, it's not uncommon for an anoretic to binge her way back to regain pounds lost. In most cases, forced starvation actually prepares the body to take full advantage of energy recovery once food restriction stops.

Dissociative-addictive BED can become much more entrenched, as the habit of reaching for food to self-soothe can start in childhood. This develops into a subconscious, learned behavior that is difficult to break. Many obese people, like Josh and Rickywayne, recognize their inability to control the amount of food they eat. For some, binges can't be counted in episodes—monumental overeating becomes a way of life.

Unclassified Eating—EDNEC/OSFED/UFED

Some severely disordered eating patterns don't fit the present criteria and are lumped together as *(Feeding and) Eating Disorders Not Elsewhere Classified*, or EDNEC. The *DSM-5* subdivides the category into *other specified* (OSFED) and *unspecified* (UFED; see page 3) to help psychotherapists, primary care physicians, and insurance adjusters make an accurate diagnosis and determine the course of treatment. If you peek in the manual, you'll find there are five classifications listed under OSFED—Atypical Anorexia Nervosa, Subthreshold Bulimia Nervosa, Subthreshold Binge Eating Disorder, Purging Disorder, and Night Eating Syndrome. UFED is the leftover cache, replacing the old EDNOS category. As their names suggest, sufferers in these categories are missing criteria that distinguish anorexia, bulimia, or binge-eating. These conditions, also referred to as *partial syndrome eating disorders*, are every bit as serious as the classic disorders. They are just as debilitating, and often more complicated to treat because sufferers may be experiencing other psychological and behavioral difficulties. Co-occurring disorders, from alcoholism to cutting to compulsive shopping to bipolar disorder commonly intertwine with all variations of eating disorders and disordered eating.

When researchers attempt to study the death rate of each type of eating disorder, the outcome of the illnesses, and the extent of patient recovery, they recognize how difficult it is to define and evaluate their subjects' particular symptoms. Serious eating issues develop into, or possibly from, an array of unhealthy practices that vary in type and intensity, even in the same person over time. The most important thing to remember is that when symptoms overlap, whether they fit classic definitions or not, they signify real psychological and physical health trouble. *No combination of symptoms is more or less serious—or dangerous—than the others.* Both OSFED and UFED classifications refer to people with severely disordered food attitudes and body image distortion.

An Oregon study of 891 eighteen-year-old women over the course of five years found that those who exhibited full and partial syndrome EDs were highly likely to develop other psychopathologies, especially depression.[42] Three years later, the same women were evaluated in terms of their overall health, self-image, and social functioning. Those with disordered eating history were equally impaired in these important areas, despite the fact that most had recovered from their eating disorders.[43]

Partial syndrome eating disorders are widespread in the general population. A 2003 study of young women noted that disordered weight control behaviors and symptoms that didn't meet psychiatric criteria for an eating disorder diagnosis were as much as twenty times more common than were behaviors and symptoms that met diagnostic criteria.[44] The incidence of partial syndrome ED cases is probably at least equal to the number of anorexia, bulimia, and binge eating diagnoses, combined. A Renfrew Center Foundation study projected, in addition to the 24 million people they had estimated with anorexia, bulimia, and binge eating disorder, 25 million *more* probably have symptoms severe enough to warrant treatment.[45] That's almost 50 million Americans with serious food issues that affect their health. Even if this figure is exaggerated, it's apparent that many more

Katherine McNeil's Memory

How "alternative" do your lifestyle eating choices have to be before we should worry that you've developed a mental disorder? One thing's for sure—you needn't be classified with a full-blown eating disorder for the issue to forever affect your life. Here's what Katherine writes:

I lost a best friend who covered her eating disorder through celiac, colitis and alcohol concerns. . . . I didn't put it together until several weeks after her passing—her refusal to see a gastro-intestinal specialist, her itchy skin rash and perpetual coldness due to malnutrition, her extensive dental reconstruction and swollen saliva glands, her taking two bites at meals and declaring herself full, and that she'd eat more later, her getting better in the hospital and rehab center, then declining within three weeks at home with neuropathy and extreme pain in her legs, feet and hands. She died of heart failure due to dehydration and low potassium after a night of throwing up. This occurred even though her doctor gave her potassium meds and other supplements. A twenty-year friendship is gone. She was so lovely, such a wonderful friend; such long-term friendships cannot be replaced. . . . I could not mandate her into treatment. She didn't think she had a problem. Her family was clueless about it, thought it was alcoholism, since they were all in AA.[i]

Eating disorders are devastating killers, Katherine concludes, and she'd like to find effective treatments for everyone affected by them.

million people than we previously thought are experiencing emotional turmoil over eating.

EDs Smell Like Addiction

The medical profession defines separate pathologies and attaches particular diagnostic criteria to the various eating disorders. It's critical from both a treatment standpoint and an insurance perspective. It's important, however, for all of us to realize three key emotional characteristics of eating disorders that bind them together. These underlying markers prove all eating disorders are different sides of the same mirror. Regardless of how a sufferer treats food, whether she is underweight, overweight, or normal, those with eating disorders show common characteristics:

- *A relentless pursuit* of their behavior
- *An intense fear* of changing their habits
- *Denial* of the seriousness of their activity

You can recognize these same emotional behaviors in all addicts, no matter which substance, or how many, they actually abuse.

Have you noticed how common it is for people to become addicted to similar substances? Consider alcohol, nicotine, pot/weed, crank/crystal meth, cocaine/crack, heroin, inhalants, or prescription medication. Eating behaviors, and possibly food itself, affect the mind in similar ways. It's not unusual to find people with EDs and so-called borderline eating disorders who also smoke and abuse alcohol and drugs. They may engage in other types of obsessions, either concurrently or sequentially, with the difficulties of their food relationships. If you've ever watched episodes of *Intervention*, the Emmy Award–winning reality series about addiction on A&E TV, you can begin to realize how much food obsession and substance abuse have in common. Let's find out why, next.

More Food For Thought

Read

Jennifer Thomas and Jenni Schaefer. *Almost Anorexic: Is My (or My Loved One's) Relationship with Food a Problem?* Center City, Minn.: Hazelden, 2013.

Watch

Real Life Teens: Eating Disorders (educational media, 21 minutes). TMW Media Group, Inc., 2002. Search local library resources for video and instructor guide. More at www.tmwmedia.com/productlisting/details/eating-disorders.

Learn

American Psychiatric Association. www.psychiatry.org/eating-disorders.
EatingDisordersOnline—Eating Disorders Support, News and Resources. EatingDisordersOnline.com.

The Joy Project: Where Hope Takes Root. News, events, links. www.joyproject .org. Follow on Twitter: @TheJoyProject. Connect on Facebook: www.face book.com/thejoyproject.

National Association of Anorexia Nervosa and Associated Disorders. www.anad .org. ANAD Hotline: 847-831-3438.

National Eating Disorders Association. www.nationaleatingdisorders.org. Follow on Twitter: @NEDAstaff. Connect on Facebook: www.facebook.com/nation aleatingdisordersassociation. NEDA Helpline: 800-931-2237.

National Institute of Mental Health—Eating Disorders. www.nimh.nih.gov/ health/publications/eating-disorders/complete-index.shtml.

Something Fishy: Website on Eating Disorders. www.something-fishy.org.

Take Action

Self-Evaluation: Eating Disorder Quiz. Klarman Eating Disorder Center at McLean Hospital, Harvard Medical School. www.mclean.harvard.edu/patient/ adult/quiz.php.

IT STARTS IN YOUR HEAD: THE SCIENCE OF MOOD, COMPULSION, AND ADDICTION

••

The person who jumped through the door and grabbed me and tied me up was,
unfortunately, me. My double image, the evil skinny chick who hisses, Don't eat.
I'm not going to let you eat. I'll let you go as soon as you're thin, I swear I will.
Liar. She never let me go. And I've never quite been able to wriggle my way free.

—Marya Hornbacher, ED survivor
Wasted: A Memoir of Anorexia and Bulimia, 1998

How do we think and feel the way we do? When does quirky eating behavior cross the line into a psychological obsession? How do we know when to eat and when to stop? What does addiction science have to say? Learn what happens in the brain during the development of compulsive eating behaviors.

Mental Obsession, Medical Addiction

Anyone can show strange eating habits, even symptoms of disordered eating, but what makes an eating disorder a medical disorder is the way it takes over your brain. Treatment specialists agree, eating disorders are elaborate coping strategies that flourish in order to deal with significant life stress. The mind-set of someone with an ED is eerily similar to someone who's abusing alcohol, tobacco, or other drugs and experiencing symptoms of chemical dependency. There are a number of real biological and behavioral parallels. Researchers who study addiction medicine have recognized signs that show when substance use crosses the line into abuse and then into dependency. Not all heavy users of drugs or alcohol reach that point, but once they do, it's virtually impossible for an addict to choose not to use. Without going for treatment, there is little hope a sufferer will spontaneously recover. Intense and prolonged substance use—the combination of the effects of the substance itself, plus the behavior associated with using it—hijacks the brain by physically altering it. This is what makes addiction a disease. Brain imaging studies suggest EDs change the brain in similar ways, but researchers still debate whether they should be considered another type of addiction. Terry Wilson is a professor of psychology at Rutgers University and member of the American Psychiatric Association's Eating Disorders Workgroup that evaluated studies and proposed changes for the *DSM-5* (*Diagnostic and Statistical Manual of Mental Disorders*, fifth edition). He argues that the evidence is clear that eating disorders are not "food addictions" or addictions to binging, purging, or dieting behaviors. "Eating disorders do not fit into our understanding of the present addiction model," he writes. "When we examine relevant studies, and in particular, those of treatment outcomes, we find important differences between the symptoms and the recovery of patients with eating disorders and those with substance use disorders."[1]

The seeds of these medical illnesses are planted early, perhaps before we are born. Below, read about twenty-two-year-old Josh, who turned to food to deal with stress in his life.

By understanding how eating disorders manifest through the brain's circuitry, we can help combat all levels of eating related problems, improve prevention screening and treatment protocols, and work to reduce the negative public health consequences and economic impact that eating disorders have on our society. So let's find out a few things about how our brains normally function, and what happens when medical disorder comes along.

Josh's Justifications

Born a normal-sized infant at seven pounds, ten ounces, Josh began using food to comfort himself at an early age. By age four, he was medically obese. Josh became the champion eater in a family of big eaters, growing up on spaghetti, chili, goulash, macaroni and cheese, pizza, scalloped potatoes, and Sloppy Joes. He grew past his father, who's also obese. "My parents would make sure we'd clean our plates before we could leave the table," Josh told the producers of the TV reality series, *Intervention*, in 2008.

"Josh's parents wanted to control every little thing in their children's lives," said Heather, Josh's former girlfriend, who is still close to him. "Josh rebelled by controlling the only thing he can control . . . by putting food in his mouth."[a]

"I always felt out of place," Josh said. "This giant guy in a world of normal people. So I felt like I didn't belong."[b] By the time he got into high school, he had stuffed himself to 300 pounds.

From grade school to high school, the name-calling was torture. "They called me Pizza tits, Joshy-poo, Fatass, Fatty, Chubby, and Fat-boy." Josh became self-conscious and withdrawn, reluctant to let anyone get close to him, physically or emotionally. "I began this cycle of being made fun of, then turning to food, then being made fun of more, because the food only made me gain more weight. A never-ending vicious cycle, completely out of control."[c]

When Josh got his driver's license, a world of freedom and fast food opened up to him. "I'd go almost every day, then when things were really bad, sometimes three or four times a day, and order three or four full meals at once," he said. "I turned to food the same way an addict turns to drugs, an alcoholic turns to alcohol. Food's my drug, my way of coping with pain, humiliation, fear, all of that. It's miserable, the most lifeless existence. It's awful. I've missed out on so much, because of my size."[d]

Josh's compulsive eating has the hallmarks of binge eating disorder. "Food addiction is so similar to heroin addiction because you do it to numb out," said Ken Seeley, the family interventionist who was called in to try to get Josh to go for treatment. "You binge eat to numb out."[e] Josh consumed from 5,000 to 8,000 calories per day, and his ED had him following in his father's footsteps. At 546 pounds, he could walk up only a few stairs before he started to sweat and his heart started to pound. Josh was at high risk for high blood pressure, heart attack, and stroke, even in his early twenties. His knees would eventually fail, and he could develop type 2 diabetes, infertility, and cancer in the future. He was killing himself, one day at a time. Luckily, Josh agreed to enter treatment where he learned to manage his feelings without depending on food.

Wild Gray Matter: A Primer on Brain Science

Your brain is the central processing unit for your body. It coordinates all its organs and systems so that you can wake up and go about your day. It takes charge of regulating automatic functions so your lungs breathe, your heart beats, and you pull back from a hot surface. It enables you to interpret the world around you, respond to what you experience, learn, grow, think, feel, believe, and do. With it, you can write a term paper, build a model rocket, drive a car, solve algebra problems, play a musical instrument. You can also enjoy a good book, a rock concert, or a meal with family and friends.

Neuroscience tells us a lot about what the different parts of the brain do and how its cells function. The brain contains up to 100 billion *neurons*, spidery-looking cells with long *axons*, arranged in a web that are constantly firing electrical impulses. This is the true representation of all our conscious and unconscious thoughts, beliefs, actions, and responses. As long as we're alive, activity is hap-

Brain Quick Facts

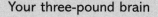

Your three-pound brain

- is about 2 percent of your body mass, but uses 20 percent of your body's oxygen and 20 percent of its blood volume
- burns approximately 40 percent of all the food energy you consume
- is made up largely of fat (up to 60 percent) and needs a steady stream of it to function well
- contains over 200 different kinds of nerve cells (neurons) that vary in size (small/medium/large/giant), shape (star/cone/pyramid/sphere/polyhedron), and color (white/gray)
- has about 100,000 miles of blood vessels
- has grown to about 95 percent of its full size by the age of three, even though you'll continue to grow for another fifteen years
- generates about 70,000 thoughts per day, not counting all the automatic signals it sends out to keep your body functioning
- attains its full capacity by age eighteen, but continues to make new and more brain cells throughout life in response to injury and learning

pening in the brain's circuits, and networks of circuits, every second of the day. Three main areas of the brain, the *brainstem, limbic* (emotional) *system,* and the uppermost part, the *cerebral cortex,* are in constant communication. They pass messages back and forth to all the brain's structures, the spinal column and the *peripheral nervous system* that exists throughout our bodies. People with eating disorders, mood disorders, and addictive behaviors have altered brain activity in these three regions.

The brainstem controls critical life functions: breathing, heart rate, body temperature, digestion, and sleeping. It's the oldest part of our brain—some form of it can be found in all animal species. It's the part of the brain that stays functioning if the body happens to be in a vegetative state, and can keep the body alive for many years.

The limbic system connects structures that determine our feelings, the end process of emotions like happiness, hurt, satisfaction, excitement, anger, fear, and love. Feelings prompt us to seek pleasure and reduce pain, which are important to our survival. When the system develops normally, we have motivation, avoid threats to our well-being, and build healthy relationships with other humans. Nature designed us to associate eating with physical sensations in order to drive us to seek food at regular intervals, except when we are under certain types of stress. Through evolution, our physical and emotional states wound around each other like vines up a tree as humans developed higher order thinking. Unfortunately, our emotional brain is easily affected by what we perceive, so the circuitry can be

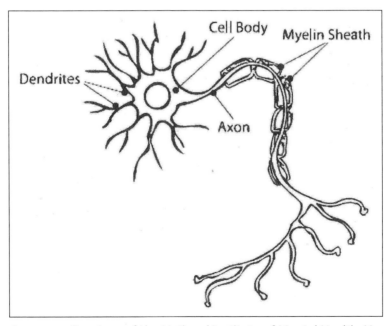

A neuron. *Courtesy of the National Institute of Mental Health, National Institutes of Health, U.S. Department of Health and Human Services.*

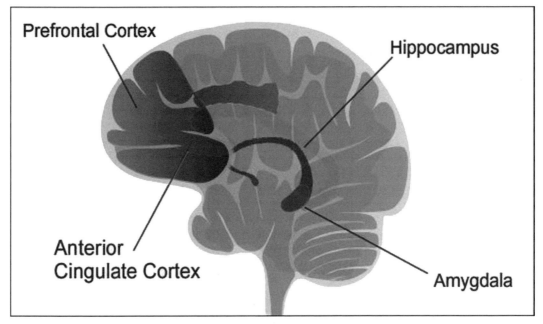

The brain (cortex connects to the limbic system). *Courtesy of the National Institute of Mental Health, National Institutes of Health, U.S. Department of Health and Human Services.*

impaired. We end up with dysfunctional thoughts and behavior about food, eating, and self-image.

The cortex surrounds the brainstem and limbic regions like a helmet. This thin layer of gray tissue is about the thickness of two coins, and is where most of our sophisticated thinking takes place. Different parts (lobes) of it have specialized functions that deal with motor coordination, problem solving, visual, auditory, and sensory information—touch, pressure, pain, and taste. The *prefrontal cortex* is the gray matter at the front of the brain. This area acts as a chief executive, giving us the ability to interpret both the emotions that arise in the limbic region, and the physical sensations that originate in other parts of the body. The *orbitofrontal cortex*, a cortical segment found near the eye socket, is strongly integrated with the limbic system. Here is where we're capable of feeling joy, focusing our attention, controlling our impulses, persevering in the face of obstacles, and caring about ourselves and others.

We need those critical brain regions to feel pleasure, perceive pain, and create and maintain bonds with other humans. To accomplish these and other critically important life activities, our brains utilize special molecules in chemical messaging systems.

Here's how most of them work. Brain and body neurons communicate by using *neurotransmitters*, protein-derived molecules that are released into the intercellular space (*synapse*) between neurons. They attach themselves to protein *receptors* on the receiving neuron. This acts like a key opening a lock, allowing the electrical signal to transmit to the next cell. Once the impulse generates, one of two things happens. Either specialized protein molecules (*enzymes*) deactivate the neurotransmitter, or *transporter* molecules from the first cell gather it up in a process called *reuptake*. This shuts off the signal between the two neurons. The transporters push the neurotransmitter back across the cell membrane of the original neuron, which recycles it for use next time. There are over sixty kinds of neurotransmitters at work in our brains, and their chemical reactions take place in a split second. Rather like trains pulling into a station together, but from different directions, when neurons transmit emotional signals, the communications happen simultaneously.

Dopamine, *serotonin*, and *norepinephrine* are three kinds of neurotransmitters that are important in enhancing pleasure and regulating mood. The brain's dopamine system (the "pleasure pathway") teaches you to enjoy whatever you are experiencing in the moment. It rewards you for something you initiate or respond to and you get the feel-good effects of dopamine transmission. It can be pushed into overdrive through the use of substances like alcohol, tobacco, and other drugs. The flood of dopamine into the synapse overwhelms the receptors and transporters, which can't pass along so many molecules or deactivate them quickly. This is how substance users get "high." After a while, normal dopamine levels no longer feel normal. The altered brain circuitry creates craving, and this is what drives susceptible people into addiction. Behaviors that bring about pleasurable consequences can be addictive in the same way. Sexual arousal has been known to

"I read too many tweets and blog comments that wonder how eating disorders can be a true illness when they're self-inflicted. It just shows how much ignorance is still out there. Everyone eats, so everyone has an opinion about food and weight, right? People who've never had an eating disorder can't understand what it's like to have a brain that convinces us it's our fault for choosing to starve or stuff ourselves, that we're hopeless and unlovable and don't deserve a better life. People who think eating disorders, or any addiction, for that matter, aren't real illness because we're in control of what we do, haven't a concept of what a 'disease' is. No one chooses to be sick. No one's to blame."

—Kelly M., writer/author
Tampa, Florida[f]

> ### ❗ Here's an Extra Scoop
>
> ⊙ Addiction, whether to food, drugs, or any type of behavior, is when you feel an irrepressible desire to repeat an activity, and you persist with it, even when it causes personal harm or trouble in your life.

increase dopamine levels by 100 percent, the same as nicotine and alcohol.[2] Eating, especially high-calorie, high-fat food, also prompts a large dopamine release, although not as much as using recreational drugs. It's believed that people who haven't been able to develop an effective dopamine system—for example, by not producing enough neurotransmitter, or because of defects in receptors or transporters—are particularly prone to eating binges, substance abuse, and developing various compulsive activities in an effort to adjust how the pathway functions and so, feel better.

Serotonin and norepinephrine are neurotransmitters that regulate our psychological state. They also function to determine our sleep and dreaming, attentiveness, appetite, body temperature, and social interaction. They share so many reciprocal connections, that when one undergoes a shift in activity, it affects the action of the other.[3] Our bodies make serotonin when the amino acid, tryptophan, reacts with an enzyme to form 5-hydroxytryptamine, otherwise known as serotonin. The production takes place in specific nerve cells in the brainstem. These serotonergic neurons are oriented so they can stretch their long axons into the frontal cortex.

Norepinephrine is also formed by brainstem neurons, which have a long reach throughout the *central nervous* system. A slightly different hormonal form of norepinephrine is produced in the adrenal medulla, a gland located near the kidneys, which releases it in response to physical stress. Both serotonin and norepinephrine induce varying effects, depending on the type of receptor they hook onto and the influence of brain chemicals. In fact, the serotonin, norepinephrine, and dopamine pathways, because of their influence on the limbic system, act as *neuromodulators*, meaning they modify the intensity of their signaling to impact many neurons at once. For this reason, they play a complex role in the neurobiology of mood disorders (i.e., depressive and bipolar illnesses), anxiety disorders (e.g., obsessive-compulsive disorder and social phobia), and various types of addictions.

Besides neurotransmission, the brain utilizes other *endocrine systems* to signal the start and end of all sorts of chemical reactions needed by the body. When the structures involved are part of the limbic system, the messages become emotionally charged. Here are some other important brain centers that regulate

Your Brain on Cake: Craving a Dopamine Release

Fresh baked bread with butter and jam. Triple fudge brownie ice cream. Creamy, rich macaroni and cheese. Crispy fried chicken and waffles. Most everyone understands what it means to have a food craving, but is it true you can become addicted? Many scientists say yes. Eating naturally prompts a dopamine release, although not as much as using drugs like cocaine and crystal meth. Like addicted drug users, binge eaters might have alterations in their brain circuitry that increase their food cravings.

Studies of compulsive eating in animals suggest that excess food intake incites changes in the brain. In an experiment on rats at the Scripps Research Institute in Jupiter, Florida, associate professor Paul Kenny and his graduate student, Paul Johnson, showed that when a test group were given all-day access to a tasty smorgasbord of food treats, the rodents overindulged to the point of obesity.[9] Their dopamine receptors changed so much, the rats had to work harder and longer to feel rewarded for doing certain tasks. In addition, they persistently overate, even when punished with electric shock. In another phase of the experiment, the experimenters showed when dopamine circuitry was initially defective, the rats were triggered to gorge.

Studies on humans point to similar findings. A brain imaging study at the U.S. Department of Energy's Brookhaven National Laboratory compared brain scans of binge eaters and non–binge eaters. When presented with the sight or smell of favorite foods, the binge eaters' brains showed an extra spike of dopamine in a brain region outside the reward center (the caudate). Lead study author and physician Gene-Jack Wang believes the dopamine in the caudate helps reinforce action potentially leading to reward. "That means this response effectively primes the brain to seek the reward, which is also observed in drug-addicted subjects."[h] The results of this study suggest the compulsion to binge might be a form of addiction.

Other studies in both lab animals and humans have shown similar areas of the brain light up in response to food cues and drug use. In 2011, a team of researchers at Yale University decided to test whether self-described food addicts actually responded vigorously to food temptation. Lead scientist Ashley Gearhardt designed a questionnaire that asked forty-eight healthy young women—average age of twenty-one at a range of body weights—to agree or disagree with statements such as, "I find that when I start eating certain foods, I end up eating much more than planned," "I find myself continuing to consume certain foods even though I am no longer hungry," and "I eat to the point where I feel physically ill."[i]

After tabulating the scores, the researchers brought the subjects back to scan their brains while they were shown a photo of a chocolate milkshake. It turned out that those with the highest food addiction scores also had the most brain activity in the same regions of the brain known to be responsive to drug craving. "I was surprised by the strength of our findings—all medium and large effects—because we excluded all [study candidates] who met a clinical threshold for eating disorders," Gearhardt told *Psychiatric News*. "If we had included such people, we would likely have had even stronger findings."[j]

our moods and influence our thoughts and subsequent behavior about what we believe we need.

- The *hypothalamus* is located deep in the center of the brain. It controls the pituitary gland, which produces and releases *hormones* that balance our drive for nourishment, letting us know when we are hungry. It helps modulate other drives as well—gratification, caretaker instinct, and stress response. It's also fundamental to body temperature regulation and sleep/wake cycles.
- The *amygdala* (pl. *amygdalae*; yes, you have two!) are almond-shaped structures located in the temporal lobe. It's considered the "heart of the limbic system" and shares connections with many midbrain and cortical structures, including the sensory cortex, hypothalamus, and hippocampus, the seat of learning and memory. It's essential in the emotional response to stress, greatly influencing the attention, perception, and memory of dangerous circumstances. It matures quickly and can record the emotional experiences of early childhood trauma, before we can become conscious of them.

- The *ventral tegmental apparatus* (VTA) lies in the midbrain and is associated with the pleasure pathway. It manufactures dopamine, communicates with the amygdalae and prefrontal cortex, and is responsible for intense feelings of desire, longing, and elation.
- The *nucleus accumbens* (NA), a brain center located on the underside of the frontal brain lobe, is linked to the VTA. It helps the prefrontal cortex assess what we like and want through the action of both dopamine and serotonin.

Evolution has allowed our brains to completely integrate what we know, what we feel, what we remember, and what we imagine. When brain circuitry relays messages from these centers to different areas of the cortex, especially our prefrontal cortex, we behave based not only on what we are experiencing in the moment, but also what we remember from the past and what we project on the future. All this complexity puts our brains at risk for disturbances. Eating disorders arise from a host of causes that we will discuss later, but there's no doubt that sufferers are experiencing altered brain chemistry. A biological tendency toward addiction is what makes people apt to develop any type of compulsive coping behaviors—eating, exercise, dieting, drinking, smoking, shooting up, gambling, gaming, shopping, hoarding, cutting, sexual gratification, Internet surfing, even working. Check out Jessie's story below, and see if you can identify the moods and feelings that drive her eating practices.

The Nature of Obsession–Eating Disordered Thinking

Jessie, twenty-one, from Corvallis, Oregon, has been seriously bulimic since she was seventeen. "I'm never not hungry," she said, "I'm never . . . not . . . hungry. I'm totally addicted to food." Her ED has trapped her in a cycle that completely rules her life. "There's something inherently wrong with me that needs to be fixed or filled or patched and I have to fill it—I have to fill up with something. It's like I need something now. Something now, now, now, now, now, now, now, now, now."[k]

Jessie's family was exasperated, amazed, and frightened. Jessie could eat three days' worth of food in three hours, binging and purging up to three times a day. She'd often resume a binge after purging. She doesn't even need to gag, just heaves directly into the toilet. "At this point, I believe she can't stop this," said her mother in the season 2 episode of *Intervention*. "It totally controls her."

As a child, Jessie got good grades in a gifted program and had friends. But she felt anxious and suffered from facial tics, panic attacks, and night terror. She always worried about impending doom. Her first binge came during her senior year in high school, when she ate all her Halloween candy, all of her brother's candy, all the brownies her mother had made, and a big plate of spaghetti. "I remember thinking, 'I am eating too much, but I can't stop,'" she said.

Jessie shifted into bulimia when she entered her sorority. She became so consumed by it, she was barely able to keep down enough calories to maintain a healthy weight. Her body continually dehydrated. "The binging and purging got worse [in college] because there was limitless, free food," she said. "I'd sleep 'til noon, wake up, eat when none of the girls were there, cuz they were in class, [then] go back to bed." Soon she had a problem she was unable to stop. She was kicked out of the sorority after a month for consuming a full pantry intended to feed seventy girls for six weeks.

She moved back home and soon family tensions escalated. Her parents sent her to a residential treatment center for sixty days, but she *relapsed* a few months after she returned. Unable to afford to feed her, they insisted she get her own apartment. Jessie took a job as a stripper, earning and spending hundreds of dollars on food to throw up. "I've lost the relationship with my family, and their trust. I don't know that I'll ever regain that. I lost school. Anything that could be lost, I have lost." She ducked her head away from the camera as tears flowed. "I've done a lot of bad things with this and I'm a really bad person, but I hope to be a good person." The TV show producers sent Jessie for treatment at Remuda Ranch in Wickenburg, Arizona.

Jessie's bulimia is classic addiction mentality. She's had cravings and relapses and the urgency to have her needs met at once. She's given up her ambition, damaged her relationships, yet feels helpless to stop, even though she's unhappy. Her anxiety and "black-and-white" thinking has given her a life of ongoing melodrama that she desperately tries to control. What's going on in her brain that compels her to binge and purge so relentlessly? Brain science tells us it's likely that the pathways that control impulse and incentive, motivation and drive, and the response to stress and pain, are the major culprits. Let's take a closer look at the role two of these systems play in the development of disordered eating.

I. Fight, Flight, or Freeze

When danger threatens, our bodies prepare very quickly to either run away or stand and confront what scares us. Our heart rate speeds up, our blood pressure rises, and our breathing is fast and shallow. Blood is diverted away from nonessential functions like tissue repair and digestion to charge up the brain and large muscle groups. *Endorphins*, the body's natural pain-relief hormones, are released and norepinephrine helps constrict blood vessels so that we are fortified against injury. A cascade of adrenaline, adrenal corticoid hormones, and neurotransmitter activity in a variety of communicating brain structures focuses our attention and prepares us to make quick decisions and take quick action. If the scare is overwhelming, we collapse. When the crisis has passed, hormones, such as cortisol, direct the hippocampus to deactivate the stress response and store the memory in a context that can be helpful later.

The stress response has always been helpful to us in emergency situations, when we need to get out of the way, defend what is ours, or come to the aid of someone in distress. The trouble is that the mechanism can also be triggered by things that aren't actually happening now, things we only remember or imagine. When you are stressed for psychological reasons—like dwelling on a time when you were embarrassed, or angry at having to do something you don't want to do, or anticipating something bad happening to someone you love—it's sometimes

The Scare That Isn't There: Emotional Processing of Stress

Because our eating behaviors are so closely tied to our emotional condition, they become scrambled due to psychological stress. Why? For better and for worse, we have many more connections running from the limbic system out to the cortex than the other way around. This means that our decision making is heavily based on how we feel, rather than perfect logic. Rarely are we conscious of the role our emotions play in any of the decisions we make when we're under stress. That's because there are actually two pathways that make us react to stressful stimuli—a long, slow, precise route from the thalamus through the sensory cortex to the amygdala, and a short, fast, direct jump from the thalamus to the amygdala.

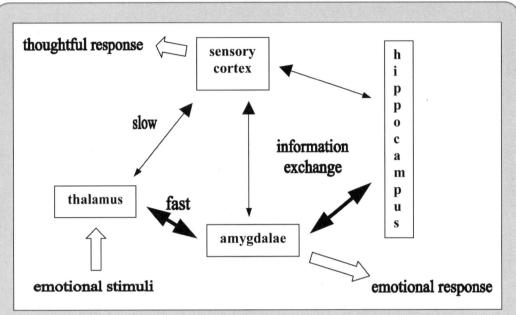

Two pathways of fear: Double-headed arrows show that communication takes place in both directions at once. Thicknesses of the arrowheads suggest the degree of relative influence the structures have on each other. *Schema adapted by the author from "The Two Pathways of Fear," The Brain from Top to Bottom ☺ thebrain.mcgill.ca.*

When we register an external stressor, the brain channels emotional information to the thalamus, which forwards the package to the sensory cortex so it can assess the nature of the stimulus and send the concept to the amygdalae. Before our minds even complete the picture of the stimulus, however, the thalamus has thrown characterizing pieces of information to the amygdalae, giving us a chance to form an immediate emotional response. Thus, if you're in a dark alley and a shadow passes close to your head, you can feel the fear and duck. If it turns out there was nothing about to hit you after all, you'll only have had a momentary scare. You can see how this would have been an advantage to our early human ancestors, who had yet to fully develop cognition.

difficult to find the off switch. And chronic stress is bad juju. Neuroscientists have shown a clear link between continued psychological stress and brain disorders like EDs.

Dr. Robert Sapolsky is a neurobiologist in the Department of Neurology and Neurological Sciences at Stanford University in California. He's well-known for studying the effects of stress on baboon troops on the Masai Mara Reserve in Kenya. He knows stress can do some pretty adverse things in your brain. "Chronic stress and chronic exposure to glucocorticoids [an adrenal hormone] can do something as unsubtle and grotesque as kill off your brain cells."[4] That'll certainly prompt changes in your eating behavior! His colleague, Dr. Bruce McEwen, director of the Hatch Laboratory of Neuroendocrinology at Rockefeller University in New York City, agrees, but believes that brains can recover, and usually on their own. "The brain . . . does change in response to stress. The good news is, these changes are . . . largely reversible. In the short run, there may be changes in the shape and conductivity of nerve cells that are part of the process of adapting to an acute [short-term] or even a chronic stress. . . . The real problem is if these changes occur and then they don't reverse when the stress is passed. Then you have what's called an anxiety or depressive disorder that needs to be treated. And it's this lack of resilience that we really have to worry about."[5]

Anxiety is common in many people with eating disorders, either as a full psychiatric condition or as a collection of various symptoms. They are an unfortunate by-product of evolution. Forty million Americans over age eighteen not only let fear and uncertainty override logic, but they also continue to feel the physiological effects of fear, even after they recognize that it's irrational. There are six main types of anxiety disorders with different symptoms, but all are based in excessive, invalid fright and worry.[6]

1. Generalized anxiety disorder
2. Panic disorder
3. Obsessive-compulsive disorder
4. Post-traumatic stress disorder
5. Social anxiety (phobia) disorder
6. Specific phobias (fear of heights, water, open spaces, flying, public speaking, etc.)

One study in 2003 found 71 percent of women with anorexia or bulimia nervosa had at least one anxiety disorder.[7] Binge eaters are more likely to have phobias than the general population. As we'll see in chapter 3, mood disorders, such as depression and bipolar disorder, are also common mental conditions in people who are susceptible to eating disorders.

Triggering Debate: What to Do about Stress

Stress is part of life and impossible to avoid completely. What kinds of situations stress you out? Do you ever use food to feel better? Do other methods work? Why might some people overeat while others restrict eating to reduce stress? Can psychological stress ever be good for you? When?

Stress can either suppress or enhance your appetite, and data from animal studies have shown both these effects. Rats and rhesus monkeys who are at the bottom of their social hierarchies (typically placing them in more stressful circumstances), eat less and have lower body weight compared to those of top rank. Yet, when given access to foods high in fat and sugar—"comfort" rat and monkey chow—these subordinate animals overeat, gain more weight than their dominant counterparts, and tend to lay down fat in the abdomen. This is a result of continually circulating cortisol, the by-product of the ongoing stress response. These same eating patterns and physiological consequences are recognizable in humans, too. A study of ten female rhesus monkeys at the Yerkes National Primate Research Center Field Station at Emory University in Atlanta tried to determine whether the monkeys' choice of a high-calorie diet actually reduced the stress levels and anxiety symptoms of those that were low ranking. The 2010 report announced that all the monkeys preferred the high-calorie diet and, after a period of isolation, had increased cortisol in their blood.[8] The subordinate animals, however, ate more than the dominant ones and became less anxious. The researchers also noted that they snacked more at night, which is also a common practice of mood-stressed humans.

II. Pleasure and Pain

We've seen the importance of dopamine on the pleasure centers of the brain, but it's not the only brain chemical that makes us feel content and satisfied. Other systems are at work as well. Endorphins are the gateway to any addiction. Besides assisting our stress response, endorphins regulate wakefulness, help us form bonds of love, and relieve us of both physical and emotional pain. Whenever we are hurting, our endorphins work as organic painkillers. They do this by binding to *opioid* receptor molecules on nerve cells throughout the body. When the binding takes place in the brain, it interferes with neurotransmitters that signal pain. This accentuates the effect of dopamine through the VTA and NA of the reward circuit. When these brain areas are stimulated in lab experiments, both rats and people find it so pleasurable, they'll ignore even painful distraction in order to continue the stimulation.[9]

Foods high in fat and sugar are well-known to raise the level of endorphins. For people like Josh, Rickywayne, Jennifer, Jessie, and others who experience enough emotional stress to cause pain, eating comfort foods provides a quick fix. It's easy for a brain to become dependent on its own soothing mechanisms.[10]

Endorphins are also the language of love. They flood opioid receptors to let infants and their caretakers establish secure connections. This is essential for an infant's survival through a long childhood. If it didn't feel good to bond with

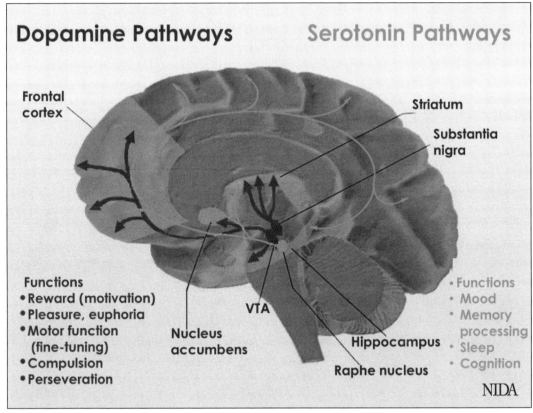

Brain reward centers. *Courtesy of the National Institute of Mental Health, National Institutes of Health, U.S. Department of Health and Human Services.*

members of our species, human civilization would be quite different. We are social creatures, and our biology has made it so. Unfortunately, we're not born with a completely wired package. Abuse, neglect, and trauma can retard children's natural bonding instincts as their brains work to develop those first relationships.

! Here's an Extra Scoop (of History)

In the early 1970s, U.S. researcher Eric Simon confirmed that receptors for opiates existed in the central nervous system.[i] This means that the human body must produce a specific *opioid* that behaves like an opiate drug. The word *endorphin* identifies the *endogenous* hormones that closely resemble the opiate drug, *morphine*. By the turn of the century, obesity researchers had begun to propose that sugar, especially in combination with fat, can be addictive. Studies into the neurobiology of eating and drug reward continue to investigate the addictive qualities of food—and not without controversy.

This leaves them vulnerable to intense cravings for an endorphin release that their minds are hungry for. Disordered eating can start easily in situations of emotional deprivation.

Endorphins are naturally secreted by the brain during strenuous and continuous exercise and while performing other ritualistic activities—think of Ruth's compulsive running. Or Josh's fast food runs. Within hours after the activity ends,

Natural Narcotic . . . Is Chocolate Addictive?

The next time you hear someone describe herself as a "chocoholic," maybe you should believe her. Scientists have speculated that of the 380 chemical compounds in chocolate, a number of them could be responsible for boosting the activity of your dopamine system. A study at the Neuroscience Institute in San Diego, California, found chocolate creates a similar brain reaction to cannabis, the active chemical in marijuana. Like endorphins, "cannabinoids" are endogenous hormones that raise levels of dopamine in the reward circuitry. It turns out that three substances in chocolate are cannabinoid mimics. One of them, anandamide, binds to many of the same receptors as THC (tetrahydrocannabinol), the active ingredient in marijuana. The other two inhibit the breakdown of anandamide, so that it stays around to affect neural synapses a little longer. Compared to THC, anandamide activity is much more localized in the brain, making chocolate-eating less of a high than smoking a joint. The National Institute of Mental Health estimates it would take twenty-five pounds of chocolate for a 130-pound person to feel any mind-altering effect.[m]

The desire some people say they have to mainline chocolate could be due to another of its substances, phenylethylamine. Like amphetamines, this compound increases blood pressure and heart rate, giving you the sense of being in love. Other stimulants in chocolate include caffeine, theobromine (toxic to dogs!), and methylxanthines, all which increase the activity in the brain's reward pathway. Most researchers point out that the amount of these stimulants is way too small to cause true dependency. Any ecstasy reported by self-professed choco-addicts is likely due to the fat and sugar—which themselves enhance endorphin activity—in their favorite treat.

they start to experience the discomfort of the painful emotions they normally feel. Soon they'll start planning another binge, or binge-purge cycle. That's how all addicts experience withdrawal and renewed desire for a hit. Loss of pleasure or freedom from painful feelings, and the desire to experience that state again, is a powerful incentive to repeat the act, regardless of the distress it causes later.

Seeking gratification and avoiding unpleasant circumstances is how we negotiate the world from the time we are infants until we reach our final day on earth. The brain's feel-good mechanisms and stress response system together govern motivation in many animal species, which is why scientists can use lab animals to test theories about what drives compulsive and addictive behavior.

When it comes to humans, simply satisfying a knee-jerk reaction to threats or desires might get us into trouble. We call on our cortical regions to assess our impulses and determine what's appropriate. Normally, they inhibit unreasonable, irrational, and bizarre behavior. Through communication with other brain structures and chemicals, they create a self-regulation system that controls our inclinations and checks our drive. But sometimes higher level brain activity does not function normally and this puts some people at risk for obsessive eating and the distorted behavior that goes with it.

Mental health develops through *neuroplasticity*; our brain directs our actions while it learns from what we do. It then chemically modifies itself. Thoughts and actions take a biochemical hold that wears patterns on brain circuits like tread marks in soft mud. When cognitive processes—specifically decision making, problem solving, and skillful interaction with others—are reinforced this way, the behavior that follows becomes habitual. A disordered mind-set can seem completely logical to those who have one. It's practically impossible for sufferers to quit a full-blown ED without help. Their brains are working against them.

Hunger—Knowing When to Say When

How do you know when to eat and when to stop? Our bodies use a variety of hormonal and physical mechanisms so that we recognize our need for food. That growling in your stomach is only one minor indication. Hormones such as glucagon (manufactured in the liver when blood sugar is low), *ghrelin* (made by the stomach when it's empty), and other hormones from the gut send their messages through autonomic nerve cells to the brain. When received by that deep-seated limbic structure, the hypothalamus, more hormones help us assess our desire for food energy. The *lateral hypothalamus* appears to handle the on switch. In turn, additional hormonal signals from the pituitary drive us to appease our hunger. We find food, we eat. Our stomachs expand, ghrelin levels drop. Blood sugar rises, and the pancreas pumps out insulin to regulate it. Cholecystokinin (ko-lay-sis' to-kye' nin), known as CCK, a hormone released by the intestine as food passes through, lets us know we've eaten enough. When these signals reach the *ventromedial hypothalamus*, we feel better and stop eating. If only it were that simple for everyone. We now know our desire for food is controlled by complex and interactive brain chemistry that both influences and is influenced by hormone balance and compulsive processes.

Since we've learned how emotional and cognitive thoughts charge up our needs and desires and determine our reality, it's easy to understand how the biological signals for nourishment can become corrupted. The input from cortical and limbic structures descends on our hypothalamus. Meanwhile, hormonal shifts take place as obsessive behaviors take hold, so we can no longer recognize when we're truly hungry or full. Chronic malnutrition—either from too little food or from a poorly balanced diet—affects the production of brain hormones we need for normal, healthy attitudes and perceptions. It becomes stressful to evaluate normal environmental cues—the sight of a taco stand or ice cream van, the smell of barbecue or baked goods wafting onto the sidewalk. We also note the time of day, memories of family gatherings, and feelings of entitlement. We worry about food availability in the future, the urgency for something n-o-w. What we choose to eat, how much, and how often are governed by all this.

Appetite, our subjective experience of hunger, is strongly influenced by our reward system, our moods, and our stress response. How we evaluate it, given our biopsychology and cultural perspective, sets up the unique behavioral patterns of disordered eating. It may be safe to say that appetite dysfunction is the number one neurochemical marker of any ED. And that it greases the wheels of addictive processes.

Jill from Gainesville, Georgia, and Johnny from Tempe, Arizona, arrived at Hilton Head Health in the summer of 2010 to do battle with their demons of compulsive eating. Both had learned from an early age that eating helped to soothe overwhelming feelings. Jill, thirty-five, struggles with low self-worth and feeling protected. "Growing up, I felt that I was never good enough and so I would then, eat," she explained in the seventh episode of *Heavy*, a discontinued series that also aired on A&E TV. When asked whether her parents would question her about the amount, she replied, "Mmm-hmm. I started hiding food, so I wouldn't feel guilty."[11] Food hoarding is a *process addiction* with underlying anxiety issues. At her initial weigh-in, Jill was shocked to see the scale register at over 300 pounds. "I thought it would be a little less than that . . . I didn't think I'd hit three hundred. I didn't think *that* was gonna be the number." Her voice wavered. "It almost felt like someone had punched me in the gut. It took all I could not to sit there and cry. And to be honest, it made me want to go eat."[12] Throughout six months of therapy at the health center, Jill denied her problem and continued to hide food in her room. It took until her final week to admit her psychological dependence on food.

A Few Bites to Feel Full, or Still Hungry after a Plate of Nachos, Six Hotdogs, and Half a Cheesecake

Choosing small portion sizes at infrequent mealtimes actually works to change the experience of hunger. The brain can learn to be satisfied with limited food, so the signals to eat become easier and easier to ignore. Eating small amounts slows food travel time, reduces stomach acid secretion, and allows gas to build up. Cramps, bloating, and stomach pain make those who are restricting food even more adverse to eating. This can happen in the early stages of an ED when an individual is toying with fasting, or during active treatment when a sufferer is having to comply with a new regimen of meals and portion sizes. People who self-starve or massively overeat, whether or not they actually have a disorder, have trouble telling when they are truly hungry. This can persist long after they return to healthier eating. "I was a hundred and three to a hundred and seventeen pounds during my entire [three decade] career," five-foot-nine supermodel Beverly Johnson told Terri Gross in an interview on National Public Radio's *Fresh Air*. "The interesting thing was that no one ever said I was too thin. . . . I was just emaciated. That's the scary part, when I look back on it. And I do think it did a lot of damage to my body. . . . I'd never get hungry. I have to remind myself to eat, because [of] whatever happens in the brain when you starve yourself like that. The brain doesn't . . . tell you when you're hungry anymore."[n]

For those who have been in the throes of any eating disorder for a while, there's little sense of how much food they really need to feel normally sated. "Even now, years after I've recovered," said Ruth. "I can be ravenously hungry, then with just a few bites, I'm instantly refueled and don't need anything more." Her friend Kelly, who struggled with bulimia, remembers how she would slam a plate of nachos, six hotdogs, and half a cheesecake after drinking Coke all day. "It's not all about the food, anyway," she told Ruth. "It is, and it isn't. It's about needing relief, and you have to have the food to get it. The high doesn't come from binging. It comes from letting it all out."[o]

Johnny, twenty, had been abandoned by his drug-addicted mother at the age of three and spent three years in foster care before being adopted. He knows he uses food as medicine. "My drug of choice is food," he said. "I've dreamt about food—it's always on my mind. I'll eat at the college cafeteria, then [go back to the dorm] and eat some more. Food's a comfort. I turn to food when I'm mad, sad, happy, everything, every emotion. I'm sad, let's go get an ice cream. I'm happy, celebrate, let's go get something."[13] At his weigh-in, he was just over 400 pounds, his blood glucose reading already in the pre-diabetic range. Johnny has food hoarding habits too, perhaps as a remnant of his earliest years when food was scarce. It was "the only thing that never abandoned" him.

Jill and Johnny feel hungry and full like normal people; it's just that they base their eating decisions on other thoughts and feelings generated in their heads. Appetite is very much a learned response. When the brain sends signals to eat that are consistently obeyed at the slightest temptation, the impulse gets stronger every time. No brain hormone will make them put down the fork if they have other reasons they have to chow down. Johnny summed it up, "It's all in my head, and I have to fix that."[14]

An Expert Weighs In: Dr. Gabor Maté— the Unitary View of Addiction

Dr. Gabor Maté is a practicing physician in Vancouver, British Columbia, on staff at the Portland Hotel Society, a field clinic ministering to Vancouver's street addicts. His practice has ranged from family medicine to obstetrics to palliative (end-of-life) care, but his most recent work has focused on examining how emotional stress relates to psychological disturbance. He has observed how early childhood experience impacts healthy brain development, affecting everything from idiosyncratic behavioral patterns to full-blown mental illness. He believes that although there are a variety of factors determining what people become addicted to, there's only one addiction process that takes place in the brain. He supports the notion that eating disorders and substance dependencies are all addictions because they fall under the definition of "any repeated behavior, substance related or not, in which a person feels compelled to persist, regardless of its negative impact on his life and the lives of others."[15] He writes,

All addictions—whether to drugs or to non-drug behaviors—share the same brain circuits and brain chemicals . . . [which] create an altered physiological state in the brain, . . . [even though] there are no circuits designated specifically for addictive purposes. . . . Addictions are not a collection of distinct disorders but the manifestations of an underlying process that can be expressed in many ways. The *addictive process* . . . governs all addictions and involves the same neurological and psychological malfunctions. The differences are only a matter of degree.[16]

Addiction, he says, is as powerful as it is because it arises out of the brain pathways that are central to our survival. Yet it's not an "equal opportunity" disease. If this were true, it would never be safe to prescribe drugs to anyone, to drink alcohol responsibly, or to have an ice cream sundae. *No substance or activity alone is inherently addictive.* Three factors are essential for any compulsive disorder to occur:

1. A vulnerable mind
2. A substance or activity with addictive/obsessive potential
3. Stress

Thus, it's not the french fries, or the pictures of airbrushed models, or inattentive, authoritative, or abusive parenting that cause eating disorders. The degree of disordered eating that someone develops depends entirely on a sensitized mind responding to the pressures that confront it. "Given [the opportunity]," writes Dr. Maté, "individual susceptibility determines who becomes an addict and who does not."[17]

Who's at Risk?

Brain science has just begun to examine the parts of the neurological puzzle that pertain to eating disorders. The interaction of hormones and the modulating activity of neurotransmitters shape the brain and suggest how process (behavioral) addictions take root. The clues are tantalizing, because one hormone might excite or inhibit neural activity, depending on the brain structure it is acting on. How other hormones are behaving in the neighborhood affects neurotransmission also. Neuroscientists understand how easily normal brain function is deterred by chemical disturbances and deficits that occur due to stress and nutrition. The science of addiction illuminates how stress-induced and reward-based eating habits might arise, as well as other obsessive behaviors that happen in those who are vulnerable.

Careful consideration of the evidence qualifies eating disorders as real and serious medical illnesses and is key to understanding the phenomenon. Thanks to the technology of brain imaging, brain scientists can now witness what is actually happening while they evaluate a particular behavior or behavioral response. This powerful tool, combined with traditional large-scale studies of heredity and environmental risk factors, is telling us more about the nature of food abuse and obsessive eating practices than was ever possible before.

The more we learn about how the brain manifests the signs and symptoms of all forms of EDs, the better we can understand why they develop and how severe they might become. "Determining when problem eating has become an eating disorder is difficult," says therapist Carolyn Costin, executive director of Monte Nido and Affiliates, based in Malibu, California. "There are far more people with eating or body image problems than those with full-blown eating disorders."[18] She points out that certain people have predispositions that make them more likely to cross the line between a borderline ED and one that's full-blown. Predispositions are risk factors that can be internal (biological) or external (environmental). When these keys rotate in just the right way, they crack open the ED vault and let it loose.

As we'll examine more closely in chapter 3, people with certain types of temperaments, who focus on food—or any other substance or ritualized behavior—to relieve stress are at great risk for developing many types of mental disorders. Given the various pressures around us, anyone may choose to skip a meal or eat cheesecake when feeling low. No one, however, decides to suffer from an eating disorder. In both a poetic and a practical sense, an ED chooses its victim. Let's discover how.

More Food for Thought

Read

Marya Hornbacher. *Madness: A Bipolar Life*. Boston: Houghton Mifflin, 2008.

Watch

Brain Development & Addiction with Gabor Maté (Internet video, 64 minutes). Heartspeak Productions, 2009. Online at YouTube.com or heartspeakproductions.ca/brain-development-and-addictio/.

Intervention (weekly cable TV series, approximately 40-minute episodes). GRB Entertainment, Inc. for A&E Television Networks. Premiered March 5, 2005. Full episodes and bonus sequences are online. More at www.aetv.com/intervention.

This Emotional Life (documentary, three-part TV series [*Families, Friends and Lovers*; *Facing Our Fears*; *Rethinking Happiness*], 339 minutes). A NOVA production with Vulcan Productions and Kunhardt McGee Productions for

WGBH/Boston, 2009. Originally aired January 4–6, 2010. www.pbs.org/this emotionallife

Learn

The Brain from Top to Bottom. Canadian Institutes of Health Research: Institute of Neurosciences, Mental Health and Addiction. thebrain.mcgill.ca.
Sara Bellum Blog. NIDA for Teens: The Science Behind Drug Abuse, National Institute on Drug Abuse, National Institutes of Health, U.S. Department of Health and Human Services. teens.drugabuse.gov/blog.

Take Action

Teen Help, Inc. Support forums, articles, videos on relationships, LGBTQ identity, mental health, EDs and addictions, lifestyle choices, and so on. www.teenhelp.org.
Yale Food Addiction Scale (2009). Rudd Center for Food Policy and Obesity, Yale University. Download from www.yaleruddcenter.org/resources/upload/docs/what/addiction/FoodAddictionScale09.pdf.

KEYS THAT TURN THE LOCK: COMPLEX AND COMBINED FORCES AT WORK

Who's at risk for an eating disorder? What factors contribute to problem eating? Let's discuss how personality traits and anxiety and depression predispose us to disordered eating patterns, and how emotional trauma, family dynamics, and chronic dieting can push someone over an ED cliff.

Sometimes is never quite enough
If you're flawless, then you'll win my love
Don't forget to win first place
Don't forget to keep that smile on your face
Be a good boy
Try a little harder
You've got to measure up
And make me prouder
How long before you screw it up
How many times do I have to tell you to hurry up
With everything I do for you
The least you can do is keep quiet
Be a good girl
You've gotta try a little harder
That simply wasn't good enough
To make us proud
I'll live through you
I'll make you what I never was

If you're the best, then maybe so am I
Compared to him, compared to her
I'm doing this for your own damn good
You'll make up for what I blew
What's the problem . . . why are you crying
Be a good boy
Push a little farther now
That wasn't fast enough
To make us happy
We'll love you just the way you are if you're perfect.

—Alanis Morissette, singer/songwriter, survivor
"Perfect," 1995

Striving to Excel

The words of Alanis Morissette off her Grammy Award–winning album *Jagged Little Pill* sum up the internal voice that lives in the heads of many with eating disorders—*be without flaw.* For some of us, the desire to be the best rises out of family culture, when winning is valued over honest effort or when parents have a need for vicarious glory and therefore push their children to succeed. Others learn through "star treatment," that the way to get attention is to be better than everyone else. We feel the pressure in comments from people we know and from media messages. The closer you get to "best," the more valuable you are and the greater your reward. People who absorb this idea develop a perfectionist personality that spurs them to compete and accomplish goals. This has both an upside and a downside.

Being competitive and setting high standards is not a problem by itself; in fact, it's a healthy way to develop self-esteem. But attempting to meet unrealistic expectations or striving to fulfill dreams that aren't yours causes mental stress and, in some, psychological harm. When you believe love and acceptance is conditional on being perfect, you begin to base your self-worth on what you achieve, rather than on other traits that make you wonderful. Those thought patterns are a dangerous construct to forming a healthy psyche. And they raise the risk for developing borderline and full-blown EDs.

A number of research teams in the last decade have explored the connection between perfectionist thinking and vulnerability to eating disorders. "We're finding that people with these disorders actually share some common personality traits," says Dr. Walter Kaye, medical director of the Eating Disorder Research and Treatment Program at the University of California, San Diego. "Both bulimics and anorectics tend to be people who are obsessive perfectionists, and they're concerned with doing things right. Things have to be done with symmetry and exactness. They tend to be people who are harm avoidant, in that they worry about the consequences of their behavior. They don't want to do things wrong."[1]

One team of researchers wondered if the drive for perfection might be a major risk for developing long-term restrictive eating. They tested the theory by recruiting 322 women with a history of anorexia and compared them to a group of women without eating disorders. All were participating in a larger international genetic study of anorexia. The subjects responded to questionnaires and interviews that rated them according to traits of perfectionism, obsessive-compulsion, and severity of disordered eating.[2] The anoretic women scored higher on all the inventories than the healthy subjects, suggesting they struggled significantly with perfectionist and neurotic tendencies. Along with evidence from prior studies, the results strongly support the idea these ingrained personality traits contribute to the slide into abnormal eating habits.

Erin's Fearful Symmetry

Perfectionism in someone with an ED isn't just about attending to small details affecting yourself, but also wanting symmetry in the world, too. Erin Meador, fourteen, was treated for anorexia at De Paul-Tulane Hospital's Eating Disorder Unit. When she was admitted in 2000, she was 20 percent below her normal body weight. "I just like everything to be controlled, in control, you know," she reported in the NOVA documentary, *Dying to Be Thin*. "Kind of like, I don't know . . . like traffic. I hate it when people try to cut in on you." She gestures with her hands to picture the vehicles moving in and out of the lanes. "They're sitting right here and the traffic's like right here and people over here because they're trying to get into another lane." She rolls her eyes. "I'm like, 'keep the lanes *straight.*'" She nods. "That's just me. That's how I am."[a]

Erin developed her eating disorder when her mother had to move overseas for a year because of her job. Feeling her world spinning out of control, Erin locked onto improving her appearance. Her deep-seated need for routine, so that she could know what to expect, combined with the personal characteristic of above average self-control is precisely what enabled Erin to restrict her eating to the point of needing hospitalization.

In a larger study published three years later, a research team at the Virginia Institute for Psychiatric and Behavioral Genetics at Virginia Commonwealth University evaluated links between specific perfectionist traits and other psychological problems. They found that people who had negative reactions to mistakes and who tended to interpret mistakes as failures were likely to suffer either anorexia or bulimia. The correlation was not present in those with other psychiatric problems, such as depression, alcoholism, or anxiety disorders. The study used standardized tests and interviews over the course of nine years to assess over 1,000 female twins ranging from age twenty-five to sixty-five.[3]

"Most patients and their parents said that perfectionism goes back to before they developed an eating disorder," said study author Cynthia Bulik, who moved

True or False

Do these perfectionist traits describe you?

T F When I take on a project, I put in 100 percent effort. I can never do less.

T F I must be better than anyone else in whatever I choose to do.

T F Nothing I do is ever good enough.

T F If I'm not very good at something, I lose interest in doing it.

T F Winning is all that matters. No one remembers who comes in second place.

T F If I'm successful at something, then I'll have to be that good all the time.

T F If I fail at something, it means I need to find something else I'm good at.

T F Making mistakes means I'm a "loser."

T F I pay a lot of attention to the details of how things get finished.

T F If someone criticizes me, I'm devastated.

T F If I get a compliment, I know it's only to make me feel good.

T F I need to always look like I have it together.

How many Ts did you circle? One or two—no worries; enjoy your life. Three to five—you probably set a high bar for achievement. Be gentle with yourself. More than five—striving for excellence may take its toll on you. Try not to be so demanding.

to the University of North Carolina at Chapel Hill, where she is both a professor of nutrition in the School of Public Health and the director of the Center of Excellence for Eating Disorders. "Many women continue to be perfectionists even after they recover from anorexia and bulimia. So perfectionism may be a trait that places an individual at risk for developing these potentially devastating illnesses."[4]

Dr. Bulik pointed out that being overly concerned about making mistakes is one particular perfectionist trait to watch. "Young girls who are highly perfectionist and punish themselves unduly for perceived failures can be helped to learn how to give themselves a break and set more realistic goals. This also could help them develop more realistic body image standards as well and perhaps prevent them from developing such extreme weight loss behaviors."[5]

Popping the Corn—Cause, Risk, and Trigger

If you search for "What causes an eating disorder?" in your online browser, you'll come up with something about how EDs are caused by a complex set of biological, psychological, and sociocultural pressures that push some people to become preoccupied with food and weight. This is not a horrible answer, but it barely begins to answer the question. Even if you ask a specialist, the conversation can get messy. After taking a deep breath, she'll probably point to a variety of internal and external pressures. She'll emphasize that causation is extraordinarily difficult to determine. Experts who have a lot of experience treating EDs are careful not to make blanket statements about them. No two people experience the onset and progression of their disorder in the same way.

Before the body of research into eating disorders really took off in the late 1990s and early 2000s, and the psychotherapeutic community began to pay closer attention, it was logical to blame authoritative parenting, defective genes, and of course, our society's commercial ideals of attractiveness that put pressure on impressionable young women. Environment, genetics, and culture play a role in all forms of disordered eating, so it's a mistake to point to any of them as the single cause of anyone's illness. They all interact to create a "perfect storm" of circumstances. Who gets an ED and who doesn't, how severe it becomes and how well one recovers, is unpredictable. Obvious symptoms such as dietary preferences and exercise obsession exist on a continuum and cannot point out who will fall off the cliff. Also, it's easy to confuse "cause" with "correlation." Someone might be extremely thin and read lots of fashion magazines. There's no definitive proof that one caused the other or that they are related at all. Practically no one, and rarely those stricken, can be objective about what is a cause and what is an effect after an eating disorder arises.

Here's an Extra Scoop

Eating disorders are *not* genetic illnesses. No single gene has ever been found to be the direct cause of any psychological disorder.

One way to think about how certain people get eating disorders is to imagine our mental state as kernels of corn. Corn is corn, but small genetic variations make some varieties capable of popping when heat is applied. The actual conditions can vary—corn can pop in a pan on top of a stove, in a microwave oven, or in an oil-free air popper. When we are stressed under various combinations of conditions, psychological kernels have the potential to erupt. Thus, brain biochemistry is what makes an eating disorder possible. As we learned in the previous chapter, our mental processes are continually adapting to sensory information received from a multitude of sources, so no one cause for EDs will ever be found. All the things that people typically mention as causing eating disorders are, strictly speaking, contributing *risk factors*. Genetics. Family dynamics. Emotional trauma. Major life transitions. Peer pressure. Media messages. Dieting. These are the types of pressures that explode minor eating "quirkiness" into full disorder.

But even some popcorn kernels are duds. Risk factors can actually minimize how severe eating problems become or even decrease the chance that any occur. When pressures work to counteract a disordered mind-set they are called *protective factors*. Thus, an especially nurturing and positive family environment, preemptive counseling, an improved life situation, contact with appropriate and supportive friends, ad campaigns promoting sound mental and behavioral health, even dietary and activity changes that further a healthy, balanced lifestyle—all can thwart an ED in someone at high risk.

The word *trigger* refers to the event or set of circumstances that took place just prior to an eating disorder—the point at which an individual's eating and weight preoccupations moved outside the range of normal. People who suffer from EDs also use the words *trigger* and *triggering* as they become aware of their illness and can identify the feeling in a given situation that urges them to binge, vomit, fast, or exercise for hours. Sometimes there is no original trigger to pinpoint, but for the majority of those that can, a diet is the one that's acknowledged most often. Surveys since the 1990s show that roughly half the U.S. population is dieting on any given day.

One literature review determined that 35 percent of "normal dieters" adopt pathological habits. Approximately one-quarter of those progress to partial- or full-syndrome eating disorders.[6] "I hadn't been terribly overweight to begin with," said Ruth, "but my pediatrician had warned me that my weight was rising faster than my height. I'd gradually made small diet and activity changes around

> "[Eating disorders] are illnesses that seem to begin by choice in the sense that most individuals [experiencing] triggering behaviors, like dieting and engaging in excessive exercise, are choices that people tend to make—often under the banner of wanting to live healthier lives. However, there is a time, under certain conditions, and for certain individuals that carry with them a significant set of temperamental characteristics, in which this effort to live better becomes an obsession. . . . This is a hallmark of mental illness . . . when an individual loses perspective."
>
> —Dr. Ovidio Bermudez, chief medical director of Child and Adolescent Services, Eating Recovery Center, Denver, Colorado [b]

the time I began high school. We had moved for my dad's job, I had to walk to a school that was a couple miles away, and I discovered running made me feel less uptight. The pounds disappeared effortlessly and I thought my weight would level out naturally. I thought I'd never have to worry about being fat. But the more weight I lost, the more I was afraid of eating. Anorexia hijacked my mind."[7]

Why do eating disorders happen to that quarter of the dieting population, but not others? "Like many medical conditions, we know it's a mix of nature and nurture," Dr. Nancy Etcoff replied to Meredith Viera on *Today*. "There seems to be genetic components, and it's also the environment. So one can have a risk factor and never have an eating disorder. Other people can be exposed to the most toxic environment, and yet not get an eating disorder, so there seems to be this volatile mix. It's the person that's vulnerable in their environment that will bring it forth."[8] This is what brain science research has been telling us is true about all addictive types of disorders. As it turns out, many risk factors for EDs are the same as those for drug and alcohol abuse. Such mental health gremlins prime people for psychological turbulence throughout their lives. Many end up nurturing mild to moderate to severe compulsions that they express through different behaviors over time. CASAColumbia (formerly known as the National Center on Addiction and Substance Abuse at Columbia University) has reported that half of all youth suffering from eating disorders also abuse drugs, alcohol, or both.[9] The examination also determined approximately one-third of alcohol or illicit drug abusers have an ED compared to around 3 percent of the general population.

We must never underestimate the complexity of the interaction of biological sensitivity and environmental pressures in determining our mental health.

Eat, Drink, Be Merry:
Food Abuse and Substance Use

Disordered eating and the use of alcohol, nicotine, caffeine, and various drugs frequently go together. This co-occurrence is known as *comorbidity*. An extensive examination by CASAColumbia® determined that individuals with eating disorders are up to five times likelier to abuse alcohol or illicit drugs. Those who abuse alcohol or illicit drugs are up to eleven times likelier to have eating disorders.[c] The National Comorbidity Survey-Replication (NCS-R) found that men and women, eighteen and over with EDs, also had high rates of substance use disorders (SUDs).[d] From a sample (*n*) of almost 3,000 interviews, researchers determined how many subjects with the three main types of EDs also abused alcohol, illegal drugs, or any other substance at some time in their lives (see table 3.1).

Table 3.1. Lifetime Comorbidity Estimates of EDs and SUDs (Hudson et al. 2007)*

Disorder n = 2,980	Alcohol Abuse or Dependence (%)	Illicit Drug Abuse or Dependence (%)	Any Substance Use Disorder (%)
Anorexia nervosa	24.5	17.7	27.0
Bulimia nervosa	33.7	26.0	36.8
Binge eating disorder	21.4	19.4	23.3

* Substance Abuse and Mental Health Services Administration (SAMHSA), "Clients with Substance Use and Eating Disorders," SAMHSA Advisory 10, no. 1 (Washington, D.C.: U.S. Department of Health and Human Services, February 2011), 5. Available at store.samhsa.gov/shin/content/SMA10-4617/SMA10-4617.pdf.

National surveys of thousands of students ages twelve to eighteen generate the data that researchers use to compare the occurrences of mental health disturbances and health-risk behaviors in teens. In the years since the publication of CASAColumbia's findings, disordered eating and eating disorders have continued to be associated with substance use and abuse. The correlation is especially significant for nicotine, alcohol (binge drinking), and inhalants among high school and college students reporting health-risk behavior. Among male students, the association is also strong for marijuana and steroid use.[e]

Scientists who investigate the biological basis for behaviors—often through family observations and comparing studies of identical and fraternal twins—have estimated that our individual biochemistry accounts for 50–80 percent of the risk of developing a psychological disorder. This percentage has been widely reported and poorly explained, so that people tend to think environmental risk factors have little impact. We still have much to learn about the genetic basis for our traits and behavior, but one thing is clear: genes aren't the secret instructions for making an eating disorder. Although comparative twin studies do suggest that *heritable* factors, including genes, contribute to psychological disorders in general, it's truly impossible to compute and separate the percentage of influence from genetic and environmental risk factors in an individual.

Nevertheless, in terms of recovery treatment, Professor Howard Steiger of Montreal's Douglas University believes gene therapy for EDs could be effective someday. "We understand that eating disorders don't occur because of moral weakness or a lack of character, they happen in people who carry real physical susceptibilities that are kind of carried by genes and then acted upon by environmental influences on those genes," he said in a 2012 interview.[10] Dr. Steiger

Hungry All the Time: Prader-Willi Syndrome

Genetic factors that lead to eating disorders are difficult to assess because of the complexity of "nature and nurture," but there is one genetic abnormality that causes a brain injury proven responsible for compulsive (binge) eating. People born with Prader-Willi Syndrome (PWS) have a faulty gene that leaves them with an insatiable appetite as well as other developmental defects. The condition—affecting 1 in 12,000 to 15,000 and equally common in boys and girls—was first described in 1956 by three German endocrinologists, two of whom gave their names to the syndrome. By the late 1960s, researchers had categorized two phases of occurring symptoms: (1) a prenatal and infancy period where the child shows lethargic fetal movement, poor muscle tone, underdeveloped sex organs, feeding problems, and an overall failure to thrive and (2) an early childhood period with developmental delays in physical growth, motor skills, cognitive processing, and speaking ability.[f] Emotional instability may come about as the child feels the stress of these handicaps. With hormone and behavioral therapy, most of these problems normalize over time. As with other genetic illnesses, PWS is a spectrum disorder, affecting some individuals more severely than others.

The source of the bottomless appetite in PWS is a malfunctioning hypothalamus due to missing or suppressed genetic material on chromosome 15. Beginning at around age two or three, Prader-Willi sufferers never feel that they've eaten enough. Seeking food is practically a constant activity. Without parents' close management of their child's food intake, constant hunger combined with an efficient metabolism leads to severe obesity by age two or three. Weight control is a lifelong burden, especially for those who struggle with diminished cognitive abilities. The American Academy of Pediatrics recommends therapy with human growth hormone to help PWS children grow taller, develop more lean muscle, and increase their energy and bone density.[g] As young adults transition from pediatric to adult health care, they should be monitored for weight stability, diabetes, hypertension, sleep apnea, heart failure, peripheral edema (swelling of hands and feet), and the use of psychotropic medications that help control behavioral issues.[h] With a structured lifestyle and supportive weight control management, people with PWS can enjoy a good quality of life and a normal life span.

thinks it might be possible someday for drugs to switch on gene proteins that help us cope effectively with stress and switch off the ones that drive the tendency for perfectionism and obsession that lead to runaway dieting. Gene therapy has the potential to help with co-occurring disorders and addictions, but we're a long way from identifying all the genetic components to target.

Jiggling the Lock:
The Keys of Anxiety and Depression

The internal forces driving an eating disorder are set into motion long before anyone can recognize symptoms. Besides perfectionism, there are other personal characteristics that foreshadow the risk of problematic eating attitudes. On a scale of one to ten, the closer to ten you rank yourself on a majority of the following traits, the higher your possibility to develop degrees of disordered eating and possibly, an ED:

- A need for safety, structure, and/or comfort
- The ability to delay gratification
- Being particularly critical of the failings of others
- Having an extraordinary sense of responsibility
- Lack of self-confidence and/or trust in others
- Desire to be exceptional at something
- Being highly disciplined and self-controlled
- Body and self-dissatisfaction
- Lack of compassion, for self and others
- Being overly concerned with how others see you
- Black-and-white, all-or-nothing thinking
- The tendency to ruminate, that is, replaying thoughts and events
- Lack of tolerance for distress

Personality traits like these often occur in people with clinically significant anxiety issues. The *American Journal of Psychiatry* has said that girls who experience high anxiety are twice as likely to suffer from an eating disorder as girls who don't.[11] Amy, twenty-four, from Toronto, Canada, is bulimirexic, binging and purging thousands of calories per day. "As Amy's personality developed, she showed more signs of being more anxious or concerned than [her sister and brother]," her mother, Wendy, told *Intervention* producers in Season 7.

Amy's older brother, Jonathan, thought Amy might have been naturally sensitive to emotional issues. Amy knew for certain she had been an anxious child. She had trouble finding her own identity. She battled with her older sister and struggled with self-confidence. "'Within the first week of high school, any scrap of self-esteem that I had left fell by the wayside,'" Amy read from her journal. "'I turned my focus on trying to look good. If I wasn't popular, cool, funny, smart, or vivacious like other girls my age, I yearned desperately to be pretty, as if that would make up for my lack of everything else.' That's when I definitely changed my food intake."[12]

Here's an Extra Scoop

Latching onto an activity or substance that soothes and calms our mood is what social psychologists call an *adaptive function*. Compulsions and addictions help us cope with stress, even though they are usually only temporary fixes, and poor substitutes for the true human needs and desires we all have.

The energy we feel from anxiety can be channeled to help us deal with whatever it is we are feeling anxious about. When you're encouraged to be open about your feelings, you feel safe about airing your troubles to a trusted listener. When you're empowered to take action to solve your problem, you learn valuable tools to handle stress. Certain families simply don't have well-developed communication skills and can't provide the kind of supportive environment a sensitive child needs to learn strategic coping skills. Girls like Amy and Jessie are at a loss when they feel stress building. Eating is a habitual activity that's natural to ritualize. Manipulating food is a way to take control of anxious feelings, and doing so relieves the pressure quite well. Intensifying a focus on eating habits serves as a distraction from sadness, despair, anger, any uncomfortable, negative emotion. It's an easy, short-term fix.

People who are anxious worry a lot about "What if . . . ?" They might have thoughts of impending doom. Jessie's parents had to calm her fears every night when she was a child—she remembers waking up with an awful feeling that something bad was going to happen.[13] Similarly, Amy's parents had to reassure her constantly. "Amy needed to be told, at this time we're going to do that, and at that time we're going to do this," said her father, Len. "Amy would get anxious anytime there was a change, no matter how small or big that might be."[14] The unknown is threatening to highly anxious individuals, who cannot tolerate uncertainty. This trait correlates strongly with the incidence of anorexia and bulimia, in particular, and we suspect it's true for binge eating as well. Researchers believe it drives the compulsions and rituals designed to gain control over fearfulness, and is therefore a likely risk factor for eating disorders.[15] Obsessive-compulsive disorder, panic disorder, social phobia, and depression have all been linked to this intolerance of uncertainty.

Like anxiety, *mood disorders* co-occur with most EDs. They affect 20 million Americans, close to 10 percent of the population, and are twice as common in women, as in men.[16] Teens experience an even higher rate—14 percent experience a mood disorder by age eighteen and 11 percent of them are severely impaired.[17] Twenty percent of Americans will experience clinically recognized mood disturbances over a lifetime. Along with anxiety disorders, mood disorders

Over and Over Again: The Link to OC(P)D

People with obsessive-compulsive disorder (OCD) engage in ritualistic behavior that they feel compelled to practice again and again. They wash hands, check locks or mechanical switches before going out, straighten objects in their living space, or hoard possessions. They take a pathological notice of the position of chairs, the relation of book heights on a shelf, the direction of tassels on a carpet. In true OCD, a state of "brain lock" occurs and sufferers are unable to will themselves out of the mental impulses. Their anxiety stems from feelings of doom, or concern about losing control over particular life situations.

People with obsessive-compulsive personality disorder (OCPD) integrate the "style" of OCD into the way they interpret social cues and how they ordinarily behave. Those with OCPD cope by adhering to rules, making "to do" lists, and setting standards for performance. People with EDs feature strong traits of OCD and OCPD, especially those doing any pathological dieting.

Multiple studies have found OCD and OCPD symptoms are highly correlated with EDs, particularly when the subjects are obsessive about contamination and compulsive about cleaning. At the University of California, Irvine in 2006, researchers looked at a population of 2,500 female inpatients being treated for anorexia, bulimia, or unclassified eating disorders. They noted that up to 65 percent of them had anxiety disorders, most commonly OCD and social phobia. They found OCD was twice as likely in those with anorexia than in those with other EDs.[i] An earlier study by Dr. Walter Kaye and his colleagues discovered that groups of anoretic, bulimic, and bulimirexic women had a higher incidence of anxiety disorders, especially OCD, compared to a group with no EDs. Forty-two percent reported that their anxiety symptoms came about in childhood, before they developed their eating disorder.[j] This was significant because anxiety in childhood is relatively rare (4–7 percent of all children) and the normal onset of OCD among women is in the early twenties. The researchers concluded that early symptoms of anxiety could be a risk factor in the development of anorexia or bulimia. Anxiety symptoms are also an early warning sign for depression.

are the most prominent mental health issue in the country and the leading cause of disability among Americans ages fifteen to forty-four.[18] By 2030, they will surpass heart disease as the most common disabling illness in the world.[19] Mood disorders are psychological illnesses and include the following:

- *Major depressive disorder*—characterized by extreme sadness, disturbances in appetite and sleep, isolation from people and activities, muscle aches and pains, and thoughts of worthlessness and suicide
- *Dysthymia*—a mild form of clinical depression that often starts in childhood or adolescence and lasts for years
- *Atypical depression*—associated with agitation and anger, rather than "the blues," and also with overeating
- *Seasonal affective disorder*—depressive symptoms that come and go with low-light winter months
- *Bipolar (manic-depressive) disorder*—periods of depression that alternate or run together with periods of mania. A milder version, bipolar II is also known as cyclothymia. (More than the other depressive disorders, bipolar disorder is associated with anorexia and underweight bulimics. This may be a reflection of anxiety components that are closely associated with this illness.)
- *Postpartum depression*—depression in women following the birth of a child

Less common forms are substance-induced mood disorder, mood disorder due to a general medical condition, psychotic depression, and premenstrual dysphoric disorder.

Because they often appear together, mood disorders and disordered eating are risk factors for each other. A mood disorder may barely be noticeable before eating becomes a problem, but it can definitely worsen as an eating disorder grows. An individual's level of serotonin activity may have a lot to do with this. Researchers suspect that serotonin levels are influenced by depression—signs of low serotonin activity have been noted in people who binge and eat compulsively. Unfortunately, there is no foolproof way to measure actual amounts that are available to the brain, and no studies have ever proven that brain levels of any neurotransmitter are in short supply when depression or any other mental illness occurs.[20] Nevertheless, we can get an idea of relative amounts of serotonin by measuring certain blood indicators.

Higher serotonin activity has been observed in people who have starved down to very low weights and then recovered. "Over-activity of the serotonin system reduces appetite," reported Dr. Walter Kaye in NOVA's *Dying to Be Thin*. He went on to explain that both human and animal studies have shown the relation-

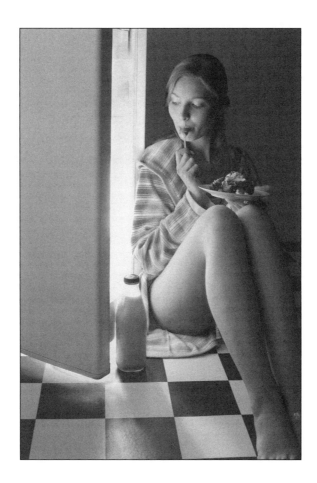

ship goes along with obsessive, anxious, and harm-avoidant behavior. Starvation diets may help certain people reduce serotonin levels, which decreases their anxiety, at least somewhat. But the brain adapts by adding new receptors. "Even a little bit of serotonin sets off these receptors," Dr. Kaye concluded. "So people have to keep starving themselves more and more to reduce the serotonin, as the receptors keep up-regulating."[21] This is one reason why undereating or cycles of binging and purging become habits that are difficult to break.

Looking at the families of people with eating disorders, not only do we find signs of anxiety and depression, but also a high rate of disordered eating and compulsive behavioral disorders among related family members. Family studies have shown that the prevalence of EDs is seven to twelve times higher among relatives of someone with anorexia or bulimia.[22] Dr. Kaye has also pointed out that if roughly 7 percent of family members have been diagnosed with an ED, we can expect another 5–7 percent of other relatives have some kind of compulsive or addictive disorder.[23] But should families accept responsibility for instigating an eating disorder? How much? Let's examine this issue, and other outside factors that work for and against us.

Everything but No One to Blame

We've come a long way since eating disorders were seen as cases of vanity run amuck in upper-class, attention-seeking young white women with low-self esteem. Once we moved away from victim blaming, we insisted it must be the fault of critical, overly demanding, and emotionally cold parents. Therapists believed eating disorders must represent an underlying dysfunction taking place in the family, something that would resolve as the conflicts were addressed in therapy. Today, we recognize there is no standard family dynamic or family member characteristic that triggers an ED or that must be eliminated if a patient is to get well. Parents are much less likely to have the finger pointed at them for mistakes in child rearing. Blaming family members for contributing to an eating disorder is not helpful. Very often, they're encouraged to be part of the recovery process. Everyone in a family can learn how to better express and interpret emotions like love and anger, and how to resolve fear. They can also exhibit positive attitudes about body weight, personal attractiveness, and mealtime rituals, through what is said and unsaid. What goes on within a family certainly has an impact on children and influences their eating behavior for better, and for worse. For people sensitive to developing an ED, family dynamics can either place them at further risk, or be able to strengthen their resistance.

Family relationships significantly affect young girls' attitudes about their body image. "Mothers have a profound influence," said Dr. Nancy Etcoff, a psychologist at Massachusetts General Hospital and faculty member at Harvard Medical School. "We asked young girls, who has the strongest influence on their body image and their beauty. They said, their mothers and girlfriends—more than 'media,' more than 'celebrities.' For the most part we found mothers were a positive influence. The girls that had the highest self-esteem and highest body image listed their moms most of all. Girlfriends could be a negative influence."[24] Fathers' attitudes and opinions also make a difference in developing their daughters' and sons' emotional well-being. We'll be discussing attitudes toward body image and the issue of self-esteem in chapter 5.

Adversity within families creates uncertainty and distress that increase the risk of developing any psychological disorder. Emotional trauma can result from long-term effects of unemployment, the ill health of a family member, as well as outright abuse. Overeaters, undereaters, alcoholics, junkies, cutters, sexaholics, compulsive gamblers, shoppers, and Internet surfers (you name it!)—all identify

Here's an Extra Scoop

When family members are willing to take part in a patient's healing process, they greatly enhance the chance for full recovery.

painful emotional experiences that took place before they were overwhelmed by their disorder. Wounds might not have resulted from severe personal abuse, neglect, or trauma, or even be terribly excruciating. Even so, the hurt is there, real, and unresolved. Settling into regimented habits, even if unhealthful, brings relief, one of many possible responses to intense feelings. Amy, with her explosive temperament, needed to feel more love and care than she got from her family. "Anorexia became my best friend," she said, "someone that never leaves me and is unconditionally there. Whether or not they're there in a positive way, they're there, and that's comforting."[25] As an adaptive function, an eating disorder rescues a sufferer from what she perceives as emotionally traumatic.

Even when parents are providing the best living situation they can for their children, there are damaging factors outside their control. An ED can lock in after major life transitions—a divorce, a remarriage, a move to a new home, the loss of a parent or close family member. Smaller ongoing stressors like bullying or competitive events can accumulate and cause a lot of emotional distress. Such toxic environments can teach us to feel helpless and hopeless, aggravating predispositions to anxiety and depression. They leave some with a warped sense of control, over both their own behavior and their effect on their world. When body weight and personal image are focal points in a person's life, it's natural to turn attention to food following traumatic experiences. Fourteen-year-old Erin revealed to her treatment team that she had been molested. "Trauma is what really hit it off," she told NOVA's documentary film producers. "Bringing up my trauma issues really made me want to . . . I just wanted to get rid of it somehow. The feelings, too many feelings, way too many feelings."[26]

Whether an eating disorder arose as a means of coping with a traumatic event or other, less tragic life stressors, there are deep psychological conflicts that need to be resolved. Some people with a history of abuse might overeat, seeking the comfort that food brings, feeding a cry for help they cannot express. Many prefer to retreat into a cloak of invisibility that comes with excess weight as a way to feel safe from unwanted attention. Others will undereat as a way to punish themselves, feeling unworthy of care. Disordered eating is also a way to seize control in the wake of runaway emotions. Whatever the extreme eating patterns that develop, an intimate relationship with food and intense body size fixation take the place of healthy human relationships.

An Expert Weighs In: Dr. Timothy Brewerton— the Intersection of Trauma

Dr. Timothy Brewerton is a clinical professor of psychiatry and behavioral sciences at the Medical University of South Carolina in Charleston, where he founded the Eating Disorders Program in 1987. He is also the executive medical director of the Hearth Center for Healing at Carolina Children's Home in Columbia, South Carolina. He's a respected researcher and lecturer in the field, has published over 125 articles and book chapters, and has made over 300 presentations to professional groups around the world. His specialized investigation into the relationship between trauma and eating disorders was awarded special commendation by the International Association of Eating Disorder Professionals in 2012. He's interested in the levels of post-traumatic stress that co-occur with eating disorders and disordered eating behaviors.

Here is how he answered a few questions in 2013:[27]

How common are traumatic experiences in people with eating disorders?

It's practically universal. More than 90 percent of women and men who reported having an eating disorder at some point in their life, also admitted to experiencing some type of earlier trauma. The same response has come from children and adolescents as well. The finding has been corroborated in a number of studies, which establishes trauma history as a risk factor for eating disorders.

What kind of trauma are we talking about?

All types of "Big T" traumas—emotional, physical, and sexual abuse; neglect and harassment; witnessing interpersonal violence or combat; natural accidents and disasters; and experiencing forms of discrimination. The data suggests that any experience that produces mild or moderate PTSD [post-traumatic stress disorder], or any form of significant anxiety, adds to the risk of developing an eating disorder.

Are some types of eating disorder behavior more often associated with traumatic stress?

As a matter of fact, yes. People who resort only to calorie and food restriction are much less likely to report significant traumas. Those with binging and bulimic-type behaviors commonly indicate traumatic histories. The association is tighter as the number of episodes increase. One 2002 study found that nearly all its subjects with bulimia had experienced multiple episodes of child abuse and were at much higher risk of having other anxiety and mood disorders.

Does an eating disorder tend to be worse in people who have experienced really terrible trauma?

There doesn't seem to be much of a relation between the extent of the victimization and the severity of the eating disorder. People with eating disorders who have experienced abuse score as less trusting and more dissociated from feelings than those with eating disorders who haven't been abused, but not necessarily as more eating disordered. One 2012 study

Triggering Debate: People as -ics

Is it wise to call someone anore(c)tic, bulimic, or binger/binge eater? Many treatment professionals, and families of people with eating disorders are unwilling to use the terms because of stigmatizing a loved one with a mental disorder. Yet sufferers closely identify with their illness and use these words without second thought. What are some advantages and disadvantages of defining yourself or someone else by a disease or disorder? How might it affect one's treatment and recovery?

did find, however, that childhood emotional abuse actually predicted the severity of disordered eating. This could be because of the effect of the abuse on self-esteem, personal drive, and ability to regulate mood.

So how can we predict whether trauma will lead to an eating disorder?

The development of PTSD or its symptoms probably points the way, along with interacting genetic factors. In looking at data from the National Women's Study, we found that women who were raped and developed PTSD were over five times more likely to develop bulimia than women who were never raped. When compared to women who were raped, but didn't develop PTSD, the ratio was the same. This indicates that it's the reaction to the trauma, rather than the trauma itself, that might predict someone will use eating habits to cope.

Teens Wired for Risk

It's risky business becoming a teenager. Brain scientists now understand that new neural pathways establish themselves well into our twenties, modifying how we learn and remember, assess social situations, and choose between alternatives. Brain circuits that work to control our emotions and check our desires—the cognitive control system—form behind those of the reward center. If you're stressed out, you feel a hard drive for relief and satisfaction. Almost every "want" and "need" can seem like a craving. If you're anxious and impulsive and are experiencing dysfunctional family, school, and social situations, you're at special risk for making conscious and unconscious choices that line the path to self-destruction.

Some deviance from normal behavior can be healthy. It's important to be able to test and explore limits—admonishments from adults to "just say no" aren't always realistic or beneficial. It's equally important to understand, though, some of us are hyperconditioned to mental stress, even mental illnesses. *Neuroplasticity*—how the brain learns from itself—makes some of us particularly vulnerable to developing eating and substance use disorders. Thought processes at work during your teen and young adult years are reinforced by behavior that then becomes highly resistant to change. For teens who are at risk and for those that succumb to emotional disorder, the long-term consequences of decisions made under such mental stress permanently affect their adult selves. When struggling with an ED and all the accompanying issues, it's hard to deepen the social connections and academic gains that are so necessary during this period. Without adequate treatment, career success and personal contentment is difficult to attain.

It's a pivotal time of life, for sure.

Has it always been like this? Modern investigation into the biological basis for behavior suggests brain development in humans has proceeded pretty much the same way, generation after generation, for eons. (Comparing DNA analyses of prehistoric human remains to people living today, paleontologists and evolutionary geneticists are certain that the human genome is virtually unchanged since the last wave of migration out of Africa around 50,000 years ago.) Whatever genetic markers for psychological disorders might exist (the result of random mutation), they've been floating among a percentage of us since at least the dawn of civilization. It's not only possible, but probable such markers put some of us at greater risk for behavioral disorders and borderline ED symptoms that usually show up in adolescence. It's part of our human destiny to struggle with emotional responses relative to cultural values and to seek to satisfy cravings by whatever means available. Any appetite can become entangled in feelings, and when food is plentiful enough, disordered eating can become a focal point. Given the delicate balance of our brain chemistry, this can spell big trouble.

Extreme eating practices have always happened in the context of personal experience, cultural pressure, and biochemical sensitivity. Anorexia, bulimia, and binge eating as we understand them today are part of a historical legacy that has its roots in human nature. Let's look back in time to find out when freaky eating was taking place, who was doing it, and why.

More Food for Thought

Read

Lauren Greenfield. *Girl Culture*. San Francisco: Chronicle Books, 2002.
Susan Nolen-Hoeksema. *Eating, Drinking, Overthinking: The Toxic Triangle of Food, Alcohol, and Depression—and How Women Can Break Free*. New York: Henry Holt, 2006.

Watch

Depression: Out of the Shadows (documentary, 90 minutes). A production of Twin Cities Public Television, Inc., and WBGH/Boston with Larkin McPhee for PBS's Take One Step series. Originally aired May 21, 2008. www.pbs.org/wgbh/takeonestep/depression/index.html.

Dying to Be Thin (documentary, 60 minutes). A NOVA production by Twin Cities Public Television, Inc., with Larkin McPhee for WGBH/Boston. Originally aired December 12, 2000. www.pbs.org/wgbh/nova/body/dying-to-be-thin.html.

Perfect Illusions: Eating Disorders and the Family (documentary, 56 minutes). A production of KCTS Television/Seattle by Peggy Case and Josh Golding, 2002. Originally aired February 24, 2003. www.pbs.org/perfectillusions.

Learn

Binge Eating and Bulimia: The Latest Psychological Research on Eating Disorders (Dr. Sumati Gupta's blog). www.bingeeatingbulimia.com.

Healthy Place: America's Mental Health Channel. Mental health community information, articles, blogs, forums, chat, streaming (online TV and radio) concerning all psychological anomalies. www.healthyplace.com.

Mental Health America (formerly known as the National Mental Health Association). www.nmha.org.

LET'S DISH ON THE PAST: THE ORIGINS OF EXTREME EATING

I ate so little in those days, my buttocks looked as knobbly as a camel's hoof. The bones of my spine stuck out like a row of spindles and my ribs looked like a collapsed old shed.

And much good did it do me.

—Siddhartha Gautama (Śākyamuni Buddha), ca. 500 BC
As quoted by Michael Wood, *The Story of India, Episode 2: The Power of Ideas*, 2007

When did people first start to force themselves to go hungry? Did people of ancient cultures overeat on purpose? Was an emotional attachment to eating as common in the past as it seems to be today? Discover the legacy of eating disorders in human culture and think about what might drive their existence in our society today.

The Best Ascetic Is a Dead Ascetic

In his quest to ease suffering, the Buddha finally understood, ya gotta eat. Having spent six years practicing *asceticism*, subsisting on drops of water and little more than one nut or grain of rice per day, the skeletal former prince abandoned starvation in his search for enlightenment. Deprivation could not bring inner peace, he thought. "My body slowly became extremely emaciated," he wrote. "My limbs became like the jointed segments of vines, or bamboo stems. My spine stood out like a string of beads. My ribs jutted out like the jutting rafters of an old abandoned building. The gleam of my eyes appeared to be sunk deep in my eye sockets, like the gleam of water deep in a well. My scalp shriveled and withered like a green, bitter gourd. Shriveled and withered in the heat and wind."[1]

On the verge of death, Siddhartha imagined there must be something else besides the extremes of self-denial and self-indulgence that could ultimately lead to serenity. Meditating in the shade of a rose apple tree, he realized that true joy, though fleeting, could be found from time to time in an imperfect world. Peace and contentment was the underlying fabric of the universe and available to all humanity. This realization didn't answer the question as to why there was suffering in the world, yet it gave him the means to define a solution for it. Accepting the offer of rice porridge from a kind-hearted peasant girl, he ate to draw strength to focus his mind. He knew he had to look within and trust himself. Washed and refreshed, he settled into a lotus position between the roots of a banyan fig—the Bodhi Tree—to meditate for supreme wisdom. Overnight, he faced his innermost fears and withstood temptation, awakening to the cosmic truth of the workings of the universe. His revelation became Buddhism's Four Noble Truths, guiding seekers to deal with discontentment. Nirvana is found within; we already have the capacity for enlightenment. To achieve it, traverse the Middle Way and find balance in the midst of overindulgence on one side, excessive restraint on the other.

Did the Buddha develop an eating disorder through his years as an ascetic and then heal himself through a gift of insight? We'll never be sure. We do know, though, humans have evolved a great physical response to periods of changing food availability, and an incredible mental capacity to handle times of deprivation and times of plenty.

First, We Got Hungry

For the greater portion of the human historical record, food has not been easy to come by. Our ancient ancestors survived for tens of thousands of years on the plants they could forage and on the animals they could chase down. Evolution has designed us to store extra food energy we consume. When lean times come, we have a better chance to survive. That's why we're (normally) tempted to take advantage of food when it's plentiful. Plus, we have a natural affinity for the creamy and the sweet. No inner bell-ringer automatically flushes calories when we've eaten more than we need. When food is scant, our metabolism ramps down to preserve our essential functioning. Our biology has let us adapt to ups and downs of food supply while our psychology has opened the window to a complicated mess of emotional eating patterns.

From the time our ancestors left off hunting and gathering to try their luck at agriculture in the Fertile Crescent, the juxtaposition of food shortages with times of plenty has determined the course of whole civilizations and the relative success of the reigning rulers. Famine is not a rare historical event—millions upon tens of millions of people have died from hunger all over the world even before the first recorded account of mass starvation in ancient Egypt around 4,000 years ago. *Food (in)security* is a continual issue for developing nations, as well as for our country and other world powers. It seems improbable that people who struggle to get enough to eat would be interested in dieting to achieve or keep a particular body shape. It's easy to assume problem eating only occurs in a society with abundant food and from modern pressures to look and feel good. Yet deliberate control of calories in, calories out is not a phenomenon only of our twenty-first-century, image-obsessed society.

Attitudes toward obesity and thinness are cultural, not period specific. Every society, economic class, and individual family has held specific notions about what sort of food and drink and how much of it should be enjoyed. Custom dictates who deserves to eat and when. Culture also creates parameters about what is attractive and desirable, and people strive to emulate the characteristics that bring them closer to the ideal. People in early human societies were not immune to such pressures. The Egyptians used *emetics* regularly for the purposes of regurgitating food they believed led to illness. Whether any of them purged over a desire to be slender is still up for debate, but it's clear that standards of beauty did exist. Egyptian drawings show slim human forms, and we know they used cosmetics and jewelry to cover and refine imperfections. Representational artwork from Persia and China indicates captivation with an ideal human face and form, while texts have described signs in medical patients that are eerily similar to descriptions of eating disorder symptoms today. It's certain the Greeks held prejudices about body size, and extremes of over- and undereating occurred through antiquity. The Romans felt the same and suffered much personal conflict over food consumption. They're infamous for eating orgies and purging practices in order to make room to eat more. Teenagers of ancient Rome, along with their mothers,

Here's an Extra Scoop

One widespread fictitious "fact" continuing to persist across the Internet (and even among experts who should know better) is the assertion that the Roman *vomitoria* were special rooms set aside expressly for the purposes of barfing after a gorge. Not true. A vomitorium is a passageway used to access a stage or playing field, or for an audience to move quickly to and from the seating area before and after the show. There's no evidence they were used for anything else.

were probably as phobic about fat as we are, and at least two emperors, Claudius and Vitellius, may have suffered full-blown bulimia.

Then, We Discovered Eating

Eating serves all sorts of purposes—few of them have had to do with nourishment. Throughout history every human civilization has seen both gluttony and deprivation used as means to ends that each culture has recognized and helped define. Want to attain greater spiritual awareness, take a political stand against injustice, or get into a size double zero? Starving can get you there. On the other hand, maintaining a larger size can enable you to feel more powerful, show off your fertility, display your community's prosperity, or serve as a layer of personal protection. If you enjoy physical challenges, you can even turn food consumption into a money-making, fame-building formula. In the last ten centuries the world has been home to ascetic monks, miraculous saints, hunger artists, fasting girls, hunger strikers, and competitive eaters. There's evidence that extreme eating and the trouble it causes has been happening for as long as we've been human.

Let's take a trip down memory lane.

2,000 Years of Funky Eating (161 BC to AD 2013)

161 BC: Size Zero Wannabes

Terence, a young North African poet, depicts the Roman Republic's contemporary emphasis on slimness and its scorn for obesity in his comic play, *Eunuchus*. Terence's character Chaerea admits that the girl he loves is not like other pinched and pressed girls of the day: "She is a girl who doesn't look like the girls . . . whose mothers strive to make them have sloping shoulders, a squeezed chest so that they look slim. If one is a little plumper, they say she is a boxer and they reduce her diet. Though she is well-endowed by nature, this treatment makes her as thin as a bulrush. And men love them for that."[2] Then he describes the girl of his dreams: "unusual looks . . . a natural complexion, a plump and firm body, full of vitality." Even the earliest cultural pressures to conform to beauty standards receive a backlash in social commentary.

Second Century: No Appetite

The Roman philosopher/physician Galen of Pergamon (AD 129–ca. 216) records his observations of "anorecktous" or "asitous," "people who refuse food and do

Body Beauty

The representation of the human form has always reflected the sentimentality of the artist and the concepts of beauty, prosperity, and goodness of the time period. During the Renaissance, the Flemish and Dutch Masters—Rembrandt, Renoir, Rubens, and Jan van der Streat (whose painting is shown here)—were especially keen to admire large, fleshy bodies. Many of the upper class flaunted their corpulent figures to physically set themselves apart from the underclass. Gradually, the tide of approval would turn again toward a leaner ideal; thin women would seem more spiritually pure, lean men as more productive.

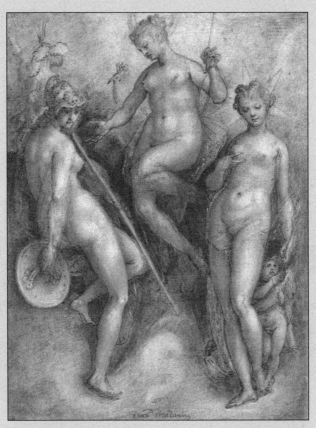

Three Goddesses: Minerva, Juno and Venus, ca. 1587 (Jan van der Straet, 1523–1605). *The Pepita Milmore Fund, National Gallery of Art, Washington, D.C.*

not take anything."[3] He thinks an abnormal stomach acid is the cause of "bulimis," an exaggerated, but false hunger signal.[4] He also knows local secrets for staying slim and recommends tonics and tinctures to use as diuretics and emetics. For the foreseeable future, *anorexia* would refer to lack of appetite as a symptom of disease, not a fully formed disorder. Variants of the word *bulimia*, describing ravenous hunger and overeating, usually followed by regurgitation, occur in texts as diverse as the Talmud and the writings of Latin grammarians.

Thirteenth, Fourteenth, and Fifteenth Centuries: Holy Anorexia!

Catholic saints of the Middle Ages, such as Margaret of Cortuna (1247–1297), Angela of Foligno (1248–1309), Catherine of Siena (1347–1380), Columba of Rieti (1467–1501), and other pious women, feed on next to nothing as they devote themselves in service to God. Everyone believes it's a miraculous sign to be freed from the necessity of eating. The phenomenon is named *anorexia mirabilis*, a "miraculous loss of appetite, divinely inspired." Although strangely invigorated with intense mental and physical energy, eventually, they all waste away. As the sixteenth century progresses, the Catholic Church frowns on severe asceticism, consigning anoretics as witches to be burned at the stake.[5] In the decades following the last of the Christian mystics, a desire for ethereality would overtake some introspective young maids in both farming villages and cosmopolitan cities of the Old and New Worlds. Under the stress of cultural expectations to control passions, and social ideals of femininity that favored the pale and lightweight, would emerge a new brand of anorexia, 'anorexia nervosa.'

1589: The Fasting Girl of Schmidweiler (Holland)

Upon her arrival home from a wedding, Katerin Cooper is taken with "a shaking" and "lost all pleasure & appetite to warm meats for a space [of] 5 years, but [would] eat cold meat." Attempting to remedy her appetite, a physician concocts a potion that causes her to suck only the juice from apples and pears. Six months later, she gives up all but water and aqua vita as a mouthwash. According to the account, Katerin "yet liveth in like disposition and state. . . without eating, drinking, or sleeping, . . . nine whole years complete."[6]

1594: The Fasting Maiden of Meurs (Belgium)

The "miraculous maid in Flanders," Eve Fleigen is poverty-stricken when she first prays to God to deliver her from intense hunger pangs. It works. Tales of

St. Catherine of Sienna (1347–1380)

Receiving her first vision of Christ as a young child, Catherine was already depriving herself of meat by the age of seven. Her first massive fast followed the deaths of two older sisters after which, to the aggravation of her parents, she confirmed herself to God. Throughout her short life, Catherine subsisted on little more than salad, regurgitating most of what she swallowed, and ignored the pleas of her Dominican sisters and other church authorities to eat more. Claiming the needs of others' salvation were so great, she had no time to think, let alone touch, earthly food, she fasted and suffered for thirty-three years.

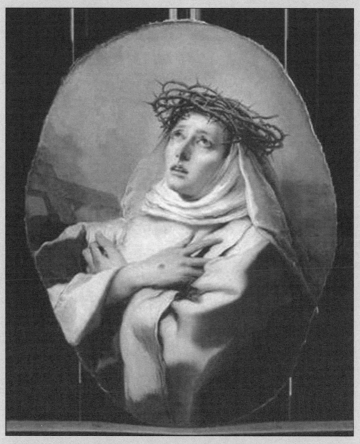

St. Catherine of Siena. *Courtesy of the Kunsthistoriches Museum, Vienna, Austria.*

St. Theresa of Ávila (1515–1582)

St. Theresa of Ávila was one of the last of the Roman Catholic "miraculous" saints. Although not as prodigious a faster as her earlier sisters, as a young nun, she attempted to follow the original Carmelite Rule by sleeping on straw, fasting eight months a year, abstaining from meat, and living in total seclusion. She also inflicted upon herself "mortifications of the flesh," making her one of the earliest "cutters."

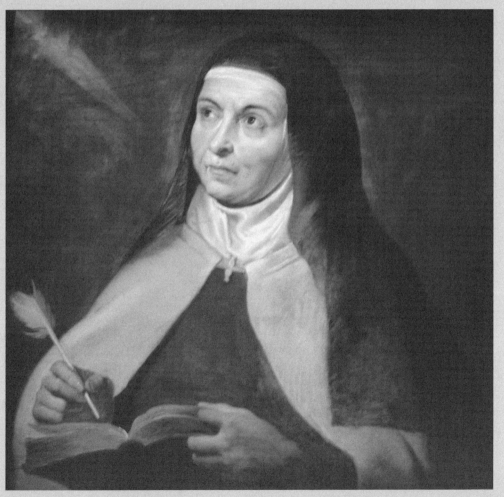

St. Theresa of Ávila. *Courtesy of the Kunsthistoriches Museum, Vienna, Austria.*

Fasting Girls: From Catherine to Karen, Part 1

Who were the "fasting girls"? Wondrous stories of miraculous maids cropped up in northern Europe during the final epoch of the last starving saints. These Anglo-Saxon girls and young women ate only miniscule amounts for months and years, an effort of inedia prodigiosa, or prodigious fasting. Some insisted their ability to survive came from divine grace, and they drew crowds of believers. Others were bedridden from serious accidents that took place prior to their abstinence and claimed to have other supernatural powers. Most were too weak to speak much, although a few put themselves on display for public entertainment. Almost all the tales end tragically—the girls either starved to death, or were called out as frauds and run out of town. A few were even executed.

Eve's ability that "din'd on a rose and supt on a tulip"[7] spread her fame far and wide. Magistrates, ministers, and noblemen devise tests to trick her into eating, which only sicken her. She manages to live for approximately fifteen years, weak and pale, complaining neither of thirst nor hunger.

1603: The Fasting Girl of Confolens (France)

After suffering a fever that temporarily took her speech, eleven-year-old Jane Balen (a.k.a. Ione Balam) refuses all food and drink for almost three years. She comes to the attention of the king's physician, Jacobus Viverius, who documents her case and checks for signs of deceit. He writes of the emaciated fourteen-year-old, "Her belly was so flat, the passages were shut, no entrance there was found . . . her privy parts were clean, thence nothing fell to ground."[8]

1668: The Derbyshire Damsel (Britain)

Eighteen-year-old Martha Taylor "hath no belly to be seen" and is "the picture of death" after a year and a week of fasting. Those around her are convinced she took nothing but a few drops of prune or raisin juice, and believe she is "a perfect and true revelation of the handy work of Almighty God."[9] A skeptic, John Reynolds, takes one look at her and pronounces that her altered state is due to illness, warning that such abstinence from food can only continue for so long.

1684–1694: A Wasting Disease of Nervous Origin

A specialist in consumptive illnesses, English physician Richard Morton, MD, examines the eighteen-year-old daughter of "Mr. Duke in S. Mary Axe" and finds her "like a Skeleton only clad in skin." He notes her loss of appetite, bad digestion, emaciation, and pale look. She also suffers from "a total Suppression of her Monthly Courses from a multitude of Cares and Passions of the Mind."[10] She had refused medical interventions for the previous two years, and was now experiencing blackouts. Despite her improvement with Morton's attempts to treat her, she soon relapses and dies within three months.

In his 1694 opus on consumption, Morton describes a second patient, "The Son of The Reverend Minister Steele," who began fasting at age sixteen as he be-

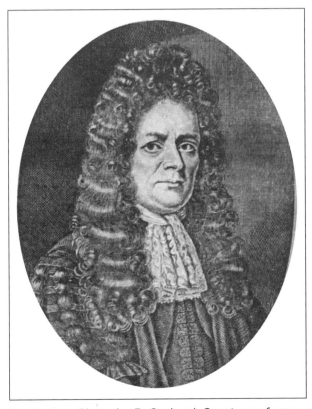

Dr. Morton. *Photo by B. Orchard. Courtesy of open-library.org. Original source: Short Biographies of the Worthies of Worcestershire by Edith Ophelia Browne and John Richard Burton (E.G. Humphreys, 1916).*

came increasingly obsessed with his studies. After prescribing various medicines to no avail, the good doctor advises him to "abandon his Studies, to go into the Country air, and to use Riding, and a Milk Diet." The young man recovers his health, somewhat, but "is not yet perfectly freed from a Consumptive State."[11] Morton is fascinated by this unique form of "Nervous Atrophy" that appears devoid of "Fever, Cough, or Shortness of Breath," and mentions that although he has observed it in England, it occurs "most frequently amongst those that have lived in Virginia."[12]

1813: The Fasting Woman of Tutbury (England)

After insisting that she had been living without food (except for the inside of a few black currants) since 1807, and having tasted celebrity in her village full of staunch supporters, Ann Moore agrees to be put under a round-the-clock watch in May. Within nine days, she is near death. When her daughter confesses she had often covertly bathed her mother in milk or gravy and transferred food morsels by mouth, Ann recants her story and admits her deception. She is disgraced and reduced to begging.

1859: Anorexia Update 1

American doctor William Chipley, in charge of the Eastern Kentucky Lunatic Asylum, publishes a paper detailing the health of adolescent girls brought to his office by anxious parents. He notes their disinterest in food and questions whether their refusal to eat might be a ploy to gain more attention. He calls their illness sitomania, believing their self-starvation a symptom of insanity. Simultaneously across the Atlantic Ocean, French physician Louis-Victor Marcé publishes his observations of hysteria affecting young Paris women who severely restrict food at mealtimes. He counsels they be cared for by medical professionals, away from the family environment.

1869: The Welsh Fasting Girl (Wales)

The farm family of twelve-year-old Sarah Jacob reports she had begun to refuse food in October of 1867, reducing her intake first to a pill-sized apple, then nothing at all. Many corroborate the story, and the Jacob family rakes in a tidy sum from the trail of religious pilgrims to Sarah's bedside. Several concerned locals, who had viewed the feeble girl, contact hospital staff, who examine her and set up a watch to discover how she was actually surviving. Convinced of Sarah's

Fasting Girls: From Catherine to Karen, Part 2

Long before the era of Photoshopping today's concave fashion models, young Victorian women of nineteenth-century America were dining on dry toast and weak black tea. New books on etiquette had set new standards for table manners and demure behavior. Health specialists advised young ladies to stay away from meat, other than tiny portions of chicken or fish, to keep carnal passions under control. Displaying any enthusiasm for food was considered vulgar, sure to offend prospective gentlemen. "People thought eating small amounts deliberately was something a good woman did," said Joan Jacobs Brumberg, author of *Fasting Girls: A History of Anorexia Nervosa*. "Having a robust appetite meant you were not a genteel woman. If you looked too robust, you looked like a working woman."[a] Girls with wasp waists could lounge on couches, not sweat in the fields.

The noose of social pressure to control desires and conform to modern standards of femininity was tightening, especially on upwardly mobile young women. Growing girls of the 1870s and '80s like Mollie Fancher, Lenora Eaton, Kate Smulsey, Lina Finch, and Josephine Marie Bedard would think they could healthfully curb their appetites with a few crackers, spoonfuls of soup, and bits of fruit and vegetable. It wasn't long before American doctors were seeing signs of malnutrition in middle and upper class teenagers. They called it chlorosis, due to the greenish cast that came over the girls' pale complexions. Known today as *anemia*, it coincided with "caprices and perversions" of the appetite, heart palpitations, lethargy, amenorrhea, and melancholy.[b] These symptoms were suspiciously similar to those of a strange wasting condition, anorexia nervosa, newly classified by doctors in Europe. The medical profession was just beginning to accept the concept of eating disorder as a psychological illness, and not just a symptom of another disease.

As most of the girls recovered and rose from their beds, the mystique of their illness together with their wan appearance became an admirable quality. Slenderness was recognized as the current Victorian image of beauty. Excess body fat was increasingly thought of as a character flaw, judged as a lack of self-control, rather than an obvious sign of prosperity.

The aspiration to saintliness was steadily morphing into a desire for thinness among girls coming of age in the earliest years of the twentieth century, just as the notion of achievement was a broadening concept for talented women. In the years to come, ideas about desire for more versus self-control and deservedness, would coexist uneasily. For a small but not insignificant legion of girls—and a few boys, too—these thoughts would spell psychological and physical disaster.

supernatural abilities and suspicious of medical intervention, her parents refuse to allow feedings without Sarah's own consent. She immediately begins to fail and within a week is dead.

1873: Anorexia Update 2

Once again, two doctors, one in Britain, one in France, treat emaciated patients and separately publish papers that add up to a full clinical picture of what they label *anorexia nervosa*. Sir William Gull originally names the malady apepsia, then changes his mind upon delivering an address to the British Medical Association. "In the [earlier] address at Oxford," he explains, "I used the term 'apepsia hysterica,' but before seeing Dr. Lasègue's paper [describing l'anorexie hystérique], it had equally occurred to me that 'anorexia' would be more correct."[13] He settles on *nervosa*, suggesting that the illness is organic, rather than a product of the female imagination. Dr. Gull, one of Queen Victoria's personal family physicians, speculates no more on the cause of the illness. He strongly believes patients, mostly young women age sixteen to twenty-three, should be treated immediately for their physical symptoms, whether or not they are agreeable, and be prevented from their "restless activity," difficult as that may be to control.[14] A nourishing diet and warmth, he observes, contributes more to recovery than prescribed medicines.

In Paris, Dr. Ernest-Charles Lasègue, a neuropsychiatrist, takes a different look at the illness he thinks is more psychological than physical. His paper on "hysterical anorexia" draws consistent parallels between his young patients' declining mental state, their family relationships, and their manipulative eating behavior. He categorizes three stages—a period of refusal where the patient becomes more and more uneasy with food items, restricting both choice and quantity, followed by a period of increasing restlessness, extended activity, and a complete lack of belief

More Wonders of Fasting: Hunger Artists

Would you, could you starve yourself for money? Fasting as a performance art was taking place in medieval village taverns as early as the mid-1500s. Watching someone sit and not eat must have been pretty fair entertainment for the late Renaissance, and "fasting wonders" were often part of seventeenth-century circus sideshows in both Europe and America. A few became famous enough to draw big crowds to special exhibitions running from thirty to forty days, usually under close medical supervision and steady relays of "watchers."

The heyday of professional fasting lasted from 1880 to 1922, but people all over the world still turn to various types of prolonged fasts for political, religious, and therapeutic purposes. The longest successful supervised fast occurred in 1965, documented by a team of Scottish medical researchers. A twenty-seven-year-old male, weighing 456 pounds, volunteered for the study designed to measure the body's biological response to a short-term fast. The patient took in non-caloric liquids and various vitamin and mineral supplements. He adapted so well to the regimen, and was so "eager to reach his 'ideal' weight," the doctors let him continue for 382 days.[c] Altogether, he lost 276 pounds and five years later had gained back only sixteen.

in the need to eat. In stage three, the patient's deterioration is evident. Family, friends, and finally the youngster herself begin to fear that she might die. Dr. Lasègue is particularly adept at describing how the illness affects the family and the stubborn difficulties of full recovery. His clinical experiences promote a behavioral explanation for eating disorders, a belief that determines the course of treatment for decades.

1890: Starving for Dollars—Giovanni Succi

From the *New York Times*, November 6, 1890:

Signor Giovanni Succi, an Italian gentleman who has attained some fame as a professional faster, began last night what he declares will be a forty-five day fast. People who would like to see how he fasts can find him in the small hall over Koster & Bial's place of entertainment, in West Twenty-Third Street, at any time of the day or night. A section of the hall has been marked off by a railing, and within that section are a bed, lounge, tables and chairs for the use of Signor Succi.

The faster dined there last evening in the presence of a score or more of ladies and gentlemen, and his repast consisted of anchovies, boiled trout, olives, celery, risotta (an Italian baked dish comprising rice, mushrooms, cheese, and wine), cauliflower, kidney stew, roast chicken, roast partridge, roast quail, grapes, pears, and a quart bottle of Chianti. It took Succi about an hour to clear the cloth, and he left few fragments. At 8:10 o'clock he lighted a cigar and began to fast. . . . The faster will undertake to exist for forty-five days without any solid food. He will drink all of the water he wants and will smoke occasionally. He has a bottle of medicine, which he says is a simple precaution to allay pains in the stomach. Of this he will take twenty or thirty drops in a glass of water every two or three days. . . . Signor Succi will pass his time in reading, conversation, fencing, boxing, and billiard playing. He will sleep whenever he feels in the mood.[15]

From the *New York Times*, December 21, 1890:

Signor Giovanni Succi finished his forty-five days' fast at 8:11 o'clock last evening with a cup of weak cocoa . . . his thirty-fifth and longest period of fasting will be his last. . . . His vitality is almost exhausted, his nerves shattered and his tissues almost gone. . . . [Doctors say] he was on the verge of collapse . . . having faithfully abstained from food. . . . He will dine in public on the stage of Koster & Bial's. . . . The bill of fare will be rice soup, sardines, chicken, roast quail, with wine, coffee and fruits.[16]

1913: Fasting for Freedom

Mohandas (Mahatma) K. Gandhi revives the practice of fasting, which had been abolished by law, to incite political change in India. Already an advocate of moderate fasts to improve general health and for religious observances, he begins his first political fast in personal atonement over an incident that occurred when he was a social activist and leader of a school in South Africa. He fasts for seven days, followed by one meal a day for four and a half months.[17] The effect on the parties he was attempting to appease is immediate, and Gandhi feels profoundly relieved.

He returns to India in 1914, seeking to help free the country from British rule through campaigns of civil disobedience using principals of nonviolence. He undertakes fasts to alleviate prejudice between Hindus and Muslims, to support labor strikes, and to protest his own imprisonment. In later years, he has only to announce a fast for peace between factions in the newly independent India and Pakistan for tensions to ease. In thirty years, Gandhi fasts in seventeen public hunger strikes and countless ones for personal reasons.[18] "They should know that I never feel so happy as when I am fasting for the spirit," he writes, referring to religious leaders during the last fast of his life to encourage peaceful relations between Delhi and Karachi.

1920s: Thin Is In

The year that American and British suffragettes win the right for women to vote is the same year the Businessmen's League of Atlantic City proposes the first Miss America Pageant. Meanwhile, Elizabeth Arden announces the return of the "natural waistline," and glorified female body images start moving away from a corseted "hourglass" style to a straighter figure. They jump out of the glossy pages of mass market advertising as the flappers smoke in speakeasies, drink gin with men, and lace up their new girdles. Industrialization is making the food supply plentiful and there's more variety than ever to choose from. The modern woman should be refined, but outgoing, demure, but independent. Womanly curves are attractive, but ought to be firm and toned. There's no lack of diet and fitness advice from companies selling "quick-fix" health products. The lid on the ED pressure cooker is set to blow.

1925–1965: Body Fixing Advice from Yesteryear

Admiration for a slim, willowy, woman's figure gains steam in the first decade of the twentieth century and advertisements for reducing soaps, salts, creams, and powders began to appear in newspapers and magazines. "Reducing has become a national pastime . . . a craze, a national fanaticism, a frenzy," observed a journalist. "People now converse in pounds, ounces, and calories."[19]

Companies market "specially formulated" supplements, clothing, and exercise equipment (everything from corsets to hypnosis recordings and Bile Beans) to slim down or beef up a body. Driven in part by a culture of consumerism, attaining body perfection is becoming a personal goal and a national pastime for men and (mostly) women. Weight gain ads target underweight people and are not uncommon through the mid-1970s.

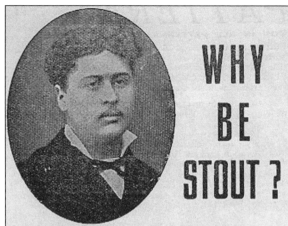

WHY BE STOUT?

Use to Lose with Obesity Soap, 1926. *Courtesy of Chris Wild @ Retronaut.com.*

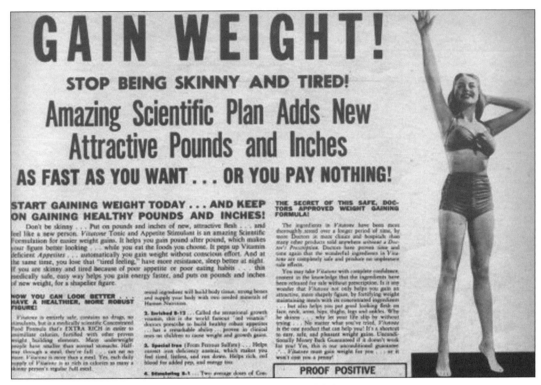

Weight gain ad from the 1930s. *Courtesy of Chris Wild @ Retronaut.com.*

1966: The Face of '66

British model Twiggy (a.k.a. Lesley Hornby) rocks the modeling world with her boyish look and angular build. "[Her] adolescent physique was the perfect frame for the androgynous styles that began to emerge in the 1960s," states a show catalogue from a 2009 retrospective at the Metropolitan Museum of Art.[20] Seventeen years old, five feet six inches and under one hundred pounds, she is the new motif of enviable body perfection. Her petite size counters the images of established models such as Jean Shrimpton and Veruschuka and opens up interest, especially in commercial print divisions, for shorter, lighter weight girls. "I was very skinny, but that was just my natural build," Twiggy (now Lesley Lawson) would tell an interviewer in 2006. "I always ate sensibly—being thin was in my genes." Her comments would come just after the reported starvation deaths of two high-profile South American models, Luisel Ramos and Ana Carolina Reston, prompting the Spanish government to ban underweight models from the catwalk during Madrid Fashion Week. (Luisel's younger sister, Eliana, also a model, was found dead in her bedroom six months later. The primary diagnosis was death due to symptoms of malnutrition.)[21] "They go on about banning size zero, but I think Hollywood stars are the worst perpetrators," Twiggy observes. "Most models are naturally long and gangly, while a lot of these young girls in Hollywood have gone on extreme diets. Their concave chests and bony arms are terrifying. It's scary to think that normal teenagers are tempted to copy them. I'd love there to be more larger models, but it's just not going to happen. Designers love to design for slim girls."[22]

1973: Hungry for Attention

Psychoanalyst Hilde Bruch publishes *Eating Disorders: Obesity, Anorexia and the Person Within*. The book is a complete volume of her findings and beliefs after over thirty-five years as a pediatrician and research into the psychological causes of eating disorders. She centers her theories on a psycho-socio-cultural model, instead of a biological one, and favors the idea that disordered eating is ego-driven and symbolic of family dysfunction. "I am convinced," she declares, "the illness goes along with the women's movement, because this [emancipation from their family] is what the girls want to show, that they are something special."[23] Bruch is recognized as the foremost authority on the treatment of EDs—anorexia, in particular. Her second book, *The Golden Cage*, would introduce millions to the illness, but would, unfortunately, drive certain misperceptions of the disease before science could uncover the biogenetic risk factors

1976: Houston, We Have a Problem

A registered nurse, Vivian Hanson Meehan had been searching for healing resources for her nineteen-year-old daughter diagnosed with an eating disorder. Unable to find specialized help, she discovers other families in her local community who also needed support and information. When the national news picks up the story, they become a cause célèbre.[24] Meehan establishes, the National Association of Anorexia Nervosa and Associated Disorders (ANAD) the first nonprofit organization in America to provide a helpline, referral service, and peer support for eating disorder sufferers and their families.

ED Stat #2

The Best Little Girl in the World, a made-for-TV movie, hits American living rooms in 1981. Based on a novel by psychotherapist Steven Levenkron, it's a groundbreaking attempt to expose anorexia and bulimia to a mass audience.

1981: Fasting for Principles

Bobby Sands is the first of ten Irish Republican Army (IRA) prisoners to die on a hunger strike protesting conditions at Long Kesh (now renamed, HM Prison Maze). After families object to the officially determined causes of death, medical certificates are amended to read "starvation," rather than "self-imposed starvation."[25] Two female IRA prisoners, Marian and Delores Price, who participated in an earlier hunger strike from the women's prison, develop anorexia and later die.[26]

1983: Superstar

Singer-drummer Karen Carpenter becomes the public face of the mortal dangers of eating disorders upon her death at age thirty-two. An immensely popular pop music artist of the 1970s, Karen had formed the Carpenters with her brother, Richard. She had crash dieted obsessively throughout her recording career, using laxatives and thyroid medication to keep her weight from rebounding. "Karen had been a little overweight as a teenager—she loved tacos and chili," Richard would tell *People* correspondent Suzanne Adelson nine months after Karen's death. "But we never teased her—to us, she wasn't that fat. When she was 17, she went on the Stillman Diet with a doctor's guidance, and she lost between 20 and 25 pounds. She was at her best weight—between 115 and 120—until 1975, when the illness first became serious."[27]

Karen weighed eighty pounds in 1982 when she checked into New York's Lenox Hill Hospital after nine months of psychotherapy. She then returned home to Los Angeles for Thanksgiving, having gained thirty pounds in seven weeks with the use of a feeding tube. She collapsed in her parent's home on February 4, 1983. The autopsy report lists her cause of death as "cardiotoxicity due to the chemical emetine, or as a consequence of anorexia nervosa."[28] Emetine is the active ingredient in ipecac syrup, a toxic substance that induces vomiting. It is meant for *one-time use*, *only*, in cases of poisoning. Repeated use can permanently damage the heart by dissolving the muscle. Karen's psychotherapist, Steven Levenkron, author of *The Best Little Girl in the World*, suspects she didn't understand

---

ED Stat #3

The 1984 Canadian Gallup Poll reports on the behavior and attitudes of Canadians with respect to weight consciousness and weight control—70 percent of women are dieting; 40 percent are continually gaining and losing weight. Sixty-six percent of women surveyed rank weight control as the most important motivator for exercise.[d]

---

the health risk and was simply using it as a means to keep from gaining more weight. "I'm sure she thought this was a harmless thing she was doing," he would tell a radio interviewer shortly thereafter, "but in sixty days, she had accidentally killed herself . . . a shocker for all of us who treated her."[29]

The sensitive, well-informed media coverage that followed Karen's passing would begin to change the view that EDs were annoying ploys of vain, spoiled girls. The door flung open for other celebrities to admit their struggles, not only with eating, but with other addictions as well. In 1990, Sonic Youth vocalist and lyricist Kim Gordon would pay tribute to Karen in the song "Tunic (Song for Karen)."

1990: Nothing Tastes as Good as Thin Feels

Corinne Day shoots an eye-popping photo spread of sixteen-year-old, soon-to-be fashion icon Kate Moss, for Britain's *The Face* magazine. Kate would become famous for her anti-supermodel stature and a raw look that would usher in the heroin chic of the 90s. Signing with Calvin Klein in 1992 for the highest paid modeling contract at that time, she'd launch into underwear (CK) and fragrance (Obsession for Men) campaigns that would tee off debates on women's body image and eating disorders. Kate tried to duck the tags. "I never weigh myself," she'd tell *People* in 1993. "I try to eat, so I won't be so waif-like. But even if I do, I'm not going to become this voluptuous thing."[30] Years later, she would admit in a *Vanity Fair* interview, her life and eating habits were, in fact, pretty disordered. "Nobody takes care of you mentally," she'd say of the industry. "There's massive pressure to do what you have to do."[31] The strain would lead Kate to other health

---

ED Stat #4

Models in the 1990s average *five* inches taller and *thirty* pounds lighter than average women.

ED Stat #5

In 1992, the American Dietetic Association reviewed surveys of middle-class children—46 percent of nine- to eleven-year-olds are "sometimes" or "very often" on diets, and 82 percent of their families are "sometimes" or "very often" on diets.[e] Eighty-one percent of ten-year-olds are afraid of being fat. Fifty-one percent of nine- and ten-year-old girls feel better about themselves if they are on a diet.[f]

abuses. During her career, she'd check herself into rehab for alcohol and drug addictions, but she steadfastly insists she was never anorexic. "I was thin, but that's because I was doing shows, working really hard," she would tell James Fox in 2012. "You'd get home from work and there was no food. You'd get to work in the morning, there was no food. . . . But I was never anorexic. They knew it wasn't true—otherwise I wouldn't have worked."[32]

1994: Food, Glorious Food

Binge eating disorder is distinguished from compulsive eating in the fourth edition of the *Diagnostic and Statistical Manual of Mental Disorders (DSM-IV)*, and introduced as a provisional diagnosis. Although recognized as a severe, life-threatening behavioral disorder characterized by recurrent episodes of compulsive overeating without any purging, it remains categorized under EDNOS (Eating Disorders Not Otherwise Specified).

1995: No One Is Immune

Television is introduced to the island of Fiji, providing a selection of entertainment that includes *Melrose Place*, *Beverly Hills 90210*, and *Xena: Warrior Princess*. By 1998, critical "fat talk" and reports of dieting and disordered eating among teenage girls rise fivefold in a culture that had long valued robust bodies and

ED Stat #6

Eating disorders in 1998 become the third most common chronic illness in adolescent girls.[g]

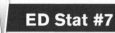

ED Stat #7

Of 1,000 women surveyed by *People* magazine in 2000, 800 said images of women on TV and in movies, fashion magazines, and advertising make them feel insecure about their looks. Only 10 percent of respondents said they were completely satisfied with their bodies.[h]

hearty eating. Parents are beside themselves with concern and agitated by the erosion of long-held traditions in just three years.

2001: Envisioning a World without Eating Disorders

The American Anorexia Bulimia Association merges with Eating Disorders Awareness and Prevention to form NEDA, the National Eating Disorders Association. The organization promotes awareness and advocacy, raises funds for research, and links sufferers and families to resources for prevention and treatment.

2003: Living on Air and Water

Illusionist and stunt performer David Blaine seals himself in a Plexiglass box suspended thirty feet above the Thames River in London. He stays forty-four days, receiving only water through a feeding tube, losing 25 percent of his body weight.[33] This modern endurance record was broken within a year. The Chinese edition of the *Epoch Times* reports Chen Jianmin of Sichaun Province maintained good health after a forty-nine-day water fast. He undertook the feat to prove the health benefits of traditional Chinese medicine.[34]

2005: The New Nor • mal

A seventy-five-minute musical theater production of a family struggling to function in the wake of a teenager's eating disorder opens off-Broadway to rave

ED Stat #8

Americans spend $46.3 billion on dieting solutions in 2004. This includes health clubs, diet pills and programs, low-cal foods, and $3.6 billion for gastric bypass surgeries. By 2008, spending is expected to top $61 billion.[i]

ED Stat #9

Hospitalization rates for eating disorders in children under twelve increased 119 percent between 2000 and 2006.[j]

reviews. Born out of Yvonne Adrian's own experience, *NORMAL the Musical* would give rise to a national tour and a nonprofit association by the same name, promoting eating disorder awareness, prevention, and recovery. NORMAL in Schools education project makes use of talkbacks and curricula for middle schools, high schools, and colleges. NORMAL also collaborates with national eating disorder organizations, researchers, filmmakers, and educators to offer more specialized programming for those at risk.

2008: Bingers, Unite

Binge Eating Disorder Association, Inc., founded by Chevese Turner in Maryland, specifically addresses the syndrome of compulsive overeating. The group advocates on a national level for the health concerns of people suffering from the disorder, and champions initiatives that reduce stigmatization and stereotyping of the obese.

2012: Major League Eating

On October 7, Tim "Eater X" Janus downs two gallons of Ben's Chili Bowl chili in six minutes at the Taste of D.C. Festival in Washington, D.C. He wins $1,500

ED Stat #10

Researchers review additional hospitalization statistics and discover there were 29,533 eating disorder–related hospital stays in 2008–2009, an increase of 24 percent since 2000.[k]

ED Stat #11

More than 40 million of the world's children under the age of five in 2010 are overweight or obese.[l]

and bragging rights over world champion pro-eater Joey "Jaws" Chestnut, who set the record the previous year. Food fascination at its finest.

2013: Make Way for the Three Percenters

Binge eating disorder, affecting over 8 million people—more than three times the number of those with anorexia or bulimia combined[35]—is designated as a distinct, diagnosable type of eating disorder by the American Psychiatric Association in the new *DSM-5*.

An Expert Weighs In:
Shan Guisinger—Adapted to Flee Famine

One of the symptoms of anorexia that Dr. Gull found most perplexing was the activity level of his bone-thin patients. Their families told him they never seemed to tire, let alone sleep. Dr Lasègue noted this as well. Both doctors were equally amazed at their patients' lack of professed appetite and lack of concern over their condition. It seemed counterintuitive that such severe starvation would be accompanied by these behaviors and beliefs. Doctors wondered,

- Where does the energy come from?
- Why should we not feel hungry enough to seek food if we are starving?
- Why would we not acknowledge how dangerously ill we are?

In 2002, clinical psychologist Shan Guisinger argued that our human biology may have benefited from an anorexia psychology to survive times of famine. "In treating anorexia, I started to wonder if their symptoms could be something that was useful in the past," she told the *Monitor* (the news publication of the American Psychological Association). "When nomadic foragers were starving, it wouldn't make sense to hunker down and just not eat. If you're starving, it means that there's no food there, and so you should move on—normal adaptation to starvation would get in the way."[36] Anorexia makes sense if we think of it in terms of an adaptive response to famine. If everybody in a tribe became sleepy and weak, preferring to stay in bed, no one would survive. A few hungry individuals with restless energy might be motivated by their group's dire situation to forage efficiently and optimistically, and be willing to travel long distances to unknown food sources. Characteristics that enable anoretics to ramp up their engines, tap into deep energy stores, function on little food, delay gratification, and unselfishly work for the good of all would have helped keep the majority of tribal members alive. Women, because of greater fat stores, could wander farther from home. When they encountered hostile communities, they were less likely to be killed than men. Rather, they'd be taken as slaves and incorporated into the new society.

"A lot of people have trouble with this theory because they think, now, in modern times, when there's so much food around, why don't anorexics [sic] just start eating again?" Guisinger noted. "But the thing about the brain is that it simply responds to body fat levels, making automatic adjustment to hunger and satiety signals. Evolution is not very elegant sometimes, and adaptations persist where they're not needed. In this case, the adaptation turns off hunger in [some] women who diet."[37]

Constructing an evolutionary reason for a recently identified illness is tricky. Ancient, nomadic tribes did not keep detailed medical reports. Philosophers and early physicians observed only anecdotal evidence for the forms of EDs we know today—they can't be scientifically verified. Nevertheless, Guisinger presents a variety of research studies across disciplines to support her hypothesis of a biological driver for anorexia—one that could likely fit all eating disorders—rather than a cultural one. Since she began investigating, three of her points are receiving growing support through genetic and physiological studies.

1. Anorexia crosses ethnic and socioeconomic lines, but arises in greater numbers in peoples who share a nomadic history—Hispanics, Native Americans, Caucasians, and Semites (Jews, Arabs).
2. Anorexia appears to develop as a response to a loss of a proportion of body fat, not as a pure result of family or societal pressures.
3. Food restriction in animals tends to generate the same restless behavior in subgroups, especially in species that naturally seek food over long distances.

The most compelling scientific support may eventually come from the Genome-Wide Association Study, begun by the National Institutes of Health in 2008 to identify common genetic factors that influence health and disease. The investigation is offering additional evidence for the biological determinants of behavior.

"It doesn't make psychotherapy irrelevant," Guisinger asserts, "but it means that more than anything, people are going to need all the help they can get from their therapist, family, doctor and dietician to fight against their body's signals in, what is to them, a very unnatural way."[38]

Get Real about Body Image and Self-Esteem

Eating connects to emotional behavior in people of all eras. Like kernels of popcorn, eating disorders lie in wait to explode when conditions are right. Triggers vary across cultures, generations, and individuals, but EDs don't discriminate between race, gender, age, or economic status. As the twenty-first century pro-

> ### ❓ Triggering Debate: An ED by Any Other Name
>
> Neuroscientists indicate the biological seeds for eating disorders go back perhaps a thousand generations. But some historians argue that religious ascetics, hunger artists, and fasting girls had different motivations and reasons for avoiding food than ED sufferers give today, so we shouldn't compare them. Do you think St. Catherine, Giovanni Sacci, or Sarah Jacob suffered from true eating disorders? Why or why not? How closely do you think past accounts of disordered eating relate to modern profiles of anorexia, bulimia, or binge eating? What do they have in common? What's different?

ceeds, EDs fester quietly, sometimes in disguise, popping up anytime, anywhere, to anybody. What kind of societal pressures push them to blossom? How do these pressures affect how we value ourselves and others as human beings? Can we learn to practice healthy responses in America, the Land of the Beautiful? Let's examine some social and cultural issues that shape our thoughts about body size, shape and weight, and think about what we might do to counteract the negative effects.

More Food for Thought

Read

Joan Jacobs Brumberg. *Fasting Girls: The History of Anorexia Nervosa*. Rev. ed. New York: Vintage Books, 2000.

Franz Kafka. *Ein HungerKünstler (A Hunger Artist)*. Berlin: Verlag Die Schmiede, 1922. English translations available in various story collections and online.

Michelle Stacy. *The Fasting Girl: A True Victorian Medical Mystery*. New York: Jeremy P. Tarcher, 2002.

Watch

Hunger (feature film, 96 minutes). A Blast! Films production for Film4 and Channel 4, 2008.

A Hunger Artist (video short, 17 minutes). Loyola Productions, Inc., 2005. Watch online at SnagFilms, www.snagfilms.com/films/title/a_hunger_artist.

The Karen Carpenter Story (made-for-TV docudrama, approximately 90 minutes). Weintraub Entertainment Group. Aired on CBS, January 1, 1989.

BOYS GET HUNGRY, TOO: CULTURE WARS ON PERFECT BODIES

Are guys concerned about food choice and physical appearance? You bet! What are some cultural values and perspectives that make us desire a personal makeover? Jump out of the box to find out some of the special challenges of males and members of the lesbian, gay, bisexual, transgender, and queer (LG-BTQ) community as they deal with critical conflicts over body image, self-love, perfection, and control. Investigate the impact of mass media on the development of a healthy self-image.

The I-Love-My-Body Pledge

I pledge to speak kindly about my body
I promise not to talk about the size of my thighs or stomach or butt, or about how
I have to lose 5 or 15 or 50 pounds. I promise not to call myself a fat pig, gross, or
any other self-loathing, trash-talking phrase.
I vow to be kind to myself and my body. I will learn to be grateful for its strength and
attractiveness, and be compassionate toward its failings.
I will remind myself that bodies come in all shapes and sizes, and that no matter what
shape and size my body is, it's worthy of kindness, compassion and love.

—Harriet Brown, mom and writer, 2009
originally posted on her blog, *Feed Me!* (harrietbrown.blogspot.com)

Eating Disorders Are Equal Opportunity Destroyers

Personal appearance is a national obsession. American culture is ripe with images of how to look and be your best along with instructions for how to carry out the mission. More than in generations past, we're exposed to a massive amount of idealized body imagery from a young age and through an increasing number of visual channels. The standards worm their way into our psyche, although everyone interprets the messages in slightly dissimilar ways due to differences in gender and family culture. Internalizing a specific standard of beauty and fitness and striving to attain a certain body size or shape can put us at war with our bodies. Research is showing this encourages militant attitudes about food, eating, and exercise in people of every race and economic class, no matter where they live. For girls and boys entering their teenage years, and for some who are younger, the normal, hormonal cascade of puberty appears to trip off disordered eating symptoms in those who have become especially sensitive to the culture of thin versus fat.

Better designed surveys are showing us you can be Hispanic, Asian, African American, Caribbean, Muslim, from Iceland, from India, or from an Indian reservation and have an eating disorder. Ethnic variation that we thought made a difference in the *epidemiology* of EDs is irrelevant. No matter what kind of a community you live in, an appetite for body perfection leaves us all open to the impact of media messages. Girls face unrelenting pressure from fashion advertisers and the dieting industry to be lithe and light, while guys are bombarded by the media with examples of chiseled male physiques. Sensitivity about body size happens in children as young as four, five, and six, depending on their exposure to perfected images and "fat talk" from family members and peers. Older people feel the pressure, too, as sixty becomes the new forty. The more intensely our personality has been shaped by issues of control and achievement, the more attuned we are to cultural standards of appearance and status. Our national obsession with image has affected our ability to relate to ourselves in a healthy way.

Diagnostic criteria for eating disorders have come about primarily through documenting female cases. Since the 1980s, however, experts have agreed that EDs are physiologically the same in men and women.[1] This is clear, even though males' motivations for body makeovers usually evolve from a desire to be more fit and muscular, rather than thin and petite. Boys, who struggle with body image concerns, reduce stress levels through diet adjustments, purging techniques, and obsessive exercise—similarly to girls.

For financial analyst Chris Skarinka of Boston, the pressures of college life at Harvard were his tipping point into bulimia. He had great expectations to succeed at both academics and sports, where he was a high achiever and varsity rower. "I didn't have the coping skills and mechanisms to deal with those in a healthy way," he said. "What was tough was that the pressures never went away. Winning a race, or doing well on an exam didn't change anything for me."[2] Chris's eating disorder weakened him gradually. "It didn't seem that debilitating," he recalled. "It wasn't until a year later, it was controlling the rest of my life. I ended up having to give up rowing because I couldn't pass the medical exam. That's when I realized I had a huge problem."

Boys who compulsively overeat are seeking the same instant gratification as girls who binge. Ron Saxen of Berkeley, California, author of *The Good Eater*, grew up in a fundamentalist household with a father who meted out corporal punishment to whomever happened to be underfoot. Ron had his first binge at age eleven, consuming almost three pounds of chocolate, fearfully sweating while waiting for his father to return home from work to whale on him. "I learned at an early age that food could take me away. It could ease the tension," he told Tanya Rivero on ABC's *Healthy Living*.[3] "Later on at nineteen, this was how I handled tension and anxiety, good or bad. When I'd get that weird feeling in my stomach, like I used to when I was a kid, food was a way to shut it down." Ron was about fifty or sixty pounds overweight by age twenty-one, and went about losing it through a range of bulimirexic behaviors. "People started saying 'Are you a model?' I said, 'Are you kidding me? I haven't had a date in two years.'" Ron's looks did get him a modeling contract, but his binging worsened under the pressure of the career. "The thing is, if you've got a problem and don't deal with it, it's not 'if' or 'when,' you're going to implode or explode, it's gonna happen for sure."

Males experience an eating disorder in essentially the same way as females and are more likely than other males to

- have had weight concerns as children (been either overweight or puny) and subject to ridicule
- adjust diet and exercise to conform to standards of male masculinity

! Ana by Any Other Name

Manorexia is the slang applied to guys who are so significantly underweight and obsessive about eating, they fit the criteria for anorexia nervosa. Unfortunately, it perpetuates the idea, even among treatment professionals, that anorexia is a different disorder in males than it is in females. Actually, clinical symptoms are the same in both genders—no eating disorder is specific to men, or to women.

- be more confused on gender identity and sexuality
- experience less sexual activity (and perhaps lower testosterone)
- be involved in an activity with body weight or aesthetic importance (wrestling, horse racing, track and field, gymnastics, dance, modeling)

Similarly to women, men with EDs are more likely to have been victimized by trauma, especially sexual abuse. Commonly, they lack a positive male role model.

How prevalent are eating disorders in males? Over the last ten years, surveys indicate that many more men have diagnosable and subclinical EDs than previously thought. Males keep quiet for fear of being stigmatized as having a "feminine" disorder, until they are so weakened and ill, they must be hospitalized. The number of young men and preteen boys that struggle in silence with eating issues is much greater than those who seek treatment, yet research has shown that they suffer as much as females. Those who binge are rarely thought to suffer from anything more than the effects of obesity. Psychology professor Ruth Striegel Weissman (formerly, Striegel-Moore) of Wesleyan University advocates for greater efforts to recruit men and boys into eating disorder research. She believes a shift in attitude is long overdue. One of her latest studies determined the medical impact and psychological distress of binge eating are just as damaging to men as they are to women. "The prevalence of binge eating has been shown to be as common in men as in women, . . . [yet] the under-representation of men in binge eating research does not reflect lower levels of impairment," she writes in the conclusion to her journal article. "Efforts are needed to raise awareness of the health effects of binge eating for men so they can seek appropriate screening and treatment."[4] The Alliance for Eating Disorder Awareness reports that as many as one in four males struggle with some type of eating disorder.[5] In 2011, a data review estimated that 10 million males in the United States can be diagnosed with either a full or partial syndrome ED.[6] Most exhibit co-occurring symptoms of bipolar disorder, obsessive-compulsive disorder, depression, and anxiety, and frequently experience companion tendencies toward substance use and behavioral addictions.

The raw numbers of eating disorder cases in males are rising along with our society's focus on everyone looking good. Standards of male beauty exist, and no ethnicity is immune. While forming their masculine identities, young men are confronted by images of buff male bodies on the beach, in the gym, and selling everything from cars to cologne. For males, who are naturally brought up to be competitive, the pressure to be strong enough, big enough, and good enough to get what they want is stressful and can play itself out in disordered behavior. Perfectionist traits in men may underlie a relentless focus on body image that feeds the development of all types of eating and exercise disorders. The pressure is particularly intense among homosexuals, a culture that has always emphasized male

Johnny Come Lately

Adolescent males are especially prone to binging to cover the effects of stress from childhood trauma. Witnessing or experiencing sexual molestation or domestic violence, or being subjected to emotional abuse or neglect can lead to forms of post-traumatic stress disorder. Nineteen-year-old Johnny Lindstrom of Tempe, Arizona, discovered how much pain he was burying with food when he entered therapy. For years he had felt unwanted, even though he had been adopted at age four by loving parents. His breakthrough moment happened when he was able to connect with his biological father and half-brother, who had cared for him briefly after his birth mother had abandoned him. The phone call, he said, "sent chill bumps down my arms. It was an amazing feeling—crazy to know that my biological family, who I hadn't talked to in so many years cared about me, loved me, missed me. It was pretty awesome."[a] Johnny discovered his father had only let his adoption go through out of his conviction that Johnny would have a better life. "I never knew about those things and had so much anger for so long," he recalled. "But I understand now what they did for me." Recognizing the connection between his binges and his emotions was Johnny's first realization that he could learn to manage his life in a healthier way.

physical attractiveness. The *International Journal of Eating Disorders* reported in 2002 nearly 14 percent of gay men surveyed seemed to suffer from bulimia, and over 20 percent appeared to have anorexia.[7] Since then, additional studies suggest homosexuality is a specific risk factor for disordered eating in men. Researchers at Columbia University's Mailmen School of Public Health found in 2007 that ED symptoms are more prevalent (15 percent) in gay and bisexual men than (5 percent) in heterosexual men.[8] They observed no such difference, however, between lesbian and bisexual women compared to heterosexual women. The study couldn't determine any values or norms of behavior within the gay community that might be responsible for the higher rates of eating disorders. This supports the theory that biogenetic factors are crucial pieces to the puzzle. It's a constellation of personality and behavioral traits, rather than sexuality per se, that predisposes certain people to EDs. Study findings indicate gay men with eating

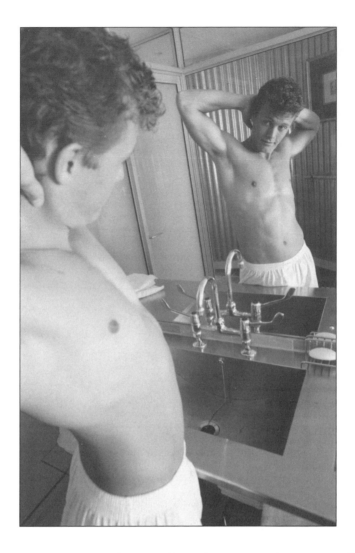

disorders have dependent, avoidant, and passive-aggressive personality styles, and likely experienced homophobic reactions from their peers while growing up.[9]

Like females, the majority of males first confront symptoms in their youth, although on average, somewhat later in adolescence. The "skinny chic" ideal of some young men in the gay community became a problem for Gabriel Perez of West Hollywood, California. "I deal with anorexia due to depression about my coming out and not being welcome in this community," he explains in a 2010 documentary on body image in gay culture. Already tall and lean, Gabriel didn't have many friends before he came out. Unconsciously, he began to imitate the behavior of the crowd with whom he felt most comfortable. "It's like the friends I hung out with were very skinny and very young and very pretty, and so we all just wouldn't eat. My diet consisted of Diet Coke and cigarettes. The pressure was on to stay skinny and fit all the time."[10]

Four of his friends admit they feel competition to look their best wherever they go. One, Nic Delis, struggles with *exercise bulimia* and works out constantly.

The rest agree their eating and body image attitudes are pretty disordered. "You're definitely conscious and aware of what you eat at all times," says DeAndre Johnson.[11]

All five young men confess they are brutally honest with each other if they think one of them is putting on weight. "We go shopping together and when we go shopping, it's the first thing we make fun of," says Nic. He pretends exaggerated shock. "'You want a what size, I heard you call for an extra pair of what size? A thirty-three? Oooh.'"[12]

"We go to underwear parties, for cryin' out loud," says Gabriel. "We have whole festivals based on nudity. Everywhere we go has ten half-naked dancers that look amazing, and we wish that we had their bodies. The whole culture is based on amazing looks."[13]

DeAndre summed it up "You walk into a club and everyone is gorgeous. You strive to be better than that. You're always striving to look better than the next person."[14]

According to a 2009 analysis from researchers at Harvard University and Boston Children's Hospital, youth up to age twenty-three who identified as lesbian, gay, bisexual, or "mostly heterosexual" had more binge eating behavior and used vomiting and laxatives to control weight than heterosexual youth. "We found clear and concerning signs of higher rates of eating disorder symptoms in sexual-minority youth compared to their heterosexual peers, even at ages as young as twelve, thirteen or fourteen years old," lead researcher S. Bryn Austin told *Reuters Health*.[15] Compared to straight girls, lesbians, bisexual, and mostly heterosexual females reported more binge eating. Only lesbians didn't report more purging. Among gay, bisexual, and mostly heterosexual males, all had much higher rates of disordered eating patterns than the straight males. In all the groups, females showed higher rates of disordered eating than males. The team took their data from a sample of almost 14,000 participants in the Growing Up Today Study, and their results were consistent with those of earlier surveys.[16] They concluded that

---

Here's an Extra Scoop

In a 2012 survey examining body image among transgender young people, 17 percent reported having an eating disorder.[b] The sixty-five respondents ranged from age fifteen to twenty-six, represented a mix of ethnicities (white, Latino, African American, Native American, Pacific Islander, Chinese, and Asian), and hailed from seven major cities across the United States. Results also indicated that higher levels of anxiety and body dissatisfaction were more likely to lead to dieting and other attempts at body fixing.

LGBTQ youth may exhibit heightened patterns of eating disordered behavior due to feelings of isolation and victimization that occur as they evaluate their identity and contemplate coming out. Other stress-related health problems are easy to find in LGBTQ communities.

Body Projects—Fixing What's Wrong

It's hard learning to become comfortable in your skin. Parents and siblings make thoughtless comments about your appearance, and you're bombarded with idealized imagery. Raging hormones, personal experience, and innate personality color your emotions and subsequent feelings. As you move into a new era of independence, you consider issues that determine your identity and develop your attitudes, which drive your desires to be who you are, have what you need, and do something worthwhile. Body image and self-esteem are important psychological properties of this growing self-awareness, whether you're male, female, or questioning your gender identity. Feeling unhappy about your body weight or shape puts you at risk for developing body image distortions, compulsive exercise behaviors, and eating disturbances. A recent eight-year study of 496 adolescents revealed that body dissatisfaction is the most robust predictor of who will develop an eating disorder.[17]

What exactly are body image and self-esteem, and how are they related to eating disorders? Body image is what you believe is true about your body and

> "To satisfy my intense need for stability, I began basing my self-worth on two things I knew could be controlled—body image and academic performance. I can remember one specific night in my dorm room, telling myself, 'Troy, you look horrible. An exercise regimen is what you need to take advantage of right now.' From that night on, the exercise regimen I planned for myself would be a burden I would carry with me the next four years of my life. After some time, I began to get positive feedback from my family and peers concerning my appearance. The attention and reinforcement became a 'high' for me. I loved every minute of it."
>
> —Troy Roness (@TroyRoness), mental health and LGBT advocate
> Minot, North Dakota[c]

how you think it's perceived by others. It's part of your total self-image, which includes the level of satisfaction you feel for yourself. Self-esteem is your overall judgment of how you compare yourself to others. Perceptions of appearance and self-worth are tightly linked, such that perceived appearance can accurately predict your self-esteem no matter your gender.[18] Body image and self-esteem develop mainly through the course of childhood and adolescence, as we process external experiences and internal feelings. Neither are static qualities—they easily fluctuate in personality types that are less bold or aggressive. Whether high or low, good or bad, the two psychologies reinforce each other. Bad body image is damaging because it compromises all aspects of self-esteem: self-worth, self-confidence, and self-respect. In certain scenarios, these can be catalysts for eating, exercise, and substance use disorders, even self-injury (e.g., cutting).

Some teens elect to alter their looks through cosmetic surgery, which has its own set of serious possible side effects and can be dangerously compelling. "I was trying to, as much as possible, imitate the Barbie image," said Jessica, nineteen, who decided to get breast implants after breaking up with her boyfriend in high school. "I thought that he would look at me differently, or want me back, even if I didn't take him back," she said. "I made the appointment when I was seventeen. Four weeks later, I had the surgery done."[19] More teens than ever are choosing to improve their appearance by any means available to them. Between 2000 and 2011, plastic surgeons more than doubled the number of breast implants and lift surgeries on teen girls. Liposuction procedures increased by 28 percent.[20]

You might lack self-esteem and suffer from poor body image, yet be motivated to improve by a sense of competition and a desire to belong. Taking on repetitive, goal-based behavior can feel like a huge relief from that insecurity. Our twenty-first-century mainstream culture universally accepts diet and exercise as focal points for self-improvement. A body project is an obvious, convenient, and responsive target on which to concentrate your energy, yet it's a potentially dangerous obsession. "I always thought like I should be little," said Brooke, eighteen. "I'm the youngest . . . the baby of the family. When I started growing up,

---

! Pretty Pennies

According to the results of a 2007 survey, women spend a total of $7 billion per year on cosmetics, and a total of $11.7 million on cosmetic surgical and nonsurgical procedures per year. Sixty-nine percent of respondents age eighteen to twenty-four are in favor of liposuction, Botox injections, tummy tucks, and breast implants.[d]

and growing faster than my brother and sisters, it just felt wrong." Brooke's ED began when she was in sixth grade. It started as bulimia, but slid into anorexia as she lost weight. "There was a time when I thought, I don't care if this ends up killing me, as long as I'm skinny when it does."[21] She's been hospitalized three times since she was twelve.

Trouble with body image and self-esteem can show up long before adolescence—since the 1990s, surveys of children ages six to ten consistently show a desire for slimness and fear of being fat. Fifty-eight percent of 494 middle and high school girls in 1992 categorized themselves as fat, whereas only 15 percent of them were actually overweight.[22] In *Wasted*, her bestselling memoir of anorexia and bulimia, Marya Hornbacher admits she never felt "normal" about her body. "It has always seemed to me a strange and foreign entity," she recalled. "I don't know that there was ever a time when I was not conscious of it. As far back as I can think, I was aware of my corporeality, my physical imposition on space."[23] She writes she was four or five when she first agonized over being fat and tearfully announced it to her parents.

Body dissatisfaction normally precedes disordered eating symptoms by a few years—we're all familiar with the decline of self-esteem and positive body image among middle school girls. Before high school graduation rolls around, practically all girls find a body part to complain about. By their late teens, males are also thinking critically about their bodies on a significant level. Those at heightened risk for obsessive and addictive behaviors are just as likely as females to engage in desperate and extreme measures of self-control, which can lead to eating and exercise disorders. In a survey of ninety-three male college students, 20 percent had weight and shape concerns. An additional 9–12 percent indicated body image disturbances. Almost half of the respondents built up self-esteem through body building, and a third felt increased anxiety if they had to miss a day of exercise.[24] Dr. Ted Weltzin, medical director of the Eating Disorders Center at Rogers Memorial Hospital in Oconomowoc, Wisconsin, insists that ED symptoms are not unusual for males and objects to the way male sufferers are often portrayed in the media. "We don't want to make it seem like it's odd and exotic," he explained. "There's a real tendency [for the media] to get spectacular with the symptoms and there's a tendency for some of the media exposure around males to see it as something kind of odd and extreme. That's really not helpful and doesn't help people seek help who have problems with an eating disorder."[25]

It's tricky to draw conclusions about the connection of body image disturbances to eating issues because it's not often obvious that someone suffering from ED symptoms has body image and self-esteem that are in the toilet. When you doubt your abilities or your value, yet are driven to succeed, it's natural to take control through what you feed your body and what you push it to do. Success-

Self-Esteem versus Self-Worth

One popular belief is that all people with eating disorders have problems with self-esteem. For some who have been violated by physical, sexual, and verbal abuse, low self-esteem is common, but it's not a universal characteristic for everybody with emotionally disordered eating. Self-esteem (how you believe you compare to others) is somewhat different than self-worth (how much you value yourself and your accomplishments). Although related parts of self-identity, they are not the same. Therapist Carolyn Costin makes the distinction in *The Eating Disorder Sourcebook*. People with eating disorders, particularly those who restrict food, are aware of their advanced capabilities, she writes. They just don't see value in their achievements. "These people feel inadequate and essentially unworthy even in the face of many accomplishments. They are unable to validate themselves internally and look for external means to do so, making them more susceptible to an exaggerated focus on appearance. . . . The goal of finding self-worth is never accomplished."[e]

Shake and bake with bad body image, and see what comes out of the oven.

ful weight loss often brings mammoth approval, elevated status, and new self-respect. The shift to healthier eating and exercise can be a wonderful boost for a self-conscious, overweight child or teenager. Amy, who emigrated with her family from South Africa to Canada, felt the rush right away. "People would notice that my lunches were healthy and they would ask me for advice, like, what should they eat or how did I stay thin," she said. "It made me feel really good. Like, oh, this

Lena Dunham's *Girls*

You find angst in teens and twenty-somethings everywhere, including Hannah Horvath and her friends on HBO's *Girls*. "She [Hannah] has that mix of complete self-confidence and no self-worth that is the trademark of most twenty-four-year-old girls, and most Jewish comedians,"[f] said *Girls* series creator Lena Dunham (@lenadunham).

is my thing. This is what I can do. I felt proud and successful and it drove me to become more rigid."[26] Amy also remarked that her idea of her own ideal size was a moving target, a goal virtually impossible for her to identify. Rather than building a positive self-image, losing weight only inflated her ego. Given her temperament, she still needed to relieve anxious self-consciousness through obsessive control over food and exercise.

Boys who are out of shape before they begin a body makeover get a genuine boost of self-esteem and body appreciation, too. In *America the Beautiful 2: The Thin Commandments*, director Darryl Roberts (@Darryl_Roberts) sat down to interview six male students who were in recovery from eating disorders that began in grade and middle school. All had been overweight and were teased about their size by their family, classmates, or both. All decided to do something about it and found themselves in a downward spiral of disordered eating. "I was this chubby kid growing up," said one, who believed that 'skinny beanpoles' could eat anything they wanted. "Why couldn't that be me?"[27]

"I didn't care about getting a six-pack or anything," said another youngster. "I just wanted to be skinny."[28]

"I was picked on for years by my brother," said a third, who got the idea of purging from a girl in one of his classes. "Then it started happening at school and no one would do anything about it. Even my doctor said I should lose weight."[29]

Each of the young men turned to compulsive activity combined with dieting to lose weight. One high school student was particularly interested in defining muscle. Two confessed they had wanted to reshape themselves to attract girls. All got more positive attention as fat disappeared. All slipped into the chasm of an ED.

Just a decade or so ago, it was much more likely for girls and women to tie together body image and self-esteem than did boys and men. Most studies from the 1990s that investigated gender differences in self-awareness found this to be true. This is not surprising considering the high value our society has traditionally placed on females' physical appearance, and how much more we value other attributes—such as competitiveness and leadership—in males. Recent research, however, suggests that neither men nor women can escape our culture's implicit message to achieve the ideal body shape. Unfortunately, as Kelly Brownell, director of Yale's Rudd Center for Public Policy and Obesity has pointed out, the body image standards to which we currently aspire are far beyond what can be achieved with healthy or sensible levels of dieting or exercise.[30] Both males and females are drilled with cultural expectations of self-control and personal discipline, and both genders are equally likely to become obsessively fixated on body makeovers. As it becomes more common for males to take their appearance seriously, and especially for those in subcultures that put Adonis on a pedestal, self-esteem and body image move together in tandem, just as they do in females.

Adonis at Work: Bigorexia Fits the Mold

For a lot of body-conscious guys, gay or straight, weightlifting is key to packing on muscle, reshaping physique, and attaining an ideal masculine image. When perfectionism and obsessive-compulsive tendencies creep into an exercise regimen, they put themselves at risk for *bigorexia*, a type of *body dysmorphic disorder*. Body dysmorphia is what makes anoretics think they're still fat. Bigorexia, otherwise known as reverse anorexia, is what leads a guy to believe he still needs to bulk up. This can accompany a number of disordered and addictive behaviors, including diet preoccupations, exercise bulimia, even steroid abuse. Melvin Myles told documentary filmmaker Christopher Hines he was out to be the big guy, the biggest muscle, the eye candy. "When I started working out I was 145 pounds. Where I'm at right now, I weigh 196 to 198. That's a lot of weight I put on. But at the same time, you see yourself for so long at 145 . . . in the mirror you feel you're still that smaller person." He then commented on others' inclination to abuse steroids. "I think it comes to a point where they don't feel they're big enough. Even though they're big, when they look in the mirror, they don't see themselves as big enough. I had that problem. Still do. Work with it."[g]

"I don't think I'll ever be happy with my body. I think every day is a starting off point. It's always a struggle. . . . I was invisible for years because I wasn't pretty enough. I very much faded into the woodwork. I started going to the gym and then I started competing in body building and that pushed me even more. To this day, I look in the mirror and I literally see myself the way I was before. It's this programming . . . I have so many years of looking in the mirror and being unhappy with how I looked, that it's just sort of ingrained in my psyche."

—Richard Klein, Los Angeles
The Adonis Factor, 2010[h]

Ryan Reconfigures

Accepting yourself as you are is part of healthy self-development. Eating disorders are often born out of that struggle for essential identity. Ryan Sallans (@rsallans) has had a rockier road than most. Born Kimberly Ann Sallans in 1979 in Aurora, Nebraska, a small farming community, Ryan never felt his female body fit his sense of self. The deep dissatisfaction played out as a full-blown eating disorder as he reached his teens and . . . well, let's hear him tell it:

There have been many moments in my life where I have questioned if I am lovable.

The discomfort I felt by all the outward attention people paid to my appearance only heightened an insecurity that I felt I couldn't tell anyone; I was a girl, but I wanted to be a boy. When my puberty began, my insecurities with my physical appearance became my obsession. As my body grew into a curvy female form I let go of the fantasy of turning into a boy and surrendered to the idea that I'd forever be uncomfortable in my own skin.

My curves made me feel fat. My curves scared me.

At the age of eighteen I decided that all of my discomfort in life would go away if I just lost weight. I believed that if I could look a certain way, then my life would align itself, my parents would love me, and my social interactions would improve. So, I set my sights on a goal that I didn't think I would be able to achieve, to be skinny.

By the time I turned nineteen, I was diagnosed with anorexia nervosa. A part of me liked my eating disorder because my body quit menstruating, my breasts were almost non-existent and I could wear boy's pants that hung off of my body. The other part of me just wanted to die and was scared of everything; people, my body, family, going out with friends, and eating outside my controlled environment.

My eating disorder caused me to live in a world that revolved around all the things I was trying to avoid; my body, food, fear and loneliness. After a year-and-a-half of torturing myself through anorexia, my spirit was ready to surrender.

As I felt the beats of my heart decrease to the point of stopping, a voice inside me said, "It's not your time." As it became silent, I felt a new rush of energy pulse through my veins and I decided it was time to quit living in fear and hiding. To do this I knew I had to be dedicated to going to therapy and seeing a nutritionist. I went to weekly appointments for another four-and-a-half years.

Ryan's ED controlled his life until he was twenty-four. Therapy helped him explore his true feelings and realize he would have to stop judging his self-worth through his body and appearance. It was then he could confront his biggest fear, his sexuality.

At the time, the logical thing for Ryan to do was come out as a lesbian. His symptoms retreated as he gradually explored his sense of self. The shadowy issues that had plagued him about his body since childhood finally crystallized when he discovered a book about transgender men. Their feelings were his feelings and their stories resonated. He knew he could fix the misalignment and transition to a life that would be true inside and out. He continues,

Through my transition I have lost relationships with some loved ones and minor friendships, but I have learned that if I would have continued to make choices in life based on what makes other people happy, then I would still be stuck in my eating disorder today.

The one thing that I am still learning is how to explore feelings without taking them out on my body. My biggest trigger is my estranged relationship with my parents. My sister tells me that my dad loves me, but that he is caught up in "appearances," his "pride" and how people see me. The ironic thing is, through my transition and my ability to state, "This is me, and this is how I am going to live my life." I've gained respect from others and have developed it for myself. I have a new found confidence, but the negative self-talk toward my body is always heightened when I learn of another comment my dad has made that hints towards his pride being more important than his kid. Because of my experiences, I work hard to help support and build self-confidence with youth while asking parents to let go of their own pride and remember how they felt as a child when the adults in their life weren't truly listening and seeing them.

For me, all I ever wanted is what I feel every kid wants, regardless of their gender: To be loved, to be supported, but also to be allowed to explore this world and let others know who we are, not what they want us to be.

There is hope for recovery. . . . [It] begins when you allow yourself to love and recognize that being lovable is about respecting oneself and allowing your inner spirit to guide your actions. It is a life-long process, but I know I wouldn't be where I am today if I wouldn't have allowed myself to do one of the scariest things in my life, to honor my truths and recognize my internal identity.[i]

Ryan's memoir, *Second Son: Transitioning toward My Destiny, Love and Life*, tells the story of his journey of self-discovery. He's a health educator and lectures widely on topics concerning LGBTQ identity, body image and eating disorders, sexuality, and social acceptance. Find out what he's up to at www.ryansallans.com.

A Universal Commandment

Our world is saturated with images of svelte and glamorous bodies. We know what the standards of beauty are and we want to measure up in the eyes of people who matter to us. "The whole world is against you and your body," said Jessica, "and you need to do everything in your power to make sure you look perfect all the time. Or you're gonna be miserable."[31] Thou shalt be thin to be attractive. Children, from all backgrounds in gender-appropriate ways, absorb this social commandment before the age of ten. Translation: Phat—*P*retty, *h*ot, *a*nd *t*empting—may be in, but fat is not.

If you're dissatisfied with your body, its size, shape, or weight, there's something you can do. If you're self-conscious, angry, uncomfortable, or ashamed about it, companies tell us we can change ourselves with a pill or a program. "I want to be good-looking, no matter what it takes," said model-turned-actor Anderson Davis, thirty. "Most men strive for that. Whether it's my body, whether it's my face. We get these pictures jammed in our face all day long, and it's like this is what's beautiful. . . . I definitely think there's power in having good looks."[32] Many people in America and all over the world would agree with him. Studies have shown better-looking people have more friends, make more money, are happier with their lives.

Advertisers capitalize on our belief in the importance of appearance to encourage us to purchase products and services. They strategically target the dissatisfied in order to sell the remedy, and they direct promotional content according to gender. Traditionally, media aimed at women have included more advertisements and articles on weight loss and "slenderizing" than those directed at men, which

Love Your Tree

Playwright, journalist, and feminist Eve Ensler has spoken to women around the world and collected their stories, sharing what they think and feel about their bodies. In her work, *The Good Body*, which she adapted for the stage in 2005, Eve recalled a conversation she had with a seventy-four-year-old Masai woman in the fields outside Nairobi. Did she like her body, Eve had asked. The woman replied, "Do I like my body? Do I like my body? I love my body. God made this body. God gave me this body. My fingers, look at my fingers. I love my fingernails, little crescent moons. My hands, my hands, the way they flutter in the air and fall, they lead right up my arms—so strong—they carry things along. And my legs, my legs are long. . . . My breasts . . . My breasts, well, look at them, they're mine."[j]

Here Eve interrupts. She can't get past her own stomach, she says. It had been flat, now it was round. Your stomach is meant to be seen, said the woman. And then,

"Eve, look at that tree? Do you see that tree? Now, look at that tree (pointing to another tree). Do you like that tree? Do you hate that tree 'cause it doesn't look like that tree? Do you say that tree isn't pretty 'cause it doesn't look like that tree? We're all trees. You're a tree. I'm a tree. You've got to love your body, Eve. You've got to love your tree. Love your tree."[k]

To discover more about Eve's activism, her writing, and her commitment to ending violence against women, visit her website: www.eveensler.org.

reflect more fitness and shape-related ideals. A comparison of men's and women's magazines in the fall of 1987 found the ten most popular women's magazines, as determined by females ages eighteen to twenty-four, had ten times more diet-related content than those most popular among males in the same age group.[33] This was practically the same ratio of eating disorders that were noted to occur in women compared to men in the 1980s. Today, among young people, EDs affect about seven girls for every boy.

In the past, women have generally indicated more preoccupation with thinness than men, but with the rising stigma associated with obesity, that gap has nar-

Triggering Debate: Just Say No

Should advertisers be held accountable and be pushed to present more honest images of people? What else do you think can be done to counteract the media's negative effect on body image? How can we practice healthy behaviors in a society that pushes us to extremes?

rowed, too. Magazines such as *Men's Health*, *GQ*, and *Instinct* now clearly market weight loss as a transformational goal. *Men's Health* has web pages devoted to losing weight, even a section called "Belly Off!" Headline blasts from January 7, 2013, read "Weight-Loss Traps," "Lose Your Gut for Good," and "Control Your Cravings." Sound familiar? It's now abundantly clear that media is intently pushing everyone's self-evaluation buttons. Men are as likely as women to have body image concerns and alter eating and exercise practices to compensate.

As a student in Philadelphia, Derek Brocklehurst, who now lives in San Francisco's Castro district, bought into the look of "pretty, smooth, tan, mostly white guys in gay magazines." "I always wanted to fit that image," he said. "I worked at Abercrombie [and Fitch] for five years. That definitely added to [my sense of] body image in America and the gay community."[34] He went on to explain the importance of visual impressions. The first thing that gets evaluated is physique, so the image of a person is what matters. It's an automatic response. "I feel like that happens to me, too," he said, "whether I'm cycling down the street, or I'm just walking to coffee with friends and wearing something tight. The pressure is on to look good, look young." Saturation of body perfect imagery in our culture diminishes our capacity to assess what is ordinarily attractive, because we're compelled to harshly compare each other. When we view our bodies, and even our personalities, through that judgmental filter, we see the parts of ourselves that don't seem to measure up. For both males and females with perfectionist traits, the "not enough" factor becomes something that should be fixed. It plays right into a relentless focus on reshaping the body and controlling its needs. Obsessively addictive behavior is just around the corner, and the comparisons easily activate the competitive side of our nature. When groups of people—friends, relatives, celebrities, reality TV show participants—are flirting with disordered eating and exercise, EDs start to pop out like rabbits.

Ruth's college roommate, "Liza," tried her first diet when she was thirteen as a part of a group challenge. They were going to see how much weight they could lose in a month. Liza's friend passed out directions for the Hot Dog Diet—you were supposed to eat only hot dogs for three days in a row and eat regular on the other four. Liza's folks flipped out and forbade her to have anything to do with it.

The Butterfly Effect in Fiji

What should have been a minor incident for a Polynesian island culture, has turned out to have far-reaching repercussions. When sociologist Anne Becker first visited Fiji in 1982, she found a remote society that had been practically undisturbed by foreign influence. A person's body size was of great interest to the people, she observed, for it represented the worth of a person in their community. Big bodies were desirable. "In some ways they were as pre-occupied, if not more pre-occupied with body size than Americans are," she told filmmaker Darryl Roberts in 2006.

> It was just in the opposite direction. The body reflects what the community is able to do, so the family and village you live in [wants to be] able to feed you well. That's why people think big bodies are beautiful. When I learned that television was going to be introduced to Fiji, I was sure [it] would have no effect on the Fijians. This is a tremendously rich culture which has been present for centuries, if not millennia. What we were able to show was that in 1995, none of the girls in our study admitted to having ever vomited as a means of controlling weight. But by 1998, 11 percent of the girls admitted this, which is incredible, because that's the same percentage you might see in a high school here in Massachusetts.[l]

Nine years later in 2007, Dr. Becker and her team assessed the impact of different types of mass media exposure on Fijian girls and whether it appeared to affect their eating behavior. They observed the more the girls engaged in social media networks, the more they increased their risk of disordered eating. Researchers continue to evaluate the connection between mass media exposure and body dissatisfaction. There's little debate that imagery does shape our thought processes, and has a sizable influence over those who strive for perfection, yet might doubt their personal value.

She wanted to win the challenge, though, so she substituted bananas, which were in the house all the time. The hardest thing was concealing that she wasn't eating anything else. But that's how she knew she was in control of her body and could keep her secret safe.

An Expert Weighs In:
Dr. Cynthia Bulik—Look in the Mirror

Psychologist Cynthia Bulik, PhD (@cynthiabulik) imagines a world where we won't define ourselves by how we think we measure up to outrageous standards of body perfection. Having practiced as a therapist and researched many issues related to EDs, she's a respected authority in the field and is passionate about translating scientific discovery for the public. Her 2012 book on body image gives practical means to start building a positive sense of self. Even though negative self-talk is hard to let go of, she suggests starting with a simple Mirror Project.

Here's what she said to feminist, blogger, and author Kjerstin Gruys (@ KjerstinGruys; www.facebook.com/pages/Kjerstin-Gruys-Sociologist-and-Author/198404800261491), who chose to go for one year without looking in a mirror (and wrote a book about it!):

> We're working hard to get women and men to change their relationship with their reflection, and each time they look in the mirror to say something positive about themselves—not necessarily about their appearance, but some affirmative statement about who they are in the world or what they have done well that day. What I noticed in writing *The Woman in the Mirror* is that women rarely smile when they approach the mirror: they walk up to it with a frown, a scowl, and with trepidation about what they might find. Then they use the mirror as a flaw detector—scanning from head to toe to catalog all of their flaws. I hope that your unveiling will allow you to do just the opposite and remind you of all of the wonderful aspects of your appearance that bring light to the world, to use the mirror to boost your self-esteem rather than bash your body esteem, and to embrace your new found reflection as a positive force in your life.[35]

Body Obsession Is a Serious Issue

Body dissatisfaction is so pervasive that psychologists have given it a name: *normative discontent*. It's normal to want a body that's sleeker, prettier, thinner, or more muscular. It might seem natural and harmless to criticize the one you have—and the ones you see—but that's how body negativity becomes a real problem. There are all kinds of negative repercussions to the fat talk you hear and say out loud. Even if the "body blues" don't propel you into the caverns of an eating disorder, it has a huge impact on your emotional life. Bad body image

- holds you back from discovering the things you like to do
- keeps you from taking risks that could change your life for the better
- reinforces insecurities and fearfulness that only worsen over time
- perpetuates self-absorption and helplessness, characteristics that make you socially isolated
- affects your self-esteem and can lead to many self-abusive behaviors

Body obsession that results from bad body image is only another risk factor associated with disordered eating. The process of correcting perceived body flaws may incite ED symptoms, or it may be a consequence of them. Just like personality, family culture, traumatic experience, and societal pressure, body image is a factor that influences the severity of eating disorder behavior. All contribute to the personal equation that makes every ED a little different for each person. Body and self-image are central issues for most, but not everyone is equally swayed by the modern myth of body beauty perpetuated in the media. That's why holding the diet, fitness, and fashion industries responsible for eating disorders is only a part of prevention objectives.

Our culture is supportive when you set out to make yourself over into a more attractive, more powerful human being. As a society, we'd never want to discourage self-improvement. Conquering fears, overcoming adversity, training to win—these are all good goals that we applaud because positive transformation is good. It's essential, however, to let the desire for change come from your core self, the self that wants to treat your body well for its own sake and not for some predetermined, arbitrary ideal.

The good news is that negative body image is fairly easy to break down. Learning to be comfortable with and even love your body no matter what it looks like can be accomplished once you stop comparing yourself to Photoshopped pictures or caring where you rank on the social ladder at school. Self-esteem can improve quickly with a little effort and attention to healthy body practices. Cheryl Haworth of Savannah, Georgia, has always been a big girl. When she was young, her family helped her come up with a way to deal with the teasing at school. "I think it was my wife who said something to her, or maybe her older sister, 'Well, why don't you arm wrestle 'em and shut 'em up?'" said Cheryl's father. "Darned if she didn't, and you know what, no more disparaging remarks."[36]

Spotlight on About-Face Media Literacy, Inc.

If we are to combat eating and exercise disorders, we need to improve our relationship with our bodies and our innermost selves. To do this, it's essential to understand the dehumanizing effects of idealized body imagery portrayed in the media, and how we internalize society's self-improvement directives. The media literacy organization About-Face conducts primary, middle, and high school programs and extra-curricular workshops on college campuses that deconstruct negative messages, promote body acceptance, and empower activism against objectionable advertising campaigns. Volunteers also give adult presentations to educate about the pressures facing young women today and what to do to strengthen their self-identities. Interns maintain a blog feed and About-Face's online presence on Facebook, Twitter, Tumblr, and YouTube. The website, www.about-face.org, provides statistics, links to research sources, and spreads of the biggest corporate offenders and winners in advertising women's images.

The San Francisco–based organization was founded in 1995 by Kathy Bruin, after she saw an ad for Calvin Klein "Obsession," featuring Kate Moss that had been plastered to a city bus. With the help of a few friends, she "spoofed" the photo with the words "Emaciation Stinks" and "Stop Starvation Imagery," plastering copies all over San Francisco. The response drew national media coverage and public support in the way of donations. The grassroots effort continued with street activism, speaking engagements, and petitions against advertisers into the next decade. About-Face became a nonprofit with a salaried director in 2008.

Cheryl grew to five feet nine inches tall, 297 pounds, and became a national champion power lifter at the age of fifteen. At seventeen she competed in the Sydney Olympics and won the bronze medal in her weight class. She placed sixth in both the Athens and Bejing games, and at age thirty, Cheryl is a role model to the young Olympic hopefuls at her home gym. "You really just have to relax sometimes, and you have to stop looking at all the magazines and what society wants you to look like. Start thinking about what you're gonna do and how you're gonna be different."[37] Instead of conforming, Cheryl decided to stand out. She admits it can be awkward, but she discovered being an extra-large female who can kick ass has advantages. Mainly, a healthy body image and self-esteem. "I train really hard," she said. "I'm fast, I'm flexible. [The size of my body] doesn't hold me back at all. As long as I can do the things that I like . . . then I'm not going to worry about it." Her story was told in the 2012 documentary, *STRONG!*

We may never get to live life in a society that is neutral about body size. But we can eat and treat our bodies well by improving how we feel about who we are. Let's hear how some girls are facing that challenge.

More Food For Thought

Read

Cynthia M. Bulik. *The Woman in the Mirror: How to Stop Confusing What You Look Like with Who You Are.* New York: Walker & Company, 2012.

Ophira Edut, ed. *Body Outlaws: Rewriting the Rules of Beauty and Body Image.* 2nd ed. Emeryville, Calif.: Seal Press, 2003.

Kathlyn Gay. *Body Image and Appearance: The Ultimate Teen Guide.* Lanham, Md.: Scarecrow Press, 2009.

Kjerstin Gruys. *Mirror, Mirror Off the Wall: How I Learned to Love My Body by Not Looking at It for a Year.* New York: Avery, 2013. www.ayearwithoutmirrors.com.

Adam Lamparello. *Ten-Mile Morning: My Journey through Anorexia Nervosa,* Lanham, Md.: Hamilton Books, 2012.

Wendy Shalit. *The Good Girl Revolution: Young Rebels with Self Esteem and High Standards.* New York: Ballantine Books, 2008.

Naomi Wolf. *The Beauty Myth: How Images of Beauty Are Used against Women.* New York: Harper Perennial, 2002.

Watch

Disfigured (feature film, 96 minutes). Launchpad Productions/Dialogue Heavy Pictures, 2008.

Do I Look Fat? Gay Men, Body Image and Eating Disorders (educational DVD, 56 minutes). Blah Blah Blah Productions, 2005. Available with discussion guide. www.doilookfatthemovie.com.

Learn

Adios Barbie: The Body Image Site for Every Body. www.adiosbarbie.com.
Binge Eating Disorder Association. www.bedaonline.com.
Eve Ensler. Watch Eve's stirring TED talks, where she throws down on her own
    body battles. www.eveensler.org; www.ted.com/speakers/eve_ensler.html.
National Association for Males with Eating Disorders. namedinc.org.

APPETITE FOR DESTRUCTION: FROM HABIT TO COMPULSION

It's very common over the course of an eating disordered life to have the A's, B's and C's of eating disorders—anorexia, bulimia, and compulsive eating. There are two types of anorectics, [those] who only restrict and [others] who restrict most of the time, then engage in episodes of binging and purging. It's not uncommon at all for women in recovery from [the restricting type of] anorexia nervosa. It's the flip side of the coin because all the underlying issues are still there and active. The disease is playing out as a different behavior.

—Dr. Kimberly Dennis, CEO and medical director
Timberline Knolls Treatment Center
America the Beautiful 2: The Thin Commandments, 2010

What do we really understand about eating disorders? Can we tell when someone crosses into one? What is the truth behind some of the myths and preconceptions? Get the skinny on flirting with starvation and hear the struggle in the trenches with anorexia, the regurgitated truth of bulimia, and the repercussions of binge eating from those most at risk.

Why Won't She Just Eat?

Anorexia. Bulimia. Binge eating. We've heard about these eating disorders for years through celebrity memoirs, reality TV shows, and whisperings about the girl on the dance team. Perhaps you were taught a special unit on body image in health class. Maybe you even researched the topic yourself and wrote a paper on some of the aspects of EDs. You can probably name someone who has displayed signs of disordered eating and compulsive exercise. Strangely, it seems the more we're presented with information on these illnesses, the slipperier the labels become.

The trouble with the *Diagnostic and Statistical Manual of Mental Disorders* (*DSM*) is that it defines psychiatric illnesses as physicians have done for centuries—by describing symptoms. Although this works well for diseases caused by viruses and bacteria, it may not be the best way for classifying illnesses as complex and gradual as mental disorders. The variation in the behavioral and physical symptoms of EDs has made it difficult for the medical profession to decide exactly what defines a clinical condition. "These problems exist on a continuum," says psychologist Cynthia Bulik, a professor of both eating disorders and nutrition, and director of the University of North Carolina Center of Excellence for Eating Disorders. "There isn't a magic line that divides disordered eating from an eating disorder."[1]

As Dr. Kimberly Dennis pointed out, people with significant eating problems slide between all sorts of behaviors. Over half of patients with anorexia binge and purge, and some patients who are initially bulimic go through periods of restrictive dieting.[2] Compulsive eating is common among those recovering from bulimia and anorexia, and may also precede either of them. Many people shift between subthreshold (less intense symptoms), partial syndrome (some defining symptoms, but not all), and full-blown conditions for years. *The majority of sufferers never fit any of the subtypes.* This is bothersome to Oxford psychiatrist and recognized ED expert Dr. Christopher Fairburn, who has pushed for a better method of classification. He has proposed a radical "transdiagnostic" solution that cancels all the subdivisions by highlighting only the extreme types of behaviors sufferers have in common. "Far more unites the various forms of eating disorders than separates them," he wrote. "The existing scheme for classifying eating disorders is a historical accident that is a poor reflection of clinical reality."[3] Other researchers have suggested a complete overhaul of the *DSM* by designating mental illnesses through personality types. The American Psychiatric Association is not expected to endorse either of the methods anytime soon.

Facts and Fictions

Myths and misunderstanding about eating disorders persist because obesity concerns and body dissatisfaction, disordered eating, and extensive exercise are so common, it's easy to deny their medical seriousness. On the flip side, it's also easy to call almost any irregular eating behavior a disorder. Fictions also persist because all misconceptions have an element of truth. Here are five big ones. What do you think?

Picky, Picky, Picky: Selective Eating Disorder

If you severely limit your food choices, you're at risk for malnourishment and *selective eating disorder* (SED). While it's normal for toddlers and young children to refuse types of food, most grow accustomed to the flavors and textures that make up a healthy diet. For some picky eaters, their small range of preferences becomes pathological and pursues them into adulthood. Josh, twenty-two, of Hacienda Heights, California, is addicted to pizza. "I crave pizza every time I want a meal," he told the producers of *Freaky Eaters*. "I don't know why I want it. I just want it."[a]

"Josh was not a picky eater when he was young," said his mom, Darlene. "The picky eating didn't start until he had money to buy his own food." When he was in third grade, Josh bought pizza for lunch at school. The lunch lady gave out extra slices on Fridays. Soon he was eating almost no other kind of food. In high school, he had plenty of energy to play volleyball and became a star player on the Los Altos Conqueros varsity team. His pizza diet eventually caught up with him—he began suffering migraines and depression and had to drop all his college classes. He couldn't believe his health was related to what he was eating, or more precisely, not eating. "I definitely forget about my problems when I'm eating pizza," he said. "For that moment, I'm not thinking about everything I lost. Whatever's going on after I eat pizza, I like how I'm feeling."[b]

People with SED suffer from anxiety and low self-worth. They show addictive cravings and withdrawal symptoms when denied their special food(s). They may even develop allergies to their food preferences. Psychologist Nancy Zucker at the Duke Center for Eating Disorders believes SED should be listed in the *DSM* as another type of ED, but more evidence is needed to determine the criteria for diagnosis. Together with a team of researchers, she launched the Food F.A.D. Study, a registry for finicky adults to assess the numbers and habits of selective eaters. "I was thinking we'd get maybe 500 responses, but when the survey went up, it just immediately went crazy,"[c] Zucker said. Over 18,000 people have taken the online survey since it began in 2010.

1. Eating Disorders Are Caused by Terrible Parenting

People with EDs might have grown up in abusive homes. Some have lazy fathers or distracted mothers. But many have normal, even wonderful childhoods. What's important is how we internalize what is going on around and inside us. "I never went without anything," said Jordana, twenty-four, who was treated for bulimia. "I grew up as an overweight child and was teased. That's about it. I stopped eating when I was in ninth grade. Once I lost weight, I became popular. . . . I felt really good. I was at my lowest weight and people thought I was pretty. I learned that being thin, people want to be your friend."[4] Family dynamics might be triggering to someone with an ED, however, no evidence proves families are the cause.[5] Therapy is no longer based on repairing dysfunctional families, but by sufferers learning alternative ways of thinking and better coping strategies to counter stressful elements of life.

2. Our Diet- and Fitness-Obsessed Culture Drives People into Eating Disorders

Images that we see in the media, comments about our appearance, training for athletic events all shape our perception of our bodies. Our cultural preference for fit and trim physiques has completely affected our ideas of what constitutes a normal weight. "My best friend died when she was almost eleven years old," said one Santa Monica, California, high school student. "We used to go buy magazines and she'd pick out a picture and say, 'By next week, I'm going to be that size.' The next week she'd pick an even skinnier girl. She'd say, 'By next week, I'll be that size.' Finally she achieved her goal, but she ended up killing herself."[6] But eating disorders don't develop simply from a drive for thinness. Research shows the risk for EDs rises significantly only when body or weight concerns combine with other inner characteristics such as insecurity, worry, perfectionism, self-doubt, and extreme fear of consequences.

3. People with Eating Disorders Choose to Have Them

"I don't think it's people's fault that they get an eating disorder, but to all my clients, I say, it is your responsibility to get yourself out,"[7] said Carolyn Costin, anorexia survivor and one of the leading treatment specialists in the country. The question of whether sufferers choose their damaging behavior is a long debate. Eating disorders "harden into a way of life," writes Dr. Michael Strober, clinical professor of Psychiatry and Biobehavioral Sciences and director of the Eating Disorders Program at UCLA. Not because people wish it upon themselves, but because it's the only way they get real relief from "life that's too painful to endure."[8] Furthermore, behavioral disorders often feel like an alternate personality run amok, and many with EDs describe their compulsions this way. On the other hand, once sufferers understand they are using eating and exercise to cope with mental stress and realize the damage they are doing, they can be helped to choose other behaviors. Believing in the power of choice is indeed part of recovery. Proper nutrition in treatment stabilized Nina's mental state so she could want to fully recover. "The biggest thing I learned here is that I can eat," she said. "I haven't purged at all because the only way I'll purge is if I binge, and that wouldn't be an option here. If you come here knowing that you want to get better and you're here because you can't take it anymore, then you're not going to do that. But if you're here because you're being forced, you're going to try to get away with as much as you can."[9]

4. Eating Disorders Are Genetic/Inherited

Unlike true genetic disorders like Tay Sachs, Huntington's Korea, or Prader-Willi Syndrome, EDs don't come from mistakes in our DNA. Psychological illnesses have inherited genetic components that make some of us susceptible, but they only account for part of the risk. Genes are simply the blueprint for forming enzymes and hormones that make chemical reactions take place. These processes are important for our personality and behavioral traits that are further shaped by the environment in which they grow. A predisposition is not a predetermination—our genes are never our destiny.

"What [gene studies] do is point us in the direction of novel kinds of biological clues that could then be targets for treatment," Jordan Smoller told Audie Cornish on National Public Radio's *All Things Considered*. Dr. Smoller is a psychiatry professor at Massachusetts General Hospital and Harvard Medical School. "This then begins a process of looking for ways to translate that information into something that might actually be helpful to folks."[10] He went on to say that genetic studies, together with studies of brain imaging and behavior, may get us to look at mental disorders in a different way and ultimately diagnose them based on their root causes, rather than symptoms.

5. Eating Disorders Are Epidemic in Our Society

Determining that EDs have become an *epidemic* is a matter of perspective. There are all sorts of clues that show more and more people are getting help for emotional eating problems, although not necessarily full-blown, chronic disorders. The Mayo Clinic has reported that the number of those entering treatment for anorexia had increased 36 percent every five years from the 1950s to the end of the twentieth century.[11] The National Institute of Mental Health indicates that hospitalization rates for eating disorders increased 18 percent between 1999 and 2006.[12] For children under twelve, hospitalizations more than doubled.[13] The number of specialized residential treatment centers in the United States has

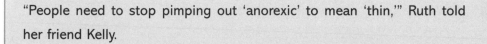

Everybody Wants One, Nobody Wants Anybody to Have One

"People need to stop pimping out 'anorexic' to mean 'thin,'" Ruth told her friend Kelly.

> Obesity is so much more common now than being skinny, it's skewed people's conception of what a healthy size actually is. Every other week it seems, the tabloids scream that this or that actor has anorexia because she or he dropped some weight for a role, or for whatever personal reason. It feeds the idea that an eating disorder is easy to get, that anyone who loses—or gains—weight is messed up in the head. But "thin" and "obese" don't mean "eating disorder," just like "binge-o-rama barfitosa" isn't a quick fix diet plan. Someone once asked me to give her "anorexia lessons." I told her I'd only do it for people who sign a waiver, that way I'd be protected when their heart failed.[d]

Kelly agreed.

> If people really understood the agony that comes from an eating disorder, they'd be a lot more careful what they wish for. I think public perception is changing, though. So many people know someone with a real eating problem now. And celebrities are falling over themselves to admit addictions because of the publicity they get. Lady Gaga and Katie Couric jumped on the bandwagon this year [announcing they previously suffered from bulimia while in their teens], because it's such a badge of honor to say you were ill and recovered. An eating disorder has become a golden challis that everybody wants to own, but no one wants to ruin their lives over food. If you've triumphed over affliction, though, that's when you prove you're super-human.[e]

gone from one to more than 170 in less than thirty years. In the last few years, many of them have seen as much as a 20 percent rise in the number of males and middle-aged women coming through the doors with moderate to severe ED symptoms.

Studies indicate, however, the forms of EDs associated with the deepest psychological issues affect only a small percentage of us. The percentages of adolescents and young adults diagnosed with clinically significant EDs worldwide have stayed about the same since the 1990s. A 2011 U.S. survey of 10,123 thirteen- to eighteen-year-olds found rates of full and partial syndrome anorexia and bulimia each affected less than 1 percent of the responding subjects.[14] Binge eating disorder and subthreshold binge eating disorder affected 1.6 and 2.5 percent, respectively.[15] A significant finding—females didn't outnumber males by a lot.

An ED for Every Color, Class, and Culture

Forming a healthy self-image is a challenging prospect for teens from minority and mixed ethnic heritages who often have to negotiate conflicting messages from family and mainstream cultures. Teenagers of color are just as likely to develop disordered eating practices as upper-middle-class white girls. Eating disorders don't discriminate and don't align on the basis of race or ethnicity—Hispanic, Asian, black, Native American, or mixed race teenagers are pushed to the brink along with whites. Of the four ethnic groups, Hispanic girls in grades 9–12 reported the highest rate of vomiting, twenty-four-hour fasting, and use of laxatives and diet pills to control their weight, according to the Youth Risk Behavior Surveillance Survey.[16] Native American high school girls had even higher rates

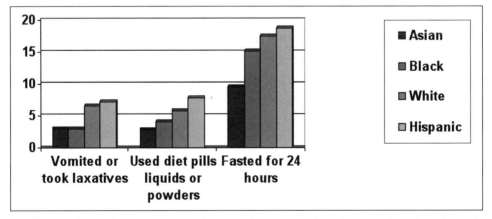

Health risk behaviors in the previous thirty days in females, grades nine through twelve. *Data courtesy of Centers for Disease Control and Prevention (CDC), 1991–2011 High School Youth Risk Behavior Survey Data, Youth Online: High School YRBSS, 2012. Available at apps.nccd.cdc.gov/youthonline (accessed March 2013).*

of these behaviors. Almost 12 percent vomited, 8 percent used diet aids, and 30 percent said they had fasted in the thirty days prior to the survey.

A study presented at the 2002 International Conference on Eating Disorders showed that women of color have many of the same abnormal eating patterns as white females.[17] Latinas in South American countries have some of the highest per capita incidence of EDs in the world. The rates in Argentina may be three times those in the United States. A poll by the Argentine Association to Fight Bulimia and Anorexia indicated that of the 90,000 teenage girls ages fourteen to eighteen who participated, one in ten suffers from an ED.[18] The Neurosiquiatrico Centre of Santiago in Chile estimated that 70,000 Chilean women between ages fourteen and thirty suffer from anorexia nervosa and that 350,000 women suffer from bulimia nervosa.[19]

Low-level disordered eating and activity patterns and *atypical eating disorders* are widely dispersed in the American population, and throughout the world, but true numbers are difficult to determine. Because so many of us have borderline issues with body image and judgmental attitudes about food choices—and observe the same in people we know—we have the impression that full-blown, long-term cases of EDs are much more common than they are. What's become evident is

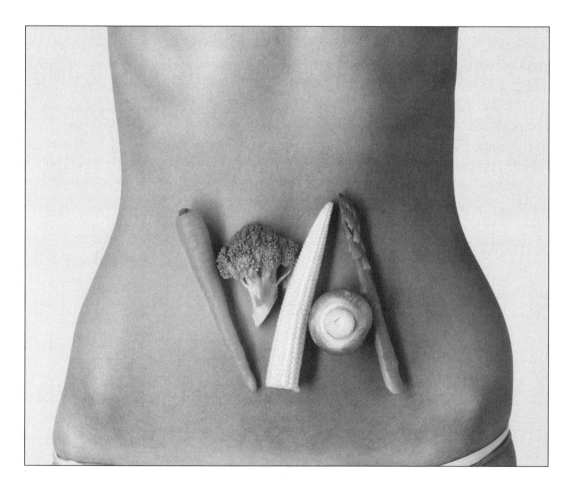

that many teens skirt around the fringes of eating and activity disorders long before college and early adulthood.

Interestingly, as awareness of an illness spreads in a society, its prevalence tends to increase. Why this happens is mysterious. It could be that greater awareness reduces stigma, prompting more sufferers to seek help. It's also possible that the balance is shifting in the factors that put us at risk, making them less protective. As social and cultural pressures grow, they can be capable of triggering eating disorders in those who might have been less vulnerable under better circumstances. The Internet and the penetrating nature of reality TV, especially, have made us more aware of all levels and types of disordered eating. Shared stories can both inspire recovery and perpetuate illness. Unfortunately, those most susceptible to addictive-type disorders can become sicker and even learn to substitute other self-abusive coping behaviors. Approximately 80 percent of individuals with anorexia and bulimia (and binge eating disorder)[20] are diagnosed with another psychiatric disorder at some time in their life.[21]

Risky Business: The Tribes of Size Zero

For some groups of people, the issue of weight and attitudes toward body size are not only a fashionable trend, but an inherent part of the job. Models and athletes must keep their bodies finely tuned if they are to succeed professionally. Although not all sink into the extreme clutches of an eating and activity disorder, the tactics to make a body the best it can be often give way to disordered behaviors. This can happen at the start of a person's training, or later in a career, as the pressure to stay competitive intensifies. *The qualities that are important to success—tenacity laced with perfectionism, intense motivation, focus, and drive, along with the ability to endure discomfort—are the same characteristics that fuel eating disorders.* Performers that enter the world of dance, modeling, gymnastics, weight lifting, wrestling, boxing—any weight-qualified sport—put themselves at increased risk for malnutrition and other

> ### ! Pushing Grandma's Buttons
>
> Middle-aged women are the fastest growing segment of the population seeking treatment for eating disorders. In a 2011 survey, 13 percent of 1,849 women over age fifty said they suffered from clinical symptoms.[f] Seven and a half percent took diet pills and 8 percent reported purging (excessive exercise, vomiting, diuretics, or laxative use) to control their weight.[g] Almost two-thirds believed that their weight or shape negatively impacted their life.

abusive health practices. Disordered eating is standard behavior for professional jockeys, who must constantly monitor their weight to satisfy racetrack limits. A study published by the U.S. National Library of Medicine surveyed the weight-loss methods for jockeys—69 percent skip meals, 34 percent use diuretics, 67 percent sweat off the pounds in the sauna, 40 percent use laxatives, and 30 percent regularly vomit,[22] or "flip," as the riders call it. The Kentucky Derby Museum, located on the track at Churchill Downs, has a memorial exhibit to jockeys who have died as a consequence of their weight-control regimens.

The statistics of models who succumb to eating disorders are grim. A report from the British Fashion Council estimated that 20–40 percent suffer from EDs.[23] A controlled study of Italian models found the girls reported significantly more eating disorder symptoms, and had a higher prevalence of partial syndrome EDs, than girls of similar age and backgrounds.[24] Sara Ziff (@saraziff), founder of the Model Alliance (modelalliance.org; @ModelAllianceNY), has noted many abuses perpetrated by the modeling industry, including drug use and the encouragement of disordered eating practices. A survey of models in New York and Los Angeles conducted by the Alliance revealed that nearly two-thirds of respondents had been asked to lose weight by their agencies. Almost half fasted or cleansed, or restricted their food intake over short periods to lose weight. Sixty-eight percent admitted they suffered from anxiety or depression.[25]

Gerren Taylor, fifteen, discovered the difficulties firsthand when she went with her mother to Europe to pursue her dreams. Gerren had begun modeling when she was discovered by a scout at age twelve. She booked a lot of work for a couple years, then left her agency to go to London. That's when she learned her hip measurement was too big for the shows in Milan. Why does a model have to be so small, *America the Beautiful* director Darryl Roberts asked New York fashion show producer Greg Moore. "It's not so much 'small,' it's just that fabric is so expensive. And the detailing. If you make a dress that's a size 4, and no one buys it, you only bought three yards. If [the model's] a size 10, you bought ten yards."[26] A designer would lose thousands of dollars in fabric costs, he explains, if they had to sew larger-size samples.

That models are at risk for the consequences of dangerous dieting is not news. The casting for runway models has been trending to younger, pre-pubescent girls since the 1980s. As the girls grow up and fill out they are compelled to stay rail thin to be competitive; thus the quest for unnatural thinness is still pursued by legions of models working full or part time in the industry. "I am six feet tall and I'm a size 2–4. I weigh one hundred and thirty pounds," one model told Darryl Roberts. "But I've already been told . . . I have to lose fifteen pounds. And there's no way around it." Concerned, Darryl asked if that would be dangerous for her health. "Health doesn't become an option in this business," she said, shaking her head slowly. "If you're going to worry about your health, go to college."[27]

Reworking the Catwalk

Plus-sized modeling is a growing segment of the overall fashion industry and many former "straight size" models, such as Kate Dillon and Anansa Sims, have built steady careers. In 2010, photos of Crystal Renn ignited her fire when she saw how much they had been retouched. Crystal, who had already gone public in *People* about her struggle with anorexia and bulimia, objected to the altering of photos taken by Nicholas Routzen for a charity. The pictures effectively reduced her from a size 10 to a size 2. The last thing Crystal wanted to do was have anybody think that she had either relapsed or fallen under industry pressure. She expressed her outrage to Meredith Viera on *Today.* "I don't want [women] to think my message isn't the same, that I think thin is the only way to be beautiful," she said. "Beauty is not a pants size; I think it's about what I have to say and how I live my life, which is in a healthy way, I believe, for me. I want them to know I'm healthy."[h] An outspoken member of the Model Alliance, Crystal suggested that models not be classified as plus or straight. "That is absolutely not the way women should look at each other. . . . I want to get rid of titles because they demean women and there's no need for that."[i]

According to Roberta Anding, registered dietitian for the Houston Ballet, most dancers weigh only 85–90 percent of what is considered ideal body weight. She says that level of (anorexic) leanness can lower the metabolic rate so that it takes fewer calories to maintain it.[28] But dancers need plenty of energy to dance. "There's people that say I'm too skinny and that I should start fattening up," said twelve-year-old Miko Fogarty of Walnut Creek, California, who placed third in her age category during the 2010 Youth America Grand Prix (YAGP), the prestigious international competition for aspiring ballet dancers. "But you have to be skinny to do ballet. You have to have lots of energy and for that you need food."[29]

"I think dancers eat a lot," insists Michaela Deprince, fourteen, who won a YAGP dance scholarship that year. "Most dancers, I think."[30]

"We're so thin because we're burning off all the calories," explains Jeanette Kakareka, sixteen. "If you didn't eat, you couldn't dance."[31]

It's not uncommon, though, for dancers to become food obsessed. As with jockeys and models, it's an occupational hazard. The structured discipline of dance attracts competitive and obsessive perfectionists, who work hard on becoming fit to do what's demanded of them. In the ethereal world of ballet, the desire to be lean and long, lithe and light, is especially keen. A dancer's job is to look picture-perfect, to hide the pushing and straining, unlike other athletes. For girls with raw talent, who start taking lessons before their bodies mature, the shift into puberty is often treacherous. Curves and bumps can jiggle and detract from the

Dancing Her Heart Out

The death of twenty-two-year-old Heidi Guenther sent the community of classical ballet reeling in 1997. The energetic ballerina had died from cardiac arrest. Family and friends believed it had occurred because of Heidi's zeal to attain the perfect dance body, and her fear of being cut from her new position as a member of the Boston Ballet's corps of dancers. Within days of the first news story, her employer was on the defensive, claiming that although Heidi had been told to lose just five pounds, she had become too thin and had been encouraged to eat more. Bruce Marks, retired artistic director of the company, emphasized that no one was ever threatened with consequences over weight control. The Ballet has always provided health counseling to all its employees. He doubted Heidi's low weight was the cause of her death. He believes it was her heart ailments. "She wasn't malnourished," he told the New York Times a few months after the incident. "Anyone here who's skinny is naturally so."[j]

Heidi's mother, Patti Harrington, acknowledged that Heidi had been diagnosed with a heart murmur as a child, and that she had occasionally experienced a racing heartbeat. She had also seen that the dancers who got the best roles most often were especially thin. "The thinner she'd get, the more roles she'd get, the more compliments she'd get," said her mother, who had always supported Heidi's dream to become a professional dancer. "There's a real subliminal message that comes with all that."[k]

According to those who knew her, Heidi had dieted by skipping meals, purging, and using diet pills and laxatives. The coroner's final report, two years later, indicated that emotional factors and disordered eating may have played a role in killing her.[l] Who, or what, was to blame could still be a matter of opinion, but in the years since Heidi's death, we are coming to realize that dieting may be much more dangerous than we thought.

look of alignment. Soon, body shape becomes more important than technique to both students and teachers, and girls begin dieting. Eating disorders are the dirty little secret no one likes to talk about in the dance profession. Even dance school graduates whose bodies fit the ballet aesthetic find it normal to justify disordered eating when they feel their career is at stake. "I counted calories so much that it upset my non-dancing friends and created barriers between us," said dancer-turned-writer Kathleen McGuire (@Katie_Mc412) of Pittsburgh, Pennsylvania. "I talked constantly about how out of shape or soft I was. . . . My refusal to eat was a distraction that caused fights in my family, spurred on by their concern for my health and my defensive stance that they just didn't understand. Birthdays, holidays, and weddings became joyless and stressful."[32] Kathleen danced around the black hole and eventually gave up the notion of becoming a ballerina. "I spent my critical training years fixated on food. My negative attitude toward eating caused me more than injury; it affected my friendships and my family as well. Even after I began to eat in a healthier way, the fear of what every bite would do to my body remained. Eventually, I found my way out of the tunnel, but I wish I had spent those years focused on what really mattered—dancing." The challenge to become slimmer yet stronger, while staying healthy and fit for work is dangerous for dancers and a serious issue for dance companies—the ballet world, in particular.

Dancers, by temperament, may be even more vulnerable to eating disorders than athletes and other higher-risk populations. A comparative study involving college and professional ballet dancers found dancers were more likely to have restricting-type anorexia than statistics show for the general public. Other ED symptoms were even more of a problem. Ten percent of them met the criteria for bulimia, while 55 percent had unclassified EDs.[33] Psychologist Rebecca Ringham of the University of Pittsburgh Medical Center led the study and reported the dancers scored noticeably higher on measures of perfectionism than non-dancers. Another study comparing disordered eating attitudes of modern dance and ballet

Tiny Dancers, *Eat*!

Taking her post as the new artistic director of the English National Ballet, former prima ballerina Tamara Rojo has said she wants to "stamp out anorexia" in ballet. "Audiences want to see beautiful and healthy-looking dancers yet there is still that pressure to be thin,"[m] she told the *Sunday Times* of Britain. "Some comes from the fashion world and that in turn affects ballet. When you are in a ballet company, you often lose perspective of reality. So you go for extremes in order to stand out and be noticed."

students at three universities showed that ballet put dancers at greater risk for eating disturbances.[34]

Starving Is as Starving Does

People who have no inclination to lose weight, but instead are forced to starve, display symptoms of anorexia. In 1944, just before the end of the Second World War, Ancel Keys and his colleagues at the University of Minnesota recruited thirty-six conscientious objectors to participate in a controlled study of human starvation. He hoped the results of the Minnesota Starvation Experiment, as it became known, would provide insight into the physical and psychological effects of extreme weight loss and be of help to aid organizations that had the task of *refeeding* hungry survivors in war-torn countries. (Keys's paper, *The Biology of Human Starvation*, was published in two volumes in 1950 and is over a thousand pages long.) After a period of three months in which researchers stabilized the participants' diet and body weight, the men were fed a "refugee menu" of potatoes, turnips, rutabagas, dark bread, and macaroni—approximately 1,800 calories per day for six months. The men took classes at the university and were assigned household duties that included cooking. They were also expected to walk twenty-two miles per week. Most lost over 25 percent of their body weight.[35] Many experienced personality and appetite disturbances, body dysmorphia, and behaviors typical of people with eating disorders—weird food rituals and hoarding, inattention, restless energy, social withdrawal, short tempers, even self-mutilation. Two showed such psychotic tendencies, they had to be admitted to the university's hospital.

The Minnesota study doesn't explain everything about the complex mental and physical processes in everyone who drops to an unnaturally low weight—and it wasn't designed to. It did prove that certain disordered eating behaviors were actually effects of the weight loss itself. Starvation alone may not kick off an eating disorder, but it's imperative to reverse it, so that "a hunger disease" has a chance to subside. Nourishing the body repairs the mind. For those with eating problems who are severely underweight, weight gain is the first step to restoring mental health.

The Role of CRF Hormones

Practically everyone can relate to food cravings to some extent at one time or another. The drive to binge comes from a deep-seated need to satisfy appetite, coming from physiological or emotional hunger, or both. Temptation, as well as

Going Hungry in the Polish Ghetto

Although history has given us recorded accounts of famine, few include detailed physical descriptions of people who starve for long periods. Even fewer experiments have been done (for obvious ethical reasons) to observe what happens to a human body deprived of food. While Keys was checking the effects of starvation in a group of healthy volunteers, Jewish doctors in the Warsaw Ghetto decided to meticulously record what was happening to the men, women, and children, whose access to food was severely restricted by the German army. Calories were officially rationed to around 300 per day—a fistful of bread and a small bowl of thin soup. A few extra vegetables and smears of butter or lard could be procured on the black market. Most Jews could find around a thousand calories a day on which to slowly starve.

Between 1940 and 1943, when the Nazis began the final deportations to the concentration camps, thousands died of hunger. The doctors watched as their patients' fat stores shrank and their skin became papery, hollowed, and dry. People complained of constant hunger at first, then of inability to concentrate or remember. Formerly happy, well-behaved children became morose and belligerent. Hair became thick on their heads and fine fuzz covered their bodies. Older teens and adults experienced hair loss. Everyone suffered from insomnia and most from some form of edema, a watery swelling in tissues and within joints as cells became less efficient in maintaining their salt and water balance. Poor blood circulation and poor immune response contributed to high rates of infection.[n] Autopsies revealed the bodies' extreme emaciation. Muscles had atrophied and all the organs were lightweight and shrunken.

The notes of the hunger disease project that survived the war became important for the medical community to realize long-term permanent features of starvation. An undernourished heart shrinks and can never quite return to its full workload capacity. As a result, blood pressure and heart rate are commonly low. The notes were also helpful because they suggested methods that would be least traumatic for a body's return to health. "Supplying adequate nutrition and food with an appropriate caloric value [2,000 to 3,000 calories a day in four to five meals] could be . . . the only rational therapy for hunger," wrote one of the doctors.° Amounts of food during the process of refeeding, though, have to be bumped up gradually to reduce the risk of cardiac arrest.

Gluttony Reigns Supreme: Competitive Eaters

The ability to consume vast quantities of food in a single sitting is fascinating to witness. Competitive eating has gone far beyond county fairs and restaurant challenges. The International Federation of Competitive Eating, now known as Major League Eating, organizes over eighty eating contests annually (www.ifoce.com). Prize money tops a thousand dollars and serious competitors travel around the world. The public spectacles draw more people than ever watched the hunger artists a century and a half ago—no doubt, there's more action to see. In 2012, more than 50,000 watched live, by either attending or tuning in to ESPN, to cheer Joey "Jaws" Chestnut at Nathan's Famous Fourth of July International Hot Dog Eating Contest. He downed sixty-eight hot dogs and buns in ten minutes, tying his own world record. Sonya "Black Widow" Thomas claimed the woman's title for the second year in a row, setting a new record of forty-five.

Although competitive eaters may not necessarily have EDs, the practices they use to train for an event can definitely be categorized as disordered eating. Joey, twenty-nine, from San Jose, California, who enters over a dozen contests per year, binges once a week on the kind of food he'll be eating next. A few days before and after an event, he'll limit himself to water, milk, and protein supplements. He eats carefully at all other times and runs for exercise. "Psychologically, I like to go in hungry," he told WebMD in 2007.ᵖ "If I see on the scale that I have dropped weight, I can easily imagine an enormous amount of food inside me."

Sonya, forty-five, originally from South Korea and now a Burger King manager from Alexandria, Virginia, slowly eats one large meal a day and does two hours of aerobics. On February 12, 2013, she ate ten and a half Fat Tuesday king cakes in eight minutes, good enough for second place and $1,000.[q] "My stomach is really normal size, but over the years it has been trained to stretch quite a bit," she reports on her website. "As far as capacity is concerned, I believe I can handle up to nineteen pounds of food and liquid overall [within ten minutes]."[r]

Health professionals worry that competitive eating is dangerous. Doctors believe overstretched stomach muscles can eventually become paralyzed, keeping the stomach from emptying normally. Dieticians are especially wary of the message competitive eating sends to spectators. "Knowing how many people don't have adequate nutrition, and how many people abuse food and overeat constantly, seeing competitive eating celebrated on TV disturbs me," nutritionist Milton Stokes told feature writer Richard Sine. "[It] sends a message to spectators that going hog wild with food is not a big deal."[s] For many, indeed, it's a very big deal.

deprivation, often makes it difficult to recognize the difference between the two. When anxiety becomes chronic in a sensitive person, it can lead to the need, as Jessie said, for "something now, now, now, now, now." The evidence suggests that this urgency, characteristic of all addictive behavior, is due to one family of hormones in particular, the corticotrophin releasing factor (CRF) system. CRF enhances appetite in a variety of ways, leading to seemingly contradictory behaviors. The activity of these hormones explains much of the motivation behind the compulsive eating of binge eaters and bulimics. It suggests why anorexia sufferers are consumed by thoughts of food—shopping, meal planning, cooking . . . everything but eating normally.

For instance, blood tests have shown that starving individuals have plenty of ghrelin, the "hungry hormone," circulating continuously, yet many anoretics claim not to recognize the signal. It turns out that CRF is elevated when the body is stressed due to starvation. CRF appears to tamper down gherlin's signal to the hypothalamus,[36] at the same time revving up anxious and depressive feelings common to almost everyone with eating disorders. This may be one reason why hunger is confounded in the depressed, leading some to deny their appetite, while others overeat. For those who feel compelled to ramp up their exercise to an extreme level, increasing physical activity raises the levels of CRF. This tends to further suppress appetite in anorexia-prone individuals while enhancing it in those susceptible to binging.

CRF also makes it hard for regular addicts to quit their drug, and brain researchers believe it works the same way in those with EDs. CRF further stimulates compulsive eating by triggering the nucleus accumbens, the structure that produces intense cravings. This is how stress can provoke bursts of binging,[37] even when a binger is not truly hungry. Besides certain types of food, cycles of binging and binge-purging might become addictive themselves because of how CRF modifies brain structures. This has been called the "dark side of food addiction." In a ground-breaking study at the Laboratory of Addictive Disorders at Boston University, researchers found when rodents were fed a diet of sugary, fat-laden food, they lost their desire for the more nutritious rat chow. Tests showed their brains generated five times the amount of CRF compared to the rats on the standard diet.[38] When returned to the tastier fare, they gorged themselves even more than they had previously. "This [CRF] punishment, [is a] negative reinforcement [that] is causing anxiety and is increasing the probability that bad behavior is [sic] performed in the future to relieve anxiety,"[39] said lead scientist Pietro Cottone. He treated the addicted rats with a CRF blocker traditionally used to help drug and alcohol abusers with substance withdrawal. The destructive eating patterns greatly improved.

An Expert Weighs In:
Carolyn Costin—Confronting the Problem

Fully recovered from anorexia, Carolyn Costin (@Carolyn_Costin) is founder and director of Monte Nido and Affiliates, renowned eating disorder and exercise addiction treatment centers in California, Oregon, Massachusetts, and New York. She has counseled people with eating disorders for over thirty years and has profound insight into the mind-set. A therapist, speaker, and author, Costin is one of the foremost ED treatment specialists, often setting the record straight on confusing aspects that are inaccurately portrayed in the media. In her book *Your Dieting Daughter*, she compiled "The Thin Commandments," a list of rules that guides eating disordered thoughts, feelings, and beliefs about food and body size.

Triggering Debate: A Twenty-First-Century Plague

A 2011 statistic puts the number of Americans with "clinically significant" eating disorders at 20 million women and 10 million men.[t] Do you think this is accurate? Are EDs common among the people you know? Do you think it's easy or difficult to actually get one? Why does it seem that way?

When does dieting become dangerous? What is going on inside ourselves and in our society that pushes so many of us to the edge of, or fully into, an ED? Costin shares some thoughts about teenagers on the brink.

When does a diet become a disorder? Basically what happens is you go on a diet like everyone else but at some point, for a variety of complex reasons, you get trapped into a vicious cycle and can't get out. One of the criteria for an eating disorder is putting an undue influence on weight and shape in evaluating self-esteem. These days, however, what young girl doesn't put too much influence on body shape and size? Being dissatisfied with one's body and going on a diet is not only acceptable but almost expected among peers. Parents actually praise you for losing weight, without even knowing how the weight loss was accomplished. Many people want to be healthier, lose weight and look better, but for some the diet becomes compelling, metabolic changes happen, and they are no longer in control. Once you begin overly restricting or purging food to control weight you find it hard to break the habit. Normal eating, or consuming food considered to be "fattening," feels so wrong, you cannot tolerate the feelings and thus continue these behaviors.

The highest instance of developing an eating disorder occurs in adolescence. That's the time when you're most struggling with identity and peer pressure. Living in our current, "Thin Is In" culture with constant influences from the media propels many of us to diet. Combine this with a genetic predisposition, such as perfectionism and anxiety and you have a perfect storm. If you want to fit in and be accepted, you might be compelled to lose weight and if you have a certain temperament, it can lead to the pursuit of thinness in an obsessive, rigid way that ends up spiraling into a disorder. Behaviors such as dieting, eliminating whole categories of food, exercising solely for weight control, constantly weighing or body checking, taking laxatives, occasionally purging, only eating diet food, having food rituals, etcetera, can lead to a full eating disorder diagnosis. It is important to note that teens can struggle with all of these behaviors and develop serious problems, even if they never meet the criteria for an eating disorder.

Unfortunately, this society idealizes the ability to control your food intake and have control over your body. I believe those who develop eating disorders can be thought of as our cultural "canaries in the coal mine." When miners took canaries in cages down into the coal mines, if the canaries died, it meant the environment was toxic, so the miners had to get out of there. People who develop eating disorders may be giving us the same message. Many of us diet, but those who develop eating disorders may be indicating that the current cultural environment is toxic. Those with eating disorders are the most susceptible to what is happening in a society where what you look like is more important than who you are.[40]

Costin strongly believes that people with eating disorders can be fully recovered. You can find more of her perspective on her website, www.montenido.com, through her YouTube channel, and on the Facebook page for Monte Nido and Affiliates.

A Creeping Madness

If we use food to cope with our emotions, how we think and feel about appetite and ourselves determine how we control our eating and exercise. Eating and not eating, exercise and puking help to fill the hole inside. Feelings quickly divorce from the habits we develop, making it impossible for sufferers to realize that anything is going wrong. As Robin Decker explained to the film crew of *Absent*, "It's kind of hard to go back to the beginning and figure out when I started to feel like there was something wrong with me and when I started to equate that feeling of something being wrong, with me being ugly."[41] Sexual molestation by her father led Robin to seek intimacy through sexual activity with eighteen- to twenty-four-year-old boyfriends while she was still in middle school. "That was the only acceptance that I found—was with the older guys," she said. "And the sex I equated to love—that's all I wanted . . . love, that's it." Robin gave birth to a son at age fourteen and then two more by the time she was in college. Her battle with anorexia began early. After her mother passed away, also a statistic of sexual abuse and an ED, Robin's eating issues worsened.[42] "I was thrown into some sick version of womanhood. You make a connection between the ugliness that you feel inside and the image you see in the mirror, and then you try and change that. Combined with, if I can't control what somebody puts in my body—by way of sexual abuse—I will control what I put in my body by counting every calorie, every carbohydrate, every gram of fat."[43] Eventually, with the help of goal-oriented strength and martial arts training, Robin, thirty-six, has learned better ways to deal with her self-hatred and insecurities. What would she say to that little girl she once was? "I would tell her not to search for her daddy's love everywhere. And that she has to somehow just believe that people love her—and that she's beautiful."

The struggles associated with food abuse vary widely and the demons of madness creep up and settle in. What are some of the consequences when weight loss, overexercising, or the need for something (everything!) now tips you head over heels into the clutches of an ED? Let's see who feels the effects, and what the rising tide of eating disorders might mean for society at large.

More Food for Thought

Read

Harriet Brown, ed. *Feed Me! Writers Dish about Food, Eating, Weight, and Body Image*. New York: Ballantine Books, 2009.

Carolyn Costin. *100 Questions and Answers about Eating Disorders*. Burlington, Mass.: Jones and Bartlett Publishers, 2007.

Roman Espejo, ed. *Eating Disorders*. Opposing Viewpoints Series. Farmington Hills, Mich.: Greenhaven Press, 2012.

Caroline Knapp. *Appetites: Why Women Want*. New York: Counterpoint, 2003.

Maine, Margo. *Father Hunger: Fathers, Daughters and the Pursuit of Thinness*. 2nd ed. Carlsbad, Calif.: Gürze Books, 2004.

Sara Shandler. *Ophelia Speaks: Adolescent Girls Write about Their Search for Self*. New York: Harper Perennial, 1999.

Kate M. Taylor, ed. *Going Hungry: Writers on Desire, Self-Denial, and Overcoming Anorexia*. New York: Anchor Books, 2008.

Learn

Eating Disorder Hope. www.eatingdisorderhope.com.

ED Bites: The Latest Tasty Tidbits in Eating Disorder Science (Carrie Arnold's blog). www.edbites.com.

Girl Zone. www.girlzone.com.

National Eating Disorders Association—Stories of Hope. www.nationaleating disorders.org/stories-of-hope.

TRUTH AND CONSEQUENCES: THE ULTIMATE COST OF FOOD OBSESSION

Today, we're told we, too, can look a certain way, if only we work hard enough at it. There's this whole myth that everyone can achieve the impossible. And that's very damaging, because if you don't achieve this look, something is wrong with you.

—Ruth Striegel Weissman, Professor of Psychology, Provost, and
Vice President for Academic Affairs
Wesleyan University, Middletown, Connecticut
Dying to Be Thin, 2000

What does extreme eating look like in the rest of the world? Is it really dangerous to be weight obsessed? Who carries the biggest burden of these mental health issues? Discover the long-term effects and repercussions of calorie restriction, purging, and overeating, and how these behaviors affect everything and everyone in our lives.

The Rising Tide

The number of people—especially young women—with eating disorders appears to be growing throughout the world, according to a 2004 data review. The study examined international reports of eating disorder prevalence and disturbed eating attitudes over the previous twenty years. A greater proportion of the population in Western countries, such as the United States, United Kingdom, Germany, Australia, and Canada, seem to suffer compared to people in non-Western countries such as Nigeria, Malaysia, Turkey, China, and Pakistan. The predominance of eating problems, typically assessed by surveying young people, also appears to be rising in non-Western populations—Iran, Israel, South Africa (among both white and non-white youth), and Fiji. Fijians show symptoms of binge eating disorder comparable to those in the United States.[1] The numbers of EDs in young women in Argentina, Brazil, and Chile might be the highest in the world. A team of Dutch researchers, who have studied eating disorder trends for over a decade, believe that although EDs are relatively rare in the general population, anorexia in young women is fairly common. They found the incidence of anorexia is rising in girls between the ages of fifteen and nineteen, the group most at risk for eating disorders.[2]

Countries in the Middle East are a varied mix of tribal and religious culture and Western influences. A 2010 study of 228 female university students in the United Arab Emirates found nearly a quarter of the sample had abnormal eating attitudes, and nearly three-quarters of participants were unhappy with their body image. Another study showed around 2 percent of a group of 900 girls aged thirteen to nineteen had a full-blown ED, a figure comparable to Western nations. Traditional Arab society is still painfully unaware of the disease's consequences. "People view it simply as 'just stop eating or don't eat,' and don't acknowledge it as a mental illness that could affect the individual medically,"[3] explained clinical psychologist Dr. Saliha Afridi to an Abu Dhabi reporter. The country's first comprehensive facility for the treatment of eating disorders opened in 2012.

Rates of eating disorders among young Asian women are alarming. They're one of the most common psychological problems in that population, yet cultural stigma prevents the majority from seeking treatment. Slim is definitely in, in Japan. Recent data indicate that over 50 percent of Japanese female college students report a history of significant and persistent dieting; 40 percent use diet pills or drinks to lose weight.[4] Some Japanese children turn to self-induced vomiting, laxatives, excessive exercise, or fasting.[5] Disordered eating problems also appear

"When I was at middle-school, girls were worried about their weight too, but I still feel that there are more slim children now. Actresses are slimmer than they used to be. There is an actress on TV sometimes who I think has suffered from anorexia. She's so thin that I feel uncomfortable looking at her. I was surprised when my students saw her on TV and told me that they want to be as slim as she is. They think she is beautiful."

—twenty-eight-year-old Japanese counselor who visits Tokyo schoolchildren[a]

to be increasing among the Chinese. Results of a study presented to the Asian Pacific Eating Disorders Conference in 2002 showed men and women college students with similar extremist attitudes about food and eating habits—in South Korea, 8.5 percent of males and females had abnormal eating symptoms.[6] Community studies in Hong Kong have indicated that 3–10 percent of young women suffer from severely disordered eating.[7]

What's going on? The more modern the country and the longer the population has been Westernized, the higher the eating disorder rates tend to be. Rapidly developing societies experience sociocultural change, which is considered a global risk factor in the development of EDs. When humans migrate, traditional culture declines. Families move into cities and are tempted to consume a greater abundance and variety of food than they had before. They're also more exposed to Western values. Worldwide, cultures are being influenced by Hollywood movies and American-style advertising. As the Fiji studies have indicated, formerly remote societies have seen a corresponding rise in drug use, teen pregnancy, and disordered eating. The obsession with body perfection reaches to the far corners of the earth and "fat phobia" is a symbol of our modern world. Some of the diagnostic criteria used in the United States might not be appropriate for defining eating disorders of every culture. Still, patterns of eating and exercise help people everywhere cope with life stress. Cultural differences exist in food restriction and binging and purging patterns, and concerns about eating and body weight may not be completely Western. Nevertheless, EDs are recognized as a mental health issue among psychiatrists and psychologists in every country.

An International Spiral

As more people affected by serious eating problems come out for support, resources grow to provide information and direct them to medical care.

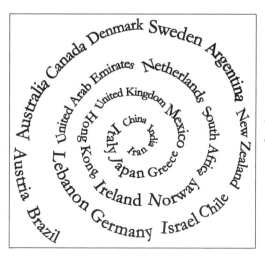

These foreign countries all have eating disorder associations and specialty clinics.

Death by Diet

According to the World Health Organization, 1,168 eating disorder–related deaths (from anorexia and bulimia nervosas and atypical forms, and from over-eating associated with psychological disturbances) occurred around the world in 2011.[8] This total reflects only youth ages fifteen to twenty-nine (671 females, 497 males). Which regions do you think reported the most? Which ones had the least?

Mortality statistics for all diseases are derived from what medical examiners list as the official cause of death on people's death certificates. Rather than being an accurate indicator of the number of deaths attributed to an eating disorder, these statistics reveal more about how a country does the reporting.[9] Comparing

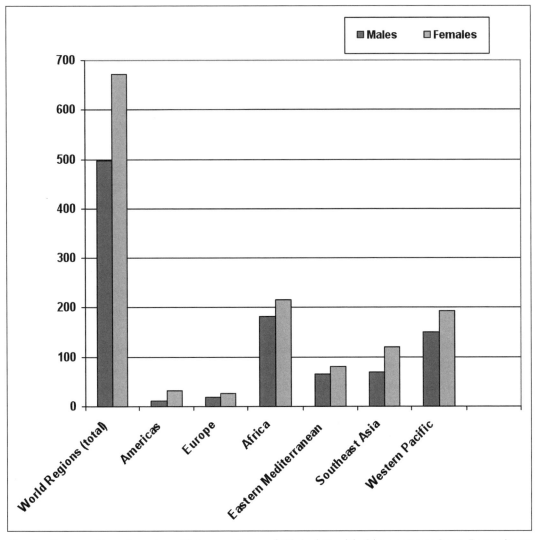

Deaths from eating disorders. *Data courtesy of Global Health Observatory Data Repository, Cause-specific Mortality for Eating Disorders, World Health Organization, 2011. Available at apps.who.int/gho/data/node.main.CODNUMBER (accessed March 27, 2013).*

the statistics between countries, they also indicate something about the level of comprehensive health care available to citizens. Studies that attempt to evaluate the death rate for the main types of EDs generally concur that the mortality risk is elevated for most of them. Reasons for death include starvation, organ failure, substance abuse, and suicide. Importantly, investigators sometimes find more deaths from natural causes, such as cancer.[10]

Unfortunately, medical examiners don't normally attribute cause of death to a mental disorder, so ED deaths are definitely underrepresented when it comes to determining public health policies. This is one reason why, on the global level, few societies understand how an eating disorder can be a medical calamity. One massive binge-purge cycle killed California teenager Andrea Smeltzer. "The coroner, he said 'it's just a mental condition, you can't die of mental illness,'" explained her mother, Doris, in *America the Beautiful*. "So I begged him. I said, 'Please, if nothing else I want my daughter to be a statistic, because, what I know, statistics, numbers, that's what determines what gets funded for research and for prevention.' My daughter needed to be one of those numbers. She needed to count."[11]

! Here's an Extra Scoop

The Eating Disorders Coalition for Research Policy and Action is a citizen-led federal advocacy organization that educates legislators on Capitol Hill about EDs and the importance to include them in public health policy. Lobby Days happen twice a year. To join the effort, and maybe even tell your story, visit www.eatingdisorderscoalition.org.

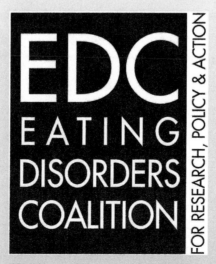

EDC logo. *Courtesy of Eating Disorders Coalition, Washington, D.C.*

"A couple of different things happen, parents bring it to the attention of their pediatrician and then people's prejudices about what looks normal gets in the way, so they're like, it's okay you lost a little bit of weight come back in six months. Don't worry about it."

—Dr. Leslie Sanders, Medical Director
Eating Disorders Program, Overlook Hospital
Summit, New Jersey[b]

Someday, Melissa: The Avrin Family Story

On a clear October Sunday in 2009, just five months after her daughter's passing, Judy Avrin stood on a stage in Foley Square in Lower Manhattan, a featured speaker for Brooklyn's first NEDA Walk, a fund-raising event for the National Eating Disorders Association. She was making a film about the life of her daughter with the support of Melissa's own journal writing. Melissa began treatment for bulimia in December 2005, Judy told the crowd, after a gastroenterologist suggested Melissa might have an eating disorder. Not fully aware of the deepening extent of Melissa's illness, the Avrins had downplayed her symptoms, which had begun in eighth grade. Judy spoke about the need for research funding and more specialized professional training. No family should have the grief that comes with losing someone to an eating disorder, she said, waving a portrait of her daughter to the assembly.[c]

Melissa's symptoms began when she started watching her weight, losing a few pounds through healthy eating and exercise. Early warning signs crept in—stomach pain, constipation, and body image concerns. By age fourteen, her bulimia was full-blown, and her sunny personality had fallen into shadows. Melissa's therapist, Danna Markson, and filmmaker Jeffrey Cobelli interviewed Melissa's friends for the documentary, *Someday Melissa: A Story of an Eating Disorder, Loss and Hope*. Her friends agreed Melissa appeared to be struggling with darker moods, and they saw less and less of her cheerful side. Nicole Kendrick met

Melissa in first grade and remained her best friend until the end of her life. She could see Melissa's torment and could sympathize because she, too, suffered from an ED. "People who knew her in the last two years never saw who she really was," she said. "She was so energetic and funny and just ridiculous but not, like, in an obnoxious way. And then, as she started to worry about what other people thought, that's when [her behavior] started to be in more of an attention-getting way. When things got really bad, . . . it just became very monotone—down. And we didn't really see that energetic, fun Melissa anymore."[d]

Tragically, the entire family, along with Melissa's older brother, Andrew, could not put the clues together, even as frozen cookie dough disappeared, along with whole pizzas and dozens of eggs. "There was no food in the house," Andrew said. "If I went out with friends, I could not bring leftovers home because they would be gone by the next morning."[e]

Although she had also previously experienced her own eating problems, her mother found some of the traces strange. Melissa would "chew and spit," leaving puzzling containers around the house. "Because I had my own struggle with bulimia, I know there was a part of me that just closed my eyes to the possibility that something could be going on," Judy said.[f]

Soon though, denial was no longer possible and at last Melissa was hospitalized, days before her sixteenth birthday. Unfortunately, once her vital signs stabilized, the family's insurance company pulled out. Melissa went home and relapsed, sinking deeper into her disorder, lying, stealing, smoking, drinking, and becoming more and more defiant.

In the midst of a divorce, her parents pulled together to send her to a second treatment center, a wilderness program in Idaho that took in teens with all sorts of combinations of anxiety-depressive disorders and addictions. She responded well to the rehabilitation. Six weeks later, she reunited with her parents, who were overjoyed to see what appeared to be the return of the old Melissa. To keep herself on track, she applied for and attended a special therapeutic high school, graduating early and returning to live with her mother in Totowa, New Jersey. Even with the loving support of her family and caring friends, Melissa found herself struggling again in a new environment. "I always believed that she really would be somebody who could recover," said Judy, tearfully, in the documentary, "even though looking back I realized the odds were stacked against her because of the level of her illness. But I never lost hope. And I still believe that she could have beaten it."[g] Melissa's heart, weakened after five years of wildly fluctuating potassium levels caused by purging, finally gave out on May 6, 2009. She had just been accepted into the film program at Emerson College, her first choice school.

Melissa's story is all too familiar to any family who loses a daughter or son, sister or brother, mother, father, grandmother, or grandfather as a result of an ED. Like Andrea Smeltzer's family, Judy Avrin decided to honor her daughter's memory by going public, hoping that by sharing her family's experience, others could learn more about the true devastation of eating disorders. "I want it to come out of the shadows," Judy told *New York Times* reporter Robin Pogrebin. "I want people to talk about it, for people to get treatment faster, to reach doctors on the front lines. I want parents to open their eyes and not be swayed by being glad that their kid fits into size 4 jeans—to stop focusing on looks."[h]

Andrea, nineteen, died in her sleep on June 16, 1999. An electrolytic imbalance stopped her weakened heart after only thirteen months of bulimic activity. "On our daughter's death certificate, it doesn't say she died of bulimia. It says unknown causes. Every parent we've talked to who's lost a child due to bulimia, I ask them, is 'bulimia' listed on your child's death certificate. We have yet to find a parent who says, 'yes.'"

Doris and Tom Smeltzer started Andrea's Voice Foundation, to warn about the dangers of obsessive eating and exercise and the need for greater awareness, quick intervention, and effective treatment of all types of EDs. Other families, who have experienced the consequences of an eating disorder through a family member, are calling for more federal and state attention to the research, education, and treatment for the disorders.

Word Up on Dieting

Fashioning yourself into an arbitrary idea of body perfection is a dangerous game, and the culture of size zero tribes can contribute to major medical problems. The long-term health effects of trying to maintain an abnormally low weight affect all

Flirting with Disaster: Wannarexia

If an eating disorder is a club that nobody wants anybody to join, why are some pounding on the door? That's how strong the desire is to fit in, to be seen not only as exceptional, but enviable. *Wannarexia* is not a diagnosis, but a cultural phenomenon that has cropped up in the last decade. Awareness of EDs—particularly, anorexia—has spread in the mainstream consciousness and a little bit of knowledge can be dangerous. Wannarexics, like Colette, seventeen, from Newton, Pennsylvania, believe a body project is the ticket to a better life. "I saw some girls with anorexia and thought that I could be popular that way too. I went on a crash diet and lost weight. At one point, I went to an eating disorders support group. I didn't fit in there either. And when I heard about the things that many of the girls went through, like missing prom because they were in the hospital, I realized I didn't want that to be me."[i] Imitating the behaviors that are connected with eating disorders can change a body's metabolism and eventually bring the opposite of the result that was hoped for. The majority of people who attempt low-calorie, food-restrictive fad diets gain back the lost weight, plus extra.

systems of the body. Metabolically, our bodies don't know the difference between a purposeful diet and an unfortunate famine. If we don't feed them enough of what is needed to take care of daily energy and maintenance requirements, they make adjustments. Diets teach the body how to become more efficient at storing energy and less willing to use it. When you start a low-calorie diet, your body breaks down muscle, in addition to fat, to get what it needs. With less muscle, it's harder to expend energy. Your body therefore needs less calories to maintain its activity—although it still requires sufficient food nutrients—and beefs up fat stores when you indulge in excess calories. A recent review of thirty-one long-term diet plans published in the *American Psychologist* found dieters gained back more weight over time than people similar to them who didn't diet.[12] The evidence convinced the authors to advise Medicare and Medicaid policy makers that diets are counterproductive for weight control. The authors even noted that at the end of the survey, the dieters were still gaining weight.

Health Food Junkies: Orthorexia

Is it possible to become so worried about your food—its nutrition, where it comes from, and how it's prepared—that you become certifiably crazy? Dr. Steven Bratman thinks so. He believes *orthorexia*, literally, "a fixation on righteous eating," should be recognized as a diagnosable eating condition. A specialist in alternative medicine, Dr. Bratman observed many of his patients were especially interested in making changes in their diet that would help control nagging health conditions like asthma. A number of them became so particular about their food choices, they obsessed constantly about food shopping and meal planning, refused to eat in social situations, and felt significant guilt when they broke their self-imposed food rules. Inadvertently they lost weight, which seemed to cause anxiety. "Among those who believe in natural medicine, the progressive view is to avoid medicine, which supposedly has side effects, and instead focus on what you eat," he explained to a WebMD health news reporter in 2000. "But everyone misses the fact that if you get obsessed with what you eat, it actually has a lot of side effects—mainly, the obsession itself."[j] Dr. Bratman guessed the obsession interfered with his patients' ability to make well-informed, careful eating decisions and instead pushed them into potentially damaging behavior.

With our growing cultural focus on chemical-free living and concern for the environment, even individuals without specific allergies have more reasons to be vigilant about what they put in their mouths. *Today*'s nutrition expert, Madelyn Fernstrom, told Savannah Guthrie in 2011 that an orthorexic may spend three to four hours a day obsessively reading food labels, worrying about everything that's in food, cutting out lots of foods, including even healthy ones like produce if she or he is worried about pesticides, or cheese because of the fat. "The way that it's different from eating disorders like anorexia and bulimia is that an orthorexic focuses on the quality of food. It's not the calories. It's not about weight loss. It's all about how they feel as a virtuous person, as a perfect person. 'I'm a better person if I restrict.'"[k]

Nutritionists and psychologists see people who have many different reasons for restricting their diets, and top eating disorder specialists suspect orthorexia is merely a symptom of anorexia nervosa. Douglas Bunnell, chief clinical officer at Monte Nido Treatment Centers of the East Coast, has pointed out that certain people are psychologically vulnerable to becoming too rigid in their eating behaviors.[i] When taken to extremes, whether a person fears weight gain or simply desires to be healthy, food restriction changes how the brain works. Bunnell, a practicing psychologist who formerly directed research at the Renfrew Center Foundation, the first residential facility to exclusively treat women and girls with disordered eating problems, believes orthorexia is an important distinction in the mind of a person suffering from it. There's no major difference from other eating disorders, though, in treating it.

As we've become aware, physiological and psychological changes that occur with dieting contribute to the complex core of eating disorders. Besides hair loss and heart failure, starvation, malnutrition, and purging techniques lead to

- brain shrinkage
- esophagitis
- osteoporosis
- muscle wasting
- joint deterioration
- dental issues
- electrolyte disturbances (causing nerve damage, arrhythmia, and cardiac arrest)

Even minor and short-term eating disturbances contribute to greater struggles with appetite and weight control in the years to come. Young people with ED symptoms are also at higher risk later in life for more significant physical and mental disorders. According to one long-term study that followed over 700 New York youth through the 1980s and '90s, those with eating disorders were more likely to have heart trouble, sleep disturbances, and problems with anxiety and mood disorders, chronic fatigue, and infectious diseases.[13]

Compulsive eating following a diet is an especially strong phenomenon for kids and teenagers because of the body's energy needs. Depriving the body of the calories and nutrients it needs to function also makes some people more likely to

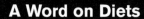

A Word on Diets

Writers Jane Hirschmann and Carol Munter are also therapists and directors of the National Center for Overcoming Overeating. They have helped hundreds of men and even more women break the yo-yo dieting cycle and their dependence on compulsive eating. In the twentieth anniversary edition of their best-selling book *Overcoming Overeating*, they emphasize how diets work only for the weight-loss corporations, not for consumers—most of whom gain back more than they lose. We've become wise to this fact, so "now even the kingpins of the diet industry avoid the word 'diet.' Instead they talk about things like 'healthy eating,' 'good choices,' and 'weight management.' [They] are using our message to sell the same product [they were] selling twenty years ago."[m]

binge on alcohol and drugs. Inadequate nutrition makes the brain more susceptible to changes in its developing reward system, some of which may be permanent. This *binge priming* has been observed in studies of animals and was noted among the volunteers of the Minnesota Starvation Experiment. During the rehabilitation phase that followed the six months of food restriction, many of the men found their appetites came roaring back. Most found this hard to control, and overeating continued to be a problem for them after the experiment was over—one, Richard Mundy, reported feasting on as many as 11,500 calories in a single day.[14] Almost all the men regained the weight they had lost, plus around thirty extra pounds in the eight-month follow-up period. Most eventually returned to their original weight. Only one kept his weight below his preexperiment level in the years afterward.

Duly given full psychological disorder status in the fifth edition of the *Diagnostic and Statistical Manual of Mental Disorders* (*DSM-5*)in 2013, binge eating had appeared in the manual as a symptom of other eating disorders since 1959. Evidence from ten years of studies convinced the American Psychiatric Association that binge eating disorder (BED) is different from other EDs and from obesity due to a unique, addiction-like profile and heritable traits. Experts are divided about whether BED is a true addiction, even though, as we saw in chapter 2, brain imaging studies have shown common circuitry lights up when drug abusers and BED sufferers think about their substance of choice. Support for the belief that at least some foodstuffs, especially junk and fast foods, are addictive for some people, is gaining ground as the nature of the food processing industry is further exposed. And of course, compulsive eating, as well as purging, feels like addiction to many patients—even their family members recognize and describe their behavior that way. So much crossover substance abuse exists in people with

Drink Your Calories: Drunkorexulimia

Drunkorexia and *drunkulimia* refer to the mix of alcohol and drug use with disordered eating and purging behavior. For students who turn to the drinking scene, swapping alcohol for food is a tactic to keep from gaining weight, despite excessive binge drinking. Alcohol consumption even becomes its own purging technique. Food restriction is a key factor in the formation of many addictive behaviors—that's why it's so common for disordered eating to co-occur with substance abuse. The Eating Disorder Center of Denver has reported 75 percent of their college age patients met the criteria for alcohol abuse.[n] Treatment centers around the country are seeing the need to tailor their programs to manage recoveries from both eating and substance use disorders.

eating disorders that mental health professionals suspect the current addiction model might have to be revised as brain science lights up more details.

People with eating disorders report a higher consumption of fast foods and snack foods and less regular meal times in childhood.[15] Years before writer Stephanie Covington Armstrong was molested by a family member, she stubbornly refused to eat her mother's uninspired cooking. The fatherless family of four rarely kept enough of anything in the cupboards and refrigerator, and Stephanie often went to bed hungry. Stephanie's bulimia erupted full force in her early twenties after a couple of romantic breakups. "Because I was a black girl with natural hair who had grown up below the poverty line, no one suspected I could be bulimic," she wrote in a National Public Radio (NPR) essay, "Digesting the Truth." "No one questioned why I ate three or four helpings per meal, why food went missing, why I never had any money or motivation, and why I never gained weight." She recalls how food—how she'd get it and how she'd avoid it—took over her thoughts, all day, every day. Restricting, binging, exercising, downing laxatives. It was not a way of life she could keep control of—or continue to live. Eventually, Stephanie found her way into a twelve-step program and then chose a therapist who taught her better coping and decision-making skills. "The pursuit of perfection took me into a very dark place that I almost didn't come back from. For a long time, I believed in silence and suffering, not understanding that one fed the other. I thought that airing my dirty laundry would humiliate me but in a safe environment, it wound up setting me free."[16]

Diet Out of Control: Shawn Colvin

Three-time Grammy winner Shawn Colvin is no stranger to alcohol abuse, drug addiction, and depression. She's also been visited by the specter of anorexia and binge eating. In a 2012 interview, she recounted how she slid into an obsessive diet without conscious intent, became dangerously thin, then proceeded to eat everything. "I was hungry," she told NPR talk show host Diane Rehm. "I was very tiny, then I was very big. Nothing fit me . . . I certainly felt better than when I wouldn't eat at all, but I made up for lost time." Shawn described the events that led up to it, how she was a mamma's girl, but finally left home in her early twenties with a boyfriend and their band. Then she began to have trouble with her voice, developing nodes on her vocal cords. "For someone who's based their identity entirely on the ability to sing . . . it sent me into quite a spin, a spiral down. I had to quit the band." She got a job in a clothing store while her boyfriend continued to tour. "I was alone in this house, for all intents and purposes, and I had to feed myself alone, which I'm still not that good at doing. . . . And I took up running, because I was bored. It was a perfect storm." After her extreme weight loss, Shawn put on sixty pounds in just three months. "It was devastating and hard to watch. I feel bad for my folks to have to see that. I don't know what I would do if that went on with my daughter. I'd be heartbroken, beyond all telling."°

Word Up on Obesity

The fear of fat, so ingrained in the minds of those with EDs, echoes in our society at large and stimulates the "What is a healthy weight?" debate. Scientists, lawyers, health policy advocates, health care professionals, health news correspondents, the diet and fitness industry, bloggers, and everyone who worries about their health and appearance, all drive a stake into the discussion. In an era where the National Center for Health Statistics determined that 78 million adults, along with more than 5 million girls and 7 million boys ages two to nineteen, are obese,[17] former U.S. surgeon general Richard Carmona (2002–2006) and officials at the Centers for Disease Control believe that obesity is our nation's biggest health crisis. Heart disease, high blood pressure, diabetes, cancer, and sleep apnea are all associated with excessive pounds. Some researchers, however, question the statistics, the

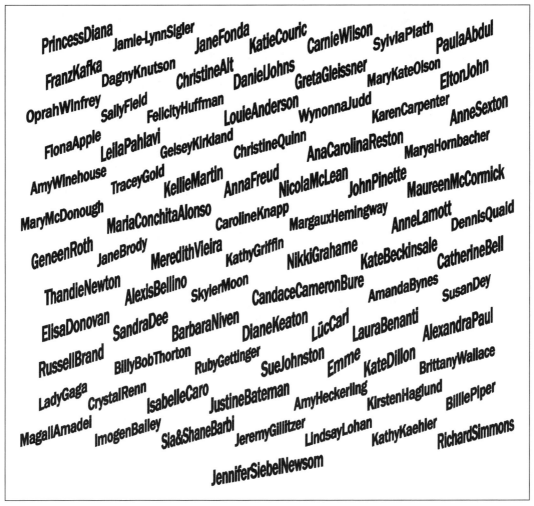

Who's Who of Who's Hungry. Actors, musicians, writers, comics, and others in the public eye who have spoken publicly about their struggles with food and eating issues. *Compiled by the author through cross-checking multiple sources, including news interviews and reports, videotaped and live performances, memoirs, and Internet sources such as EDReferral.com.*

methods of body weight assessment, and the wisdom of government-sanctioned messages to lose weight.

There's no question our culture holds weight biases. Our attitude toward obesity may be fueled less by a desire to be healthy and more by fear of the discrimination that overweight bodies endure. Westernized countries have upheld body perfect standards for so long, people of every heritage look down on the obese. By the time you're in first grade, you're well aware of how large bodies are treated in our society. Overweight people are preliminarily judged as being lazy, unintelligent, and gluttonous. If you're between the ages of twelve and twenty-five, this is a big deal. (And truthfully, it's a big deal, no matter what your age.) Losing weight is seen as the key to not only getting fit, but also to a totally improved self.

"Most people who lose weight will ultimately regain it. If you do this over and over and over again, you develop a nation of weight-cyclers, a yo-yo dieting society. And there are risks associated with yo-yo dieting that are every bit as hazardous as the risks associated with just being fat."

—Glenn Gaesser, PhD

Director, Healthy Lifestyles Research Center

Arizona State University, Tempe, Arizona

Author, *Big Fat Lies: The Truth about Your Weight and Your Health*[p]

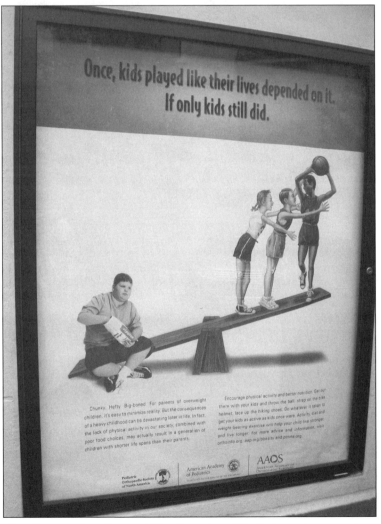

Obesity warning! "Once, kids played as if their lives depended on it. If only kids still did." *Photo by the author.*

The "Baloney" Mass Index: BMI

Overweight, or overfat? Underweight, or underfat? A bathroom scale tells you how many pounds you're carrying but it doesn't tell you anything more. A calculation called the body mass index (BMI) is supposed to help medical professionals identify potential weight problems that are associated with serious health conditions. The trouble with the BMI formula is that it can under- or overestimate the actual amount of fat on your body. By itself, it isn't an accurate indication of overall health risks. So how did the BMI number become the holy grail of health insurers and public health authorities?

$$BMI = \frac{Mass\ (lbs)}{Height\ (in)^2} \times 703$$

The BMI was devised by a nineteenth-century Belgian researcher, Adolphe Quetelet (Ket'-e-lay), in order to average the body sizes of different human populations. A century later, when Ancel Keys investigated the biology of starvation in his Minnesota lab, he used the formula to compare the loss and regain of body mass in his subjects. The BMI number was never intended to predict disease risk. Nevertheless, the National Institutes of Health recommends it so that doctors can simplify patients' health profiles.

Colorado law professor Paul Campos has criticized the way obesity is accused of causing the nation's worsening health crisis. He is angry about how the BMI is used to justify evidence of an "obesity epidemic" in this country. "The index has become [a] false scientific tool," he says. "Because it's a mathematical concept . . . that makes it seem more scientific . . . to then label people as overweight, obese, or underweight.[9] It's like the science of phrenology in the 1800s, when it was thought that by mapping bumps on the skull, we could tell if someone was a criminal. We're dealing with the same nonsense today."

But what if thinner isn't necessarily better? What if extra weight actually benefits long-term health and mortality? What if you could be fit and fat? In fact, studies support the notion that there is a wide range of weight that is healthy for people. Ragen Chastain (@danceswithfat) is an international dance champion. She is also morbidly obese. "I went to the doctor, and he looked at me and without doing any tests tried to diagnose me with type 2 diabetes, which I do not have," she said in *America the Beautiful 2: The Thin Commandments*. "[He] told me I needed to start walking, ten minutes a day, five days a week. I said, 'well, you know, I work out and dance about twenty hours a week. I'll be happy to cut down if you think that's the way to go.'"[18] Her diabetes test came back negative. The doctor still told her to lose weight. "The studies that show anything between disease and weight are correlational," Ragen told Darryl Roberts. "Which means all they know is that disease and weight happen at the same time, sometimes, but not all the time. They're not causational, so they don't prove the weight causes disease." She went on to explain that studies of cultures where there is no stigma against obesity, also show no negative health outcomes. Ragan is at the top of the body mass index chart—type 3, super obese. "But I'm metabolically in perfect health. I can do the splits. I can press a thousand pounds with my legs, and I dance at a professional level."

Stressing about how your appearance measures up to others' puts you at risk for developing disordered eating and exercise habits, which are probably at least as dangerous as the health risks of being overweight. Dieting leads about one-quarter of us into pathological behavior patterns, and many more into years of struggle with food and weight preoccupations. That's what happened to Ragen, who's been a cheerleading captain, multisport varsity athlete, class valedictorian, a National Merit Scholar, an author, and an entrepreneur.[19] She went through a period of disordered eating and compulsive exercise so severe, she was hospitalized. Even though she had not been underweight, she was extremely malnourished. Dieting hadn't worked, so she decided to go about regaining her health with a fresh attitude. "So I thought, well, what if I just accept that I'm going to be whatever size I'm going to be?" she asked, "But I'm going to practice healthy behaviors and see what happens. It was sort of an experiment where I would end up. And where I ended up was a big, fat, healthy girl."[20] Ragan campaigns for size acceptance and blogs at danceswithfat.wordpress.com. She also continues to dance and choreograph.

An Expert Weighs In:
Lynn S. Grefe—It's Time to Talk about It

Lynn Grefe is president and CEO of the National Eating Disorders Association. Her job is to bring national attention to the problems faced by struggling individuals and

Barf Online

When pop culture critics are quick to criticize people in the public eye for their portliness, they can feel the burn. A *New York Times* Arts critic and a *Marie Claire* blogger each got an earful in 2010 when they tore down a principal ballerina and the stars of the *Mike & Molly* sitcom. After attending a performance of *The Nutcracker*, Alastair Macauley "snarked" that New York City Ballet's Jenifer Ringer had bitten into extra sugarplums. Ringer, who had previously divulged her struggles with fasting and compulsive eating, immediately felt a groundswell of support from the blogosphere. "OMG! This is terrible! We thought reviewers were supposed to review the dancing, not someone's stomach," wrote celebrity follower, Perez Hilton, on FitPerez.com. "Not cool, man."[r]

Maura Kelly, author of the blog *A Year of Living Flirtatiously*, slammed the actors of *Mike & Molly*, claiming she'd "be grossed out if I had to watch two characters with rolls and rolls of fat kissing each other . . . because I'd be grossed out if I had to watch them doing anything. I find it aesthetically displeasing to watch a very, very fat person simply walk across a room."[s] Then she insisted she wasn't "some size-ist jerk." Nearly 160 return comments and a thousand tweets later, both Ms. Kelly and her *Marie Claire* editors realized she had to issue an apology. Kelly seemed truly chagrined. "A few commenters and one of my friends mentioned that my extreme reaction might have grown out of my own body issues, my history as an anorexic, and my life-long obsession with being thin. . . . I think that's an accurate insight."[t]

Founder of the Body Image Council and retired plus-size model Emmé told Meredith Viera on *Today* that she thought the question of fat acceptance was an important one to have in the public dialogue. "It's great to hear what perhaps is an underbed of predjudice," she said. "Take a look at all the comments this particular blog got. The voices of American women and men are actually making things tip. . . . This might have been the way that a lot of people felt, but not anymore."[u]

their families, address the negative messages of body image and size discrimination we find in our culture, and promote access to sources for recovery. She's well aware of the consequences of these illnesses on people and society, having traveled the country, speaking and listening to the stories of those seeking help. Her own family has also been personally affected. When asked about the repercussions of eating disorders for young people in 2013, here's what she had to say: "I've met people who have lost so much valuable time of their life, as a result of an eating disorder. Yet, once they are in recovery it's like the world opens up to them, and they regret the time lost. For us, we ask every day, why are we letting people get so sick? And allowed to lose valuable living time? It motivates us to try to steer people to help much sooner, before they do get so sick."[21] Grefe also answered these questions:

How are families coping with the effects of such illnesses?

I know families that are in a quandary, and just don't know how to help their child. Treatment is not affordable for the average person. For difficult cases, the cost of residential treatment is twenty-five to thirty thousand dollars. Per month. People take second mortgages on their homes. They deplete their retirement accounts. If somebody has a serious eating disorder, a stay can be three to four months. Thankfully, if we diagnose at the earlier stages, there are other alternatives such as outpatient treatment, and also family-based treatments that are becoming more available and advisable in some cases.

Parents are pretty much handcuffed when it comes to forcing an adult child to go into treatment—that's a special, and tough situation as they watch their loved one deteriorate. When a sufferer is under eighteen, it's not necessarily easy, but at least parents can take control.

How might our nation better address the needs of those affected?

Some things that need to happen in our country are educating parents and educators of the early signs and symptoms of eating disorders, encourage screenings, and make quality help affordable and available. The government should, in fact, force insurance companies to cover these illnesses. Beyond that, I find it unacceptable that the federal government spends so little per year on research for eating disorders treatments and cures, while we know that eating disorders have the highest mortality rate of any mental illness. That must change.

What could the rest of us do to help stem the tide?

Most eating disorders start with a diet, so we really need to be careful when considering changing eating or exercise behaviors. Moderation is the key. I worry when parents talk about not letting kids have a cupcake at a birthday party or not allowing candy at Halloween. It is really a world gone

> **? Triggering Debate: Extreme Makeovers, Transforming Ideals**
>
> What are some of the costs of self-transformation? When is it vital? How far should you go to become someone different? What are the consequences of accepting yourself as you are? What are some strategies that you can use to improve self-image and trust your appetite(s)?

wild when we look at those extremes. We were born with birthday suits of all shapes and sizes, and if we're smart, we will take care of these suits and wear them well. It is not one size fits all!

Here Come Cowboys

The consequences of eating disorders and the results of poor self-image are devastating on many levels. Health complications that occur from malnutrition and starvation are terrible for anyone who experiences them. Families are traumatized by having to deal with emotional upheaval and the financial burdens of treatment that can last many years. The contributions to society that so many sufferers could have made are forever lost and impossible to measure.

Thankfully, many are riding to the rescue. Through the advocacy work of concerned professionals, affected families, and recovered individuals, people are coming together to lasso the pressures that swing open the gate to an eating disorder.

Here are some laws currently enacted or proposed that deal with mental health or police the marketers of body perfect imagery. How well do you think they address the problems of eating disorders?

- Mental Health Services Parity Act—This historic legislation, in effect since 2010, has meant that people in most group health plans can be insured equally for both mental and physical health. "With the passage of this bill, insurance companies can no longer arbitrarily limit the number of hospital days or outpatient treatment sessions, or assign higher copayments or deductibles for those in need of psychological services,"[22] said Katherine Nordal, executive director for professional practice at the American Psychological Association. The act also extended mental health services to 82 million Americans not protected by state laws. Unfortunately, certain mental health disorders, such as eating disorders were not specifically included, leaving each state to decide how private insurers cover treatment.

- Affordable Care Act—According to the National Women's Law Center, nothing has changed with the passage of the newest health care reform, in full effect in 2014. Insurance companies may still determine how much eating disorder treatment to cover, or whether to cover any at all. States that insist anorexia and bulimia be covered like any other mental health condition include California, Connecticut, Delaware, Maryland, Massachusetts, Minnesota, New Jersey, Vermont, Washington, and West Virginia.[23] All other states have either no laws concerning treatment coverage, or list exceptions to required coverage.

- The FREED Act (HR 2101)—The Federal Response to Eliminate Eating Disorders Act comprehensively addresses eating disorders research, treatment, education, and prevention.[24] Passages from the bill have been included in other health care policy legislation, due to lobbying efforts of the Eating Disorders Coalition on Capitol Hill. On May 23, 2013, congressional representative Ted Deutch of Florida introduced the entire bill on the floor of the House.

- Media and Public Health Act (proposed January 2012)—Formerly known as the Self-Esteem Act, the proposal would require all national ads and editorial content featuring an altered human body to carry "truth-in-advertising" labels.[25] In 2012, state representative Katie Hobbs sponsored a similar bill that would force Arizona advertisers to put a disclaimer on ads with altered or enhanced photos.[26]

When fourteen-year-old SPARK Summit blogger Julia Bluhm collected 85,000 signatures on a Change.org petition protesting the practice of Photoshopping models' photos in teen magazines, she had no idea the editor of *Seventeen* would take her seriously. *Seventeen* editor Ann Shoket did indeed sign on to Julia's "Body Peace Treaty," agreeing not to misrepresent bodies or faces and to feature only healthy-sized girls and models in the magazine's pages. Only a few months earlier, *Vogue* icon Anna Wintour announced the magazine would no longer cast underage, or decidedly underweight models.[27] And both the Council of Fashion Designers of America and the British Fashion Council have adopted new guidelines to ensure the health of runway models. Are the tribes of size zero actually turning over a new leaf?

Is it possible to have a world where no one is lost to an eating disorder? When images of extreme emaciation or corpulence aren't taken as something to strive for or against? Where anyone experiencing symptoms can find the support they need to recover? Let's look at what is being done to prevent the spread of EDs and what friends and families are doing to help sufferers in need.

More Food for Thought

Read

Laurie Halse Anderson. *Wintergirls*. New York: Viking, 2009.

Paul Campos. *The Diet Myth: Why America's Obsession with Weight Is Hazardous to Your Health*. New York: Gotham Books, 2005. (Originally published as *The Obesity Myth* in 2004.)

Nancy Etcoff. *Survival of the Prettiest*. New York: Anchor Books, 2000.

Frances Kuffel. *Eating Ice Cream with My Dog: A True Story of Food, Friendship, and Losing Weight . . . Again*. New York: Berkley Books, 2011. (Originally published as *Angry Fat Girls: 5 Women, 500 Pounds and a Year of Losing It . . . Again* in 2009.)

Courtney E. Martin. *Perfect Girls, Starving Daughters: How the Quest for Perfection Is Harming Young Women*. New York: Berkley Books, 2007.

Geneen Roth. *Feeding the Hungry Heart: The Experience of Compulsive Eating*. New York: Plume, 1993. www.geneenroth.com.

Michelle Simon. *Appetite for Profit: How the Food Industry Undermines Our Health and How to Fight Back*. New York: Nation Books, 2006.

Watch

Girl Model (documentary, 90 minutes). An Ashley Sabin & David Redmon production for First Run Features, 2011. Aired nationally for POV's twenty-fifth anniversary season on March 24, 2013, on PBS stations. www.pbs.org/pov/girlmodel and girlmodelthemovie.com.

Soul Food Junkies (documentary, 64 minutes). A Byron Hurt production for the Independent Television Service (ITVS), 2012. Aired nationally on PBS's Independent Lens, January 14, 2013. www.pbs.org/independentlens/soul-food-junkies.

Learn

Andrea's Voice Foundation. www.andreasvoice.org.

Food Politics—blog by Marion Nestle (@marionnestle). www.foodpolitics.com.

National Association to Advance Fat Acceptance. www.naafaonline.com.

National Eating Disorder Information Centre (Canada). Information on eating disorders and weight preoccupation. www.nedic.ca.

Someday Melissa, Inc. www.somedaymelissa.org.

Take Action

Eating Disorders Coalition for Research, Policy, and Action. www.eatingdisorders
coalition.org.

National Eating Disorders Association—STAR (Solutions through Advocacy
and Reform) Program. www.nationaleatingdisorders.org/get-involved/star
-program.

WHO CAN YOU CALL? PRACTICAL ADVICE THAT MAY HELP

··

*I think that half the women in this world who are plus-size
would not be if they never went on a diet.*

—Christine Alt, plus-size model and wellness advocate
to Sally E. Smith for *BBW Magazine*
"Christine Alt: Not the Girl Next Door," ca. 1999

What can be done to help prevent the slide into an ED? How can sufferers relieve stress and stabilize their mood and behavior? What kind of reaction should be expected from trying to help someone struggling with an eating disorder? Learn how you can advocate to eliminate eating disorders.

Body Image Revolution

In November of 2009, six of the top-working, full-figured models posed for a photo spread in *Glamour*. With them was Lizzi Miller, a newcomer to the industry. The up-and-coming, size 12–14 model had posed in the September issue, for an article on feeling comfortable in your own skin. *Glamour* has been proud to feature a diverse array of body sizes, and often runs photos of larger size models. But the reader response to that snapshot of Lizzi Miller, with her obvious, natural belly roll, astounded editor Cindi Leive. After receiving more than a thousand joyous e-mails and blog comments, followed by appearances on *Today* and CNN, Cindi decided to up the ante. Crystal Renn, Amy Lemmons, Ashley Graham, Kate Dillion, Anansa Sims, and Jennie Runk were featured au naturel in a two-page photo spread with Lizzi. The resulting feedback—online comments continued for two years—proved that size still matters to us in a big way. (To view the Matthias Vriens-McGrath photo, visit the magazine article, "These Bodies Are Beautiful at Every Size" by Genevieve Fields, at Glamour's website: www.glamour.com/health-fitness/2009/10/these-bodies-are-beautiful-at-every-size. You can link to the earlier photo of Lizzi there as well.)

Embracing the beauty of all women, no matter what their size, still breeds a lot of divisive opinions. "There were women . . . saying they were like a size 12–14, but still were saying, how dare *Glamour* put these women . . . on there," said Anansa Sims. "It really shows you how society has messed with our minds, to make us take something so great and find some type of way to think like it's negative."[1] Anansa knows something about trying to make a body become something it's not. "I'm a size 12 to 14, and I'm fit, happy and healthy," she later told reporter Ginny Graves in 2012.

> I wasn't always this way. In fact, the most unhealthy I've been was when I was 40 pounds lighter. [When] I decided I wanted to be a model . . . I starved myself, took laxatives and over-exercised to fit into the clothes that models wear, and then signed with a major agency. People said I looked great, but I felt miserable because I was depriving my body of nutrients, and the more weight I lost, the more my self-esteem fell. Now I'm a plus-size model, and I'm the size I was meant to be. Everyone's body is different; you can be unhealthy if you're skinny or heavy. The key is to find the weight that's best for your body and stay there.[2]

While it's true that eating disorders are more complicated to fix than finding a good weight and staying there, it's smart to be concerned about size obsession and the draw to dieting solutions when it comes to prevention. Studies show girls and women with high levels of body satisfaction are less likely to diet for the sake of improving appearances and are protected from the risk of developing an ED. A three-year, Australian investigation of approximately 2,000 secondary school students found food restriction was the most important predictor of new eating disorders. Girls who severely cut back calories were eighteen times more likely to develop one.[3] Two-thirds of the participants who ended up with an ED had dieted moderately. Mental health status was also important. The girls with eating disorders had the highest rates of early dieting and greatest indications of psychiatric problems. Daily exercise seemed to lessen the risk of experiencing full-blown symptoms. This led the researchers to agree with evidence from animals studies—calorie restriction, not exercise, is the danger factor for those most at risk.

"I know women who are producers who are surviving on nothing but juice and almonds. Even though they are not on-camera talent, they feel that to fit in this industry and in this town, you have to have a frail, bird-like physique. It's not even enough to be thin. You actually have to look ill. And I'm not interested in that. I never have been.

"People cannot process the fact that a woman could be sexual and funny and brilliant and sensitive and flawed and beautiful and all of those things. Women are typically objectified in this business. [They're] used to being put in boxes and compartmentalized. People are more comfortable when we stay in our box. The primary job for women in Hollywood is still super-attractive actress. That is the most high-profile women's job in Hollywood. So you can see why it would be challenging for a writer or a director who is attempting to sell her ideas and not her sexuality or looks or charisma."

—Diablo Cody, screenwriter/producer[a]

Sport Gone Bad: A Triad for Female Athletes

We know regular exercise is good for our health. Aerobic activity combined with strength training improves the function of our heart and lungs, hormonal balance, and bone density. Physical fitness is also good for self-confidence. Whether you play a team sport or simply exercise for fun, you can enjoy the benefits of an active lifestyle. For those at risk for EDs, however, the drive to excel in a sport, especially one that emphasizes a stereotypical body size or shape—gymnastics, ballet, diving, figure skating, rowing, martial arts—can lead to a combination of symptoms called the *female athlete triad*, a term coined by the American College of Sports Medicine (ACSM). When active girls

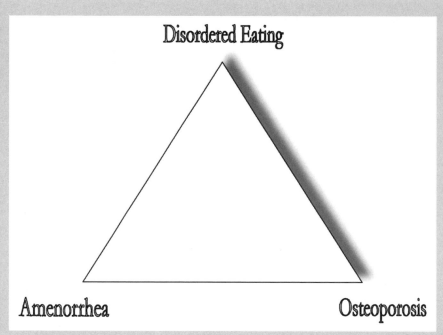

The female athlete triad.

and women don't get enough nutrition and calories to match their energy expenditure, they can disrupt their menstrual cycle and lose bone mass. The ones who exercise prodigiously can easily fall into the triad and be classified with an *atypical eating disorder*.

Studies in 1999 and 2002 found at least one-third of female college athletes showed atypical eating disordered behaviors.[b] The ACSM recommends coaches, trainers, parents, and sport administrators to be on the lookout for the early warning signs of EDs and resist pressuring athletes to achieve excessive leanness. Team members should not be pressured to weigh-in outside the regular season, and guidelines that encourage an unrealistically low body weight should be revised or eliminated.[c] The ACSM strongly advises that individuals be required to seek medical attention if they show any signs of an eating disorder. Recovery from the triad usually involves at least three health professionals—a primary physician, psychologist, and nutritionist—as well as support from family, friends, team members, and coaches. For more information contact the ACSM, www.acsm.org, and visit the website of the Female Athlete Triad Coalition, www.femaleathletetriad.org.

Prevention Intention

When scientists uncover genetic evidence for our behavior, the information is usually passed along to the public in a way that makes it seem as if an eating disorder is unavoidable. In fact, the opposite is true. Eating disorders are environmentally triggered by factors in society and culture and are therefore preventable. Strategies for prevention are helpful for shouldering anyone away from all types of behavioral addiction. None are foolproof, but all are commonsense means to develop a strong body image and self-esteem, fortify our brains against intense stress, and channel healthy coping mechanisms that lessen obsessive tendencies.

Experts speak of three kinds of prevention programs, universal, selective, and integrated, which differ mainly according to whom they are targeted for:

1. Universal—A public health style of prevention for the general population to improve the overall psychological health of all kids, teens, and adults. The philosophy is to change the environment in order to minimize the influence of social and cultural factors that put people at risk for behavioral disorders and substance abuse. Such programs enhance the development of a healthy body image and self-confidence and teach us how to get along with others. Limiting children's exposure to TV and Internet advertising, getting families to participate in community improvement activities, and broadcasting public service announcements against bullying are examples of universal preventions. So is encouraging the medical profession to take a health-centered approach to weight management.
2. Selective—Programs aimed at groups at heightened risk for developing eating disordered behaviors, for example, elementary and middle school girls, especially those involved in pageants, modeling, dancing, or other athletic pursuits. The philosophy is to strengthen protective factors that can provide greater resiliency to the pressures that drive us into disordered eating. Examples of selective prevention might be a girls' class on deconstructing media messages, or participating in an awareness event for body image and eating issues.
3. Indicated—A means of prevention targeted to specific individuals who already show preliminary signs of body dissatisfaction, food and weight obsessions, and abnormal eating and activity behaviors. The goal of such programs is to turn the tide before treatment for a full-blown eating disorder is necessary. Prevention for indicated teens focuses intensely on positive messages of self-care and the development of personal interests. Warnings about the health consequences of EDs may be important to share with people who are beginning to struggle, but they need to be

> ## ! Here's an Extra Scoop
>
> ⊙ Eating disorder therapists have clients actually destroy their bathroom scale in session to give them a sense of power over the tyranny of numbers. The private "scale bashing" or "smashing" has become a public event during National Eating Disorder Awareness Week on college campuses and through clinic-sponsored events. You can find plenty of images and videos all over the Internet.

incorporated carefully to keep from glamorizing illness (e.g., "anorexia chic").

Prevention works. According to a recent review, more than half of the eating disorder prevention programs studied successfully lowered risk factors, and over a quarter showed participants reduced their symptoms.[4] The best programs for teenagers were conducted by professional interventionists who presented interactive and multiple sessions having to do with body acceptance or questioning of media and cultural messages.

While indicated preventions are mostly utilized in private, mainly clinical settings (family and individual counseling, for instance), many other programs work at changing our social institutions and cultural practices. Thus, anyone can

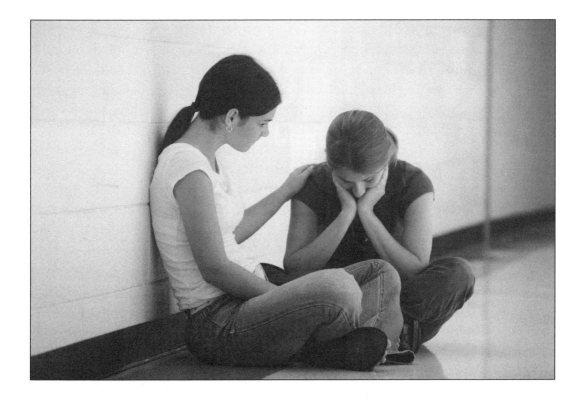

contribute. When you refuse to engage in "fat talk" or "body snarking" (your own or anyone else's); when you appreciate someone for what he can do, rather than what he looks like; when you reach out to the quiet, shy, awkward kid in class and include her on your team, you are helping to prevent EDs and possibly other forms of mental illness.

Even as researchers point out possible early warning signs, one difficulty for most families is that the potential for EDs continues to defy recognition. Behavioral patterns come about much earlier than physical health trouble and often fall in the range of what we consider normal weight and body-focused behavior. Disciplined dieting is still recognized as an enviable aspect of self-control. The people closest to someone who might get an eating disorder are the ones in the best position to interrupt the progression of symptoms. Family members, friends, teachers, and health care professionals must increase their knowledge of EDs, learn to adjust their attitudes about body size, and change their conception of what is normal teen behavior.

R U OK? Eight Ways to Help a Friend

Besides being hard to detect, another difficulty with EDs is that sufferers rarely acknowledge they have a problem and resist any idea that they ought to get help. If you suspect your friend is on the brink of an eating disorder, there are things you can do to be supportive and nonthreatening.

Do:

1. Express concern about her well-being. Share your experience *only* if you, too, have struggled with addictive behavior and can truly relate to the underlying feelings that drive the need to restrict, purge, binge, and so on.
2. Make yourself available to listen whenever she feels the need to connect. Or check in regularly, if she doesn't object. Always assure her that she can feel safe talking to you, and do it only where you know you won't be distracted.
3. Educate yourself about EDs. Break down the myths and misconceptions. If you present information to your friend, do it casually and nonjudgmentally.
4. Consult someone you trust for your own peace of mind, and certainly if you believe your friend is in imminent danger. Encourage your friend

to speak to a resident adviser, school counselor, or health professional whom she trusts.

Never:

1. Comment on or express any feelings about weight loss, weight gain, food choice, or physical appearance.
2. Promise to keep a secret, or that you won't go to someone else, if you think she's about to self-destruct. Do not agree or attempt to be her therapist.
3. Agree to assist in anything that perpetuates disordered behavior. No pig-out nights, protecting the bathroom door, sharing dieting tips, and so on.
4. Lose your temper, make her feel ashamed, or attempt to trick her into eating something she doesn't feel safe about.

Above all—be respectful, supportive, and caring, and remember, if you honestly believe you must choose between having the friendship and saving your friend's life, a living, former friend is always better than a dead one.

Online Congregations

People with eating problems can all relate to each other. The online universe is the most popular place to go to find people of like minds. Social media gathers people together who are feeling isolated with their eating problems. Those who join in the discussions are of all ages and at various stages in the continuum of their ED. Parents and treatment professionals are troubled, and with good reason. According to a study published in 2010 by the *American Journal of Public Health*, 83 percent of 180 ED support sites openly advised visitors how to start and maintain an eating disorder.[5] Social networking sites are still the wild and woolly frontiers of disordered camaraderie. People with eating issues have long had a subculture of their own, even before the World Wide Web.

Sixteen-year-old Sara described her experience in 2008 for a PBS *Frontline* episode: "It's weird because I have this one life that's fake . . . all happy-go-lucky, whatever, and then I have the real me. When I'm online . . . I'm completely 100 percent me. I'll talk about anything to these people because I know they won't

How to Talk about It

The National Eating Disorders Association (NEDA) makes these three suggestions:[d]

1. Use "I" statements. "I'm concerned about you because you refuse to eat breakfast or lunch." "It makes me afraid to hear you vomiting."
2. Avoid accusatory "You" statements. "You have to eat something!" "You're out of control!"
3. Avoid giving simple solutions. "If you'd just stop, then everything would be fine."

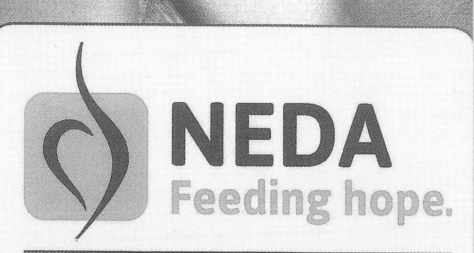

Feeding hope. *Reprinted with permission from the National Eating Disorders Association. For more information visit www.NationalEatingDisorders.org. or call NEDA's Helpline: 1-800-931-2237*

judge me. Sometimes, it makes me feel better because it's like, 'Oh, there's people out here like me,' or, I have a little niche of my own, a little comfort zone. But sometimes it makes me feel worse because I know how many people are suffering like me."[6]

Sara had been successfully hiding her anorexic tendency from her parents and frequented *pro-ana* web rings, forums, and blogs. "I'll look for something called '*thinspiration*,' which is basically inspiration to stay and become thinner than I am now. And it's just like, here's other people who can do it. 'Look, this woman, she did it, I can do it, too.'" Posts on pro-ana and *pro-mia* sites are frank about how to hide binges and purges and maintain a low weight. "I'll be talking online to these people and I'll be the anorexic person that I am," she says. "And I'll just go on and I'll see, 'Oh, like wow, this person hardly eats. Mad props to them. Congratulations. I wish I was like that.' But then, sometimes, certain days . . . the other side of me will kick in and be like, 'This is disgusting. These people shouldn't be living like this. What's wrong with them?' It's like, part of me is completely Ana and part of me is anti-Ana. So it's a complete struggle every day."[7] As a result of the conversation with the documentary producers, Sara talked to her parents and agreed to see a therapist.

Pro-ana, pro-mia, and *thinspo* have become universal code for the glorification of the drive for thin and for EDs as lifestyle choices. Medical associations and eating disorder organizations in both the United States and United Kingdom have urged providers of social networks to clamp down on such communities, but the web is a difficult place to police. In 2013, the ED community continues to thrive on Tumblr, Pinterest, Twitter, and Instagram, despite efforts to ban specific search terms and hashtags. Not all ana/mia sites have content that militantly promotes disordered eating—many are moderated and prohibit posting diet tips or weight goals. But any type of discussion forum with people who are in the midst of their illness is often damaging to minds that are skating with obsessive behavior. A key trigger is active engagement—ruminating with others over the very thoughts and feelings that stimulate you to control your eating. Even so-called pro-recovery sites are not the best places to direct someone who wants to open up about eating issues, because they are usually peer operated by members in various stages of their own illnesses (and with vastly different degrees of insight!). A 2006 survey of 698 patients ages ten to twenty-two revealed slightly over half of them had visited either pro-ED or pro-recovery sites, or both, prior to their hospitalization. Forty-six percent of the pro-recovery visitors learned new techniques that favored the growth of their eating disorder. Treatment stays were longer for the patients who had visited online sites, compared to those who did not.[8]

Treatment teams at recovery centers have become so familiar with patients' reported use of technology to deepen their symptoms that they refer to an "e-triggers" trend. Besides social networking, sufferers use game consoles, computers,

Reality TV Takes the Cake

What happens when the small screen brings EDs into your living room? Can reality TV help sufferers recover by opening the door of their closets? Do YouTube videos help erase ED stereotypes, or do they only glamorize and promote disease? In 2005, the cable channel FX debuted a TV series, *Starved*, that portrayed the tragically comic lives of four twenty-something friends, Billie, Dan, Sam, and Adam, in New York City. It was an intense, and unpleasant, behind-the-curtain look at characters struggling with binging, purging, obsessive dieting, compulsive exercise, alcohol abuse, and gender identity. Eric Schaeffer, the show's writer, director, and executive producer, who also played Sam, drew on his own food and compulsive issues to create the controversial sitcom.[e] Coincidently, each of the other cast members—Laura Benanti, Del Pentecost, and Sterling K. Brown—had themselves suffered from various degrees of disordered eating and lent their own experiences to the script. Eating disorder specialists were concerned that the show ridiculed a serious medical condition. NEDA did not laugh and compelled advertisers to pull the plug after only seven episodes. "Just because you've had an experience doesn't mean you have anything interesting to say about it, or are able to articulate whatever interesting thing you have to say,"[f] said Robert Lloyd in his *Los Angeles Times* review.

Reality TV executives have continued to exploit people's eating issues for entertainment, much to the distaste of professionals in the field. *What's Eating You?* premiered on E! Entertainment Television in 2010. Offering "true stories of food, fear and obsession," the producers introduced Melissa, Amanda, Mona, Gaby, Marc, and Adrienne; profiled their struggles; and encouraged them to enter treatment. Although the show is no longer in production, bonus clips are still available to view online. *Starving Secrets*, developed for the Lifetime Network in 2011, is hosted by anorexia survivor Tracey Gold, best known for her role as Carol Seaver in the 1980s sitcom *Growing Pains*. The show enters the lives of chronic anorexics, bulimirexics, and others with severe EDs and offers therapy at the production's expense. Lynn S. Grefe, president of NEDA, along with many eating disorder therapists, doubt the "television recovery process." "We do not support putting people who are ill on television,"[g] Grefe told Margaret Wheeler Johnson of the *Huffington Post*. Gold, who publicly battled her ED from the age of eleven until her mid-twenties, answered the concern through the British tabloid *Daily Beast*, "It's not an easy show to watch, but it's riveting and it really lets you know what it's like."[h] She thinks that turning the public spotlight on the participants will be a strong motivator for them to recover. Treatment specialist and former NEDA board member Carolyn Costin, who is featured on the show, understands the role that reality TV plays in the public perception of any psychological disorder. She hopes that the producers, who are also responsible for the Emmy-winning series *Intervention*, present the participants and the subject respectfully and responsibly and give reason for hope.

On the other side of the scale, there seems no end to the public fascination with the obese. *Too Fat for Fifteen: Fighting Back* (Style Network), *Thintervention* with Jackie Warner (BravoTV), *Heavy* (A&E), and *The Biggest Loser* (NBC) have tackled the much more common difficulties people have with overeating and underactivity.[i] Although most participants do not have full-blown eating disorders, all have unhealthy relationships with food and their bodies and express many variations of disordered thinking about eating and body size.

tablets, and iPhones to track calories or compute lost weight from exercise formulas. "These triggers can simply kick-start one behavior that may be taken to an extreme, and they can serve as enablers for unhealthy food- or exercise-focused behaviors that have already begun," said Dr. Ovidio Bermudez of the Eating Recovery Center in Denver. "An important part of the mindset of individuals struggling with eating disorders is a desire to learn how to 'do it better' and how to compete with others. Both of these can be cemented by accessing information related to losing weight."[9]

Despite the pitfalls, finding helpful, "anti-ED" advice online is possible. NEDA moderates a public, fee-free forum at www.nationaleatingdisorders.org for anyone returning to wellness. There are separate sections for those contemplating treatment, those in active recovery, families and friends who want to be supportive, and males with EDs. The site is secure, but what you discuss is not confidential. Read the community guidelines before adding your two cents.

Lively, real-time discussions happen quickly. If you participate, keep in mind, people deep into their disease are often not rational. Their thought process is circular, and they can be self-absorbed, whiny, and belligerent. Be as kind and sympathetic as you would to a friend in the room with you. Never let yourself get frustrated.

Parents and adult caregivers find excellent advice and support in the wealth of resources at www.feast-ed.org. F.E.A.S.T. (Families Empowered and Supporting Treatment of Eating Disorders) is great for friends, family members, and those in recovery looking for information—research studies, treatment evaluations, a news blog, book reviews, even a glossary of ED terminology. Membership is free, and F.E.A.S.T. hosts local support systems for members and live conferences that bring families and clinicians together. Task forces have been internationally established in Canada, Great Britain, and Australia. The online forum, Around the Dinner Table (www.aroundthedinnertable.org), has been active since 2004.

Spotlight on Something Fishy: Website on Eating Disorders

The online world is full of body-obsessed health and fitness blogs and YouTube videos where everyone has an opinion and anyone can hang a shingle as a health reporter or nutrition expert. Something Fishy (www.something-fishy .org) is one of the best known and most comprehensive ED sites on the web. In operation since 1995, it disseminates accurate information on all forms of eating disorders. Anyone in trouble with disordered eating and seeking support from others will find the site worthwhile. Friends and families of sufferers are also welcome. Something Fishy features breaking news feeds from around the world, basic facts and statistics, as well as a moderated community forum—still going strong as of this writing—and a treatment finder. The most unique and heart-wrenching part of the site is the memorial section. The pages, highlighted with candles, list names of those who have perished. There are over 600 final resting dates of women and a few men, most with short eulogies from a loved one. Over 300,000 people have joined the online support forums (www.some thing-fishy.org/online/options.php) since 2000.

Read 'Em and Weep: Personal Stories of Hell and Hope

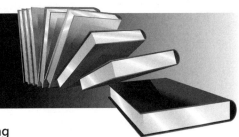

Although those who are touched by an eating disorder have many similar feelings, actions, thoughts, and insights, the journey into and (hopefully!) out of a disorder is an individual one. Whether the struggle took place for a year, five years, or forty, telling one's own story can be surprisingly therapeutic, plus help other sufferers and the ones who love them. Memoirs even let treatment professionals better understand the illness. Besides the publications mentioned at the end of the previous chapters, here are some authors with clear voices, who will add to your knowledge. (Note: Even the most inspiring writers sometimes share details that can be triggering to sensitive readers with eating issues. For this reason, these books are recommended only for family and friends, and those working at recovery.)

Marianne Apostolides, *From Inner Hunger: A Young Woman's Struggle through Anorexia and Bulimia*, 1998.

Kim Brittingham, *Read My Hips: How I Learned to Love My Body, Ditch Dieting and Live Large*, 2011.

Frank Bruni, *Born Round: A Story of Family, Food and a Ferocious Appetite*, 2010.

Stephanie Covington Armstrong, *Not All Black Girls Know How to Eat: A Story of Bulimia*, 2009.

Marya Hornbacher, *Wasted: A Memoir of Anorexia and Bulimia (PS)*, 1998.

Caroline Knapp, *Drinking: A Love Story*, 1996.

From seven celebrities:

Shawn Colvin, *Diamond in the Rough: A Memoir*, 2012.

Portia de Rossi, *Unbearable Lightness: A Story of Loss and Gain*, 2010.

Jane Fonda, *My Life So Far*, 2006.

Tracey Gold with Julie McCarron, *Room to Grow: An Appetite for Life*, 2004.

Jenny Lauren, *Homesick: A Memoir of Family, Food and Finding Hope*, 2004.

Crystal Renn with Marjorie Ingall, *Hungry: A Young Model's Story of Appetite, Ambition and the Ultimate Embrace of Curves*, 2010.

Ron Saxen, *The Good Eater: The True Story of One Man's Struggle with Binge Eating Disorder*, 2007.

And three more from moms:

Lorri Antosz Benson and Taryn Leigh Benson, *Distorted: How a Mother and Daughter Unraveled the Truth, the Lies, and the Realities of an Eating Disorder*, 2008.

Harriet Brown, *Brave Girl Eating*, 2010.

Doris Smeltzer, *Andrea's Voice . . . Silenced by Bulimia*, 2006.

"Part of the reason I wrote the book [*Unbearable Lightness: A Story of Loss and Gain*] is because I wanted people to know it was the worst time of my life. Being that concerned about how much I weighed was the biggest waste of time in my life . . . if I could take it all back, I would."

—Portia de Rossi to Cynthia McFadden
ABC News Nightline, November 4, 2010[j]

And the Survey Says . . .

One of the quickest ways to identify the potential for eating disorders and other mental illnesses is to screen for them. Screening tests are designed by mental health professionals and conducted by community mental health services or primary care professionals to identify one's level of risk for illness. What's involved in a screening? Answering a series of questions gauges your perception of your body and health, your relationship to food and exercise, and your activities concerning them. The survey might be short, with only a few yes-or-no questions, or lengthy, with multiple-choice answers. It may be presented to you at a doctor or dentist's office, or released online for you to take as a self-evaluation quiz. Different styles of assessments are offered by mental health screening providers to health care professionals in hospitals, clinics, and schools, and to associations involved in mental

It's Good to SCOFF

The SCOFF questionnaire is a newer screening test developed for non-specialists by three British researchers in 1999. The team wanted to create a short and simple assessment tool that would address the core features of anorexia and bulimia, without judging the severity of symptoms.[k] The SCOFF questions have not been validated for children, but are appropriate for teenagers and adults. The five questions are surprisingly effective in determining the possible existence of any type of ED.

1. Do you make yourself *S*ick because you feel uncomfortably full?
2. Do you worry that you have lost *C*ontrol over how much you eat?
3. Have you recently lost more than *O*ne stone (fourteen pounds) in a three-month period?
4. Do you believe yourself to be *F*at when others say you are too thin?
5. Would you say that *F*ood dominates your life?

Every "yes" reply scores one point. A total score of two increases the likelihood a responder is experiencing eating disorder symptoms.

SCOFF is extraordinary because it's an excellent indicator for symptoms of binging, even though there's no formally agreed-upon definition of a food binge. The *DSM* (*Diagnostic and Statistical Manual of Mental Disorders*) describes a binge as a large amount of food—considered much greater than the amount eaten by a normal person—consumed in approximately two hours. It's clear that binging is distinct from general overeating, but what truly constitutes a binge is in the eye of the eater. For an anoretic, it could be anything more than three bites of steak, six peas, and a slice of tomato. The key is how you perceive your behavior, your own sense of obsessive thinking, loss of control, and level of distress.

health advocacy. Survey modifications depend on who is actually answering the questions, male/female, child/teen/college student/adult, parent/friend/self. You might come across some popular ED screening inventories such as the Eating Attitudes Test (www.eat-26.com), the Bulimia Test—Revised (BULIT-R), and the Eating Disorders Inventory (EDI-2). Two face-to-face interviews that clinicians use are the Eating Disorder Examination (EDE) and the Interview for the Diagnosis of Eating Disorders (IDED-IV).[10]

The difficulty of defining and assessing food binges has made it hard for doctors to screen overweight patients for binge eating disorder (BED). Wesleyan University professor and psychologist Ruth Striegel Weissman recommends asking a few direct questions in a sensitive, yet straightforward manner. She suggests starting with "Do you feel you have a problem with your eating?"[11] If the answer is yes move on to the next question:

- Do you feel driven to eat even when you're not hungry?
- Do you eat a large amount of food all at once?
- Do you feel as if you can't stop?
- Do you feel as if eating is escaping from your feelings?
- Do you eat until you're uncomfortably full?
- Do you feel guilty or depressed afterward?
- Do you hoard food to eat when you can be alone?

Excess body weight alone, of course, is no indication of an eating disorder. Far less than half of all overweight and obese people have psychological eating issues. Nevertheless, eating disorder specialists would like health care professionals who treat patients for obesity to become more familiar with appropriate BED screening questions like these.

There are places online where you can go to take an ED screening test. Some are offered through the websites of treatment centers. NEDA has partnered with Screening for Mental Health, Inc., to offer a National Eating Disorders Screening Program (NEDSP), a confidential, anonymous ED self-assessment (MyBody Screening.org) to college students and members of the public. Even though the results can't prove you have or don't have an ED, they give an idea if your eating behaviors are inside or outside the range of normal, and whether you should contact a treatment professional for follow-up. The online tool evaluates your level of risk for actual ED symptoms, not just disordered eating. After a few background questions for demographic purposes, the questionnaire proceeds through a short series covering obvious eating and body image issues. Clicking "submit" at the bottom immediately presents you with a recommendation for further action.

The NEDSP launched in 2013, to coincide with National Eating Disorder Awareness Week (NEDAW), a yearly event held in the final week of February.

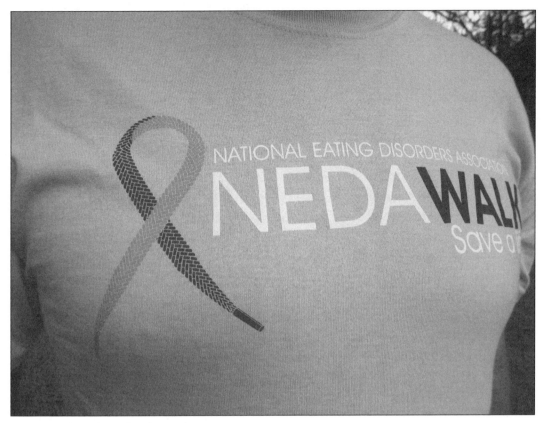

NEDA walks. *Photo by the author.*

NEDAW attempts to turn public attention to the health needs of ED sufferers and their families and promotes greater understanding of the severity and long-term effects of the illnesses. The effort also directs those at risk to local resources. During NEDAW, in-person screenings are made available at over 500 colleges and 100 community sites across the country.[12] In addition, many local mental health services offices conduct ED seminars and symposiums for mixed professional audiences while offering public film screenings, candlelight vigils, and the NEDA fund-raising walk. Even though there are no national screening guidelines for eating disorders, the American Psychiatric Association, American Psychological Association, American Academy of Pediatrics, and National Collegiate Athletic Association all endorse the NEDSP event and recommend routine mental health checkups for all adolescents.[13]

A positive screen from any tool is *not* a diagnosis! If your score gives reason to believe you may have some type of eating disorder, you should be fully evaluated by a medical practitioner, and particularly a psychiatrist. They'll combine their evaluations with the physical exam findings and a patient history. The purpose of screening is to open up communication with individuals about the nature of EDs and prompt early intervention by directing them to avenues of treatment.

Be a Mental Health Advocate

One of the best ways you can make a difference in preventing the spread of EDs is to advocate for legislative action. Volunteers around the country take part in NEDA's Solutions Through Advocacy and Reform (STAR) Program. Through letter writing and talking to local state and federal legislators, advocates work to increase funds for research, education, and preventative programs, and improving access to treatment for all. In 2012, NEDA initiated the National Eating Disorders Awareness Caucus to lobby Capitol Hill. Two congresswomen, Nita Lowey (Democrat–New York) and Renee Ellmers (Republican–North Carolina) served as co-chairs. In 2013, victorious STAR volunteers in Virginia watched Governor Bob McDonnell sign a bill to implement ED screenings in the public schools, and to have information about eating disorders sent to parents of Virginia public schoolchildren. In Missouri, STAR volunteer advocates succeeded in the passage of legislation that authorizes state funding for an actuarial study into the costs of insurance coverage for EDs. Find out what NEDA's STAR Program is doing in your state and get involved. Visit NEDA's website to watch the free, archived webinar "Advocacy and Lobbying: Using Your Voice for Change," and contact star@myneda.com to find out more.

An Expert Weighs In:
Dr. Michael Levine—EnD the Insanity

Michael P. Levine, PhD, taught psychology at Kenyon College in Ohio for thirty-three years. He became interested in the field of eating disorders in 1983 as a result of volunteer work as an educator and advocate for the Mental Health Association of Knox County, Ohio. Now retired, he's still an active advocate for understanding and preventing EDs, writing articles and books, and speaking at conferences around the world. He's been particularly interested in the prevention of eating problems through education, public health initiatives, and the control of mass media.

In 2013, Dr. Levine shared some of his thoughts when asked about ED prevention:[14]

Would you tell us how we might counteract those tendencies we have to obsess on food choices and eating habits?

Teenagers can combat this spectrum of "body disregard"—as body image expert Dr. Jennifer Muehlenkamp calls it—by working on developing a positive body image, by learning to acknowledge, tolerate, and cope with distress, and by focusing attention and effort on helping others in the community. It's important not to limit and distort your sense of self in the world by focusing solely on yourself and your looks.

How can parents, school programs, and national initiatives be effective in promoting sound mental health and normal eating behavior?

We must, first and foremost, make it clear to each other and to the schools that we care about these topics. Parents and other citizens can work with the schools and with various community organizations—religious institutions, the scouts, YMCA or YWCA, for example—to promote experiences that create what Dr. Richard Lerner calls the 6 Cs of positive youth development: *C*ompetence (life skills), *C*onnection, *C*haracter, *C*onfidence and positive sense of self, *C*aring (compassion), and *C*ontribution to community and society.

How can programs designed to prevent obesity keep from triggering disordered eating behaviors in those who are vulnerable?

Obesity prevention efforts should promote (a) a more active, less sedentary lifestyle; (b) less time in front of the television or the computer; (c) eating more fruits and vegetables, so as to be better nourished; (d) exercise and playing for the purposes of fun, fitness, function, and friendship (the "4 Fs"), rather than weight control; and (e) media literacy in regard to advertising and other forms of propaganda.

Obesity prevention efforts should never introduce (a) irrational fears about fat; (b) hostile, unjust attitudes about fat people; (c) moralistic attitudes about "good/safe" and "bad/dangerous" foods; (d) calorie-restrictive

Triggering Debate: Pounds Aweigh

Some early prevention programs indicated that raising awareness of the dangers of EDs actually helped to promote them. Why might this be so? How might you design a program to teach girls and boys to value their health, put diet and exercise in proper perspective, and encourage them to develop a positive self-image? Do you think it's risky to get overweight and obese people to lose weight?

dieting; or (e) beliefs that weight and shape are totally under one's control and that slenderness will completely transform one's life.

Never Say Die(it)

Whether or not people can actually be deterred from all levels of disordered eating is an open question. For people who do develop clinically diagnosable EDs, the disease has such strong biological components laid so early in a patient's lifetime that many professionals doubt every ED can be eradicated in the foreseeable future. Our society is not moving en masse toward a greater acceptance of portly figures, even though many Americans are losing the battle of the bulge. "I have seen *no* good news on changing attitudes of body weight and size, actually just the opposite," Lynn Grefe, president of NEDA, wrote in an e-mail. "I witness body size discrimination all around us, as airlines propose 'fat tax' and diet advertising is allowed to blatantly stereotype people and tell everyone they need to diet, and ads are permitted to alter images of people without disclosure to make everyone look thin."[15]

Despite the bleak prognosis, studies that have evaluated prevention programs suggest reasons for optimism. Many show improvements in knowledge and attitudes pertaining to body image, which is a first step in producing sustained changes in behavior. No one short-term curriculum or other intervention is likely to be sufficient.[16] The more that anorexia, bulimia, binge eating, and all forms of EDs are understood as major health risks and the more they are discussed openly, the more we all see the need for intervention. If those at high risk for EDs can experience positive environments that generate good self-care, they can be protected from the most devastating effects of EDs, which can be extraordinarily difficult and expensive to treat. The American Psychiatric Association has noted that the patients that have the best prognosis for recovery are the youngest ones.[17]

Here are five organizations that are making a difference in the lives of many girls (and boys) that you should know about:

1. Saving the Adolescent Selves: Girls Inc. Teaching girls the ropes of self-reliance and self-sufficiency for over sixty years, Girls Inc. chapters involve 125,000 girls, six to eighteen, in 350 cities across North America. Programs address media and financial literacy, substance abuse and early pregnancy prevention, leadership and community volunteerism, health and physical fitness, and skills-building for math, science, technology, and engineering careers. With corporate and private donations, Girls Inc. has awarded over $3.3 million in college scholarships to high school graduates. www.girlsinc.org.

2. Kind + Creative + Strong = Beautiful: Rewrite Beautiful. Art instructor and ED survivor Irvina Kanerek thought that the spontaneous style of street art could help ED sufferers find the road to recovery and keep young girls from falling onto the path. She started Rewrite Beautiful in 2009 in Huntington Beach, California, by taking pictures of her Facebook friends, combining them with affirmative statements, and leaving the work in public spaces. Her mission now involves teams of girls and boys who focus on the creative talents they have to change their communities, rather than their bodies. Beautiful Action Clubs are underway across the country for junior high, high school, and college students. www.rewritebeautiful.org.

3. Confidence Is Contagious: Proud2BMe. When Dutch university student Scarlet Hemkes created an online social network as an alternative to the pro-ana and pro-mia websites she was shocked to find on the Internet, she had no idea how popular it would become. Soon she was overwhelmed with e-mails from young girls, looking for her advice and help to deal with eating and body issues. Scarlet, who had struggled with anorexia and bulimia herself, launched Proud-2BMe in 2009 in collaboration with Dr. Eric van Furth, director of Rivierduinen, the largest specialized center for EDs in the Netherlands. The site is now published by NEDA and is a completely interactive forum for sharing stories, health information, and resources for recovery. proud2bme.org.

4. No Body Bashing: Fed Up Inc. ED survivor Bridget Loves founded this Los Angeles nonprofit in 2009 to improve self-esteem, perceptions of media imagery, and eating habits. A six-hour classroom program and the one-hour "No Body Bashing" workshop is directed toward girls and boys age six to eighteen. Teens who have completed Teen Leader training can work with certified adult instructors to bring the curriculum into schools and community centers. The program also features top experts in the field, plus celebrities and people in the entertainment industry willing to share their stories. www.facebook.com/fedupinc.

5. Ending the Drama Years: Girl Talk. Celebrating ten years of programs in forty-three states and in countries around the world, Girl Talk is a structured mentoring partnership between high school students and middle school girls. Fifteen-year-old Haley Kilpatrick envisioned the organization as a response to

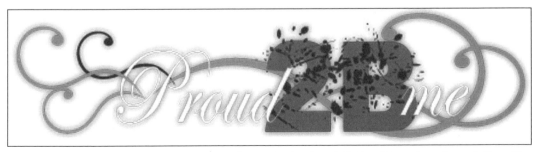

Proud2BMe. *Reprinted with permission from the National Eating Disorders Association. For more information visit www.NationalEatingDisorders.org or call NEDA's Helpline: 1-800-931-2237.*

the drama she had faced during her own tween years. Her friendship with an older high school student had helped her maintain her self-esteem and taught her the ropes of building effective relationships. Haley came to recognize that what girls need to fortify themselves against bad body image, low self-esteem, and bullying is

- an anchor activity
- a stable role model
- a community project with group involvement

Girl Talk rose to the national level as a volunteer-run nonprofit in 2002, setting up fee-free chapters under an adult adviser. Led by one, or a team of high school girls, weekly meetings involve discussion and activities around the important topics of middle school girl life. Girl Talk also hosts summer camps and workshops for additional leadership building and community activism. www .mygirltalk.org.

Up next, intervention and treatment.

More Food for Thought

Read

Annie Fox and Ruth Kirschner. *Too Stressed to Think? A Teen Guide to Staying Sane When Life Makes You Crazy*. Minneapolis, Minn.: Free Spirit Publications, 2005.

Kids Peace Corporation. *I Have This Friend Who . . .* Center City, Minn.: Hazelden Publishing, 2007.

Jessica Weiner. *Do I Look Fat in This? Life Doesn't Begin Five Pounds from Now*. New York: Simon Spotlight Entertainment, 2006. www.jessweiner.com.

Watch

Miss Representation (documentary, 90 minutes). Girls Club Entertainment, LLC. Premiered on the Oprah Winfrey Network, October 2011. Screenings information at www.missrepresentation.org. Director/Producer Jennifer Siebel Newsom spoke at TED^xWomen in 2011. www.tedxwomen.org/speakers/ jennifer-siebel-newsom.

Real Women Have Curves (feature film, 90 minutes). HBO Independent Productions/LaVoo Productions/Newmarket Films, 2002.

Learn

Bulimia Anorexia Nervosa Association (Canada): A Centre for Eating Disorders, Health and Wellness. www.bana.ca.

Feministing. A blog for young feminists. feministing.com.

KidsPeace—TeenCentral. "Totally real. Totally anonymous. Totally yours." Interactive sections include "Weight Aware!" "Anti-bullying," "Quit Smoking!" and more. www.teencentral.net.

National Alliance for the Mentally Ill. www.nami.org. Information Helpline: 800-950-NAMI (6264).

National Hopeline Network (Kristin Brooks Hope Center). www.hopeline.com. Crisis Center phone network: 800-SUICIDE.

National Suicide Prevention Lifeline (U.S.): 800-273-TALK (8255).

IT GETS BETTER FROM HERE: INTERVENTION AND TREATMENT

· ·

But I feel fine!

—Ruth at age seventeen,
seventy-two pounds,
and 5 percent body fat

What's an intervention and how do you do one? What's the difference between residential and outpatient treatment, and how do they work? What can you expect from an intake exam? Are there any medications that are effective? Read how integrated programs with behavioral therapies and family treatment offer the best hope for recovery.

Reaching the Bottom of the Rock

The body has incredible adaptive potential. That's a fancy way of saying it can manage to live on limited food . . . up to a point. When forced to function on less energy, inadequate nutrition, or both, the body conserves what it can. It down-regulates its systems and starts breaking down less essential parts of itself, so to not completely sacrifice its sustaining organs. Our bodies hate to operate this way, and the mental and physical consequences can be enormous. One legacy of Ancel Keys's Minnesota Study (see chapter 6, p. 140) established that nutrition directly and predictably affects minds as well as bodies. A difference, though, between having an eating disorder and ordinary malnourishment—or some other medical issue—is the sufferer's perception of the problem. Dr. Joel Jahraus, medical director of Oliver-Pyatt Centers in Miami, Florida, contrasts the attitudes of people he sees in his office. "The individual . . . who tells me, 'I don't know what's wrong, I'm losing weight, everybody's getting frustrated with me because I can't put on weight, and I'd like to get them off my back and just gain some weight, but I can't seem to do that and I'm working hard at it,' as opposed to the individual who says, 'Weight loss? Not a big deal. I'm not really concerned about it. I don't see why other people should be concerned about it.' *That's* the individual that I'm more concerned about having an eating disorder."[1] Attitude is one of the aspects that Dr. Jahraus and other specialists use to diagnose an ED in their clinical practice.

The paradox of anorexia is the restless energy that tends to make the sufferer feel well, or at least not sick. Combined with deep suspicion that a medical specialist's job is to make them fat, anoretics famously resist treatment. Bulimics are also reluctant, perhaps more so, because they are not obviously starving to death and believe purging is necessary to control their weight. For everyone with eating problems, the desire to be seen as normal prevents them from seeking help. The stigma of mental illness comes from the belief that victims are doomed to a life of unrelenting, debilitating psychosis that forever prevents them from living regular, productive lives. The truth is otherwise. "They can recover," says Dr. Thomas R. Insel, director of the National Institute of Mental Health (NIMH). "Most women do recover. But one of the great obstacles to that is the lack of access to long-term care."[2] Healing the brain from an ED and training it to acquire the skills leading to recovery takes much longer than healing the body from the effects of low or excess weight.

Treatment delays have also come from the medical establishment. Families whose teenager is toying with disordered eating habits are too often counseled not to interfere. "Parents are still advised by therapists not to pressure their child to eat, not to talk about food, not to be the 'food police,'" writes mom and author Harriet Brown, in her family memoir. "They're told to butt out, stand down, give their teenager space and autonomy."[3] The problem isn't about the food, parents have been told; it's about control. It's because of ordinary issues of adolescent

Here's an Extra Scoop

While a majority (approximately 75 percent) of teens with eating disorders reported contacting special services for emotional or behavioral problems, only a minority (less than 28 percent) actually talked to a professional specifically about an eating or weight problem. According to the NIMH-funded study published in 2011, most do not receive treatment for their specific eating condition.[a]

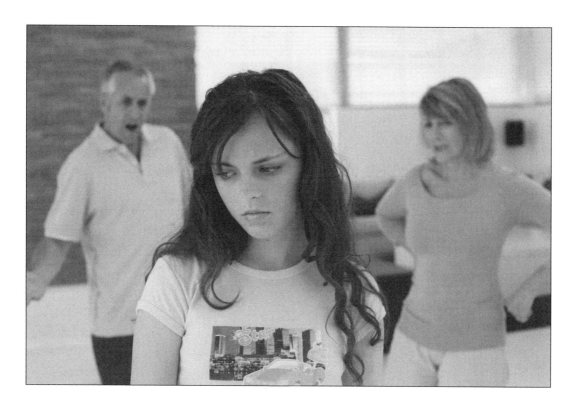

identity and independence. Disorders will vanish when the psychological difficulties that force the starving, binging, purging, and so on have resolved. The
problem with this, says Brown, is that people die before this happens. The longer
the patterns of food and body abuse continue, the more permanent damage they
can do. Early interruption, particularly in young children, gives the best chance
for complete recovery.[4]

Older teens and young adults struggling to cope with emotional issues through
eating, substance use, and self-abuse, fight to appear "in control" and "normal."
They also benefit from quick intervention. Despite disordered thinking, they're
often expected to rationally evaluate their health situation and choose to go for
treatment when they feel ready. In traditional cases of chemical dependency, general consensus used to be that addicts had to hit "rock bottom" before they would
enter rehab. The idea behind an intervention is to create that bottom, so the sufferer can see no other option but to agree to enter a recovery program. Interventions create consequences so that sufferers are motivated to change the present
state of affairs. The best outcomes occur when family members stay involved.

Intervention Convention

Planned interventions make it possible for sufferers to accept treatment. For
young adults, it may be the only means to get them to go. It's not necessary to

attempt an intervention on people under eighteen, because minors are not legally responsible for themselves and can be placed in a facility by parents and doctors. Involuntary treatment should be a last resort, however. Convening an intervention for underage teenagers is smart because it respects their autonomy.

Interventions aren't designed to bully a person into therapy. They are an opportunity to mirror the best qualities of the person and confirm a family's love and support. An intervention can be informal and low key, even when a lot of caring people participate. It can be as simple as a series of individual conversations, with concern expressed to the sufferer over days, weeks, even months, or done in a one-time family meeting. Professional interventionists may act as a remote consultant, or may arrive in person to coordinate the sit-down. The presence of a professional is only necessary if a family is under incredible strain and thinks a third party will make success more likely.

Some teens describe themselves as misfits in their family, among their peers, and generally in their community. This alienation feeds their resistance to the idea of therapy. Those with ED symptoms can feel instantly triggered when facing a confrontation where food-related impulses come up. Jenny Graham, an interventionist with Carefrontations, in Camano Island, Washington, suggests taking the following steps:[5]

1. Invite your loved one to meet in a safe and confidential environment.
2. Express your specific concerns without judgment or threat.
3. Suggest making an appointment with a specialist to evaluate the need for treatment.

If the sufferer answers "yes," facilitate the action as soon as possible. If the answer is "no," or if your loved one rebels against the initial conversation, revisit steps 1–3 at a later date. Of course, if disordered behavior is so severe you believe there is immediate danger of life-threatening consequences—and this may well be the case, especially if drugs, alcohol, or threats of suicide are involved—Graham strongly recommends meticulous planning with a treatment team.

A professional interventionist can help a family whose communication skills are shaky. A formal, supervised intervention carries a special kind of momentum, says Graham. "When you put [one] together, you want to ride on the . . . hope that this is gonna work. People who care, who are significant to your loved one, they're probably willing, so go ahead and ask. It'll take two days of their time."[6] The intervention itself may take twenty minutes to an hour, two hours, tops, she says, and the weight of the outcome is not on any one set of shoulders. Go with your gut in deciding which interventionist will relate best to your loved one and will provide a plan that helps the entire family on a path of recovery. "In my experience as an eating disorder intervention specialist, I have learned that they are

KatherineMcFee Divine KaseyChambers ShaneSellers JanetJackson AudreyHepburn LilyAllen JohnCandy JoshRamsey
AllisonKriegerWalsh CassElliot DemiLovato TerriSchiavo StacyLondon Mo'Nique ChrisFarley MauraKelly
JohnPrescott DavidCoulthard MikeHuckabee CarréOtis ShawnColvin CatherineOxenberg SharonOsbourne
JennyLauren JoyNollenberg AllegraVersace MarielHemingway Luisel&ElianaRamos VictoriaBeckham GeriHolliwell
MelanieChisholm CathyRigby AmandaBeard JacquelynEkern KellyClarkson NancyKerrigan ShelliYoder AnnaWestin
AlanisMorissette HeidiGuenther JohannaKandel ChristyHeinrich ZinaGarrison PortiaDeRossi CalistaFlockhart
CourtneyThorne-Smith BethennyFrankel RalphieMay NadiaComaneci KateyTracey CynthiaFrench
Nicole"Snooki"Polizzi ScarlettPomers PaulaMeronek StephaniePratt JaimePressly TaraReid ChristinaRicci
JoanRivers GretchenRossi NicoleScherzinger LaceySchwimmer AllySheedy AshleeSimpson YeardleySmith
PetaWilson KateWinslet BrittanySnow KateThornton JeffGarlin EvannaLynch TinaNodlund KatherineJenkins
CrownPrincessVictoriaOfSweden

Who's Who of Who's Hungry (a second helping). More celebrities who have acknowledged their battle with food and eating issues. *Compiled by the author through cross-checking multiple sources, including news interviews and reports, videotaped and live performances, memoirs, and Internet sources such as EDReferral.com.*

most successful when the individual struggling cares deeply for the person who initiates it. Your relationship may or may not be thriving, but the bottom line is, they [*sic*] might accept an invitation to get together with someone they [*sic*] care about, and ultimately say 'yes' to the offer of help."[7] Despite what you may have seen on A&E and TLC—for example, *Intervention, Addicted, Freaky Eaters, My Strange Addiction*—someone doesn't have to be completely out of control, or at rock bottom, for an intervention to work.

Sweet Surrender—What to Expect from the Docs

I. Acquiring Treatment

The avenues of treatment for an eating disorder involve nutritional counseling and levels of psychotherapy and medication, depending on a sufferer's age, medical condition, family situation, finances, and the diagnosis. It may take some time for all the issues involved to come to light, but a preliminary treatment plan should be put in place as soon as possible once a sufferer agrees to, or is brought in for, an evaluation. Specific eating assessment by an experienced specialist is wise—primary care physicians may or may not have a good understanding of ED symptoms, or may not want to confront the person about it. Often patients are evasive about offering details, minimizing their problems out of shame or because of their ambivalence about recovery. When the sufferer is a minor or when an individual is so compromised by illness she's unable to take the initiative, family members or other concerned individuals can take the lead by locating care providers. Medical regulations protect adult patient privacy, so while family and friends can assist and lend support in navigating the issues of acquiring treatment—locating a facility, determining insurance coverage, deciding between in- and outpatient programs, and so on—all consent rests with the patient. No one over age eighteen can be forced into treatment against her will, unless she is considered a danger to herself or to others.

Finding the right setting can be like a game of Where's Waldo? There are hundreds of options and every situation will have its limitations. If your regular family physician is not able or available to direct your search, start by visiting either NEDA (National Eating Disorders Association) at www.nationaleatingdisorders .org or F.E.A.S.T. (Families Empowered and Supporting Treatment for Eating Disorders) at www.feast-ed.org. These two organizations provide complete guidance on the basics of securing care, including criteria for evaluating treatment settings and individual professionals. The Academy for Eating Disorders (www .aedweb.org) and the International Association of Eating Disorder Professionals (www.iaedp.com) offer directories of certified ED treatment professionals who are practicing in the United States. All members of the treatment team should have a good rapport and should establish a trusting relationship with the client-patient and involved family members.

Here are some questions to ask when contacting care providers:

- What kind of experience do the health care professionals and treatment center have in treating EDs? What are the professional credentials and licensing? What is the philosophy and approach to treatment?
- What is the assessment process like? Is a medical evaluation required to enter the program? To what extent is family involved?
- Will the program address other mental health issues? Does it offer "step-down" levels of follow-up care? How is it determined when treatment ends?

Jenny's husband, Scott Graham, is also an interventionist and a certified mental health counselor. He's visited hundreds of treatment centers for all kinds of addictions. "I talk to everyone, 'from the top to the bottom.'" he said. "I eat their food. I want to know, does it feel right. Beyond that, I want to look at the clinical staff . . . [that it's] solid. There's a lot of programs that tout themselves as co-occurring, or dual diagnoses programs, and really, they're not. They might have a contract doctor that comes in, or a therapist [who's] just doing . . . medication management, they're not really treating the people. So I want to look for programs that have master's level, PhD people, doctors who are here, employed five days per week at a minimum."[8]

Most people with ED symptoms make individual office appointments with a psychotherapist, primary care physician, nutritionist, and any other necessary specialists after they receive their diagnosis. If a patient is medically unstable with severe weight loss, depressed vital signs, lab results that show an acute health risk, or complications from other medical problems, such as diabetes, he or she'd be admitted as an inpatient. A doctor will insist on it if symptoms rapidly worsen or if there is a risk of suicide. Residential placement or partial (day) hospitalization is advisable when no progress has been made with outpatient appointments. As long as the patient is relatively stable without needing medical monitoring, outpatient programs offer the least traumatic and least expensive forms of therapy.

II. Medical Management

Evaluating someone for an eating disorder, according to ED specialist Carolyn Costin, "takes patience, empathy and finesse."[9] It may also require a fair amount of detective work to reveal the true nature of the illness. A clinician wants to determine which diagnostic criteria are being met, how severe the symptoms are, and what other complicating factors may be present. Patients' attitudes about body weight and food, their level of concern over gaining or losing, and their actual eating obsessions are only a small—although important—part of the assessment. Because EDs are a unique combination of mental health and physical issues, medical exams, lab work, and psychological screenings are all necessary for an accurate diagnosis.

So what can you expect when you walk in for an evaluation? A specialist, or a primary care physician with experience in treating or referring people with eating disorders, will ask about the following behaviors to help determine the reasons for medical complications:

- Eating patterns (severity of restrictive eating, frequency of binging or binging and purging)
- Changes in weight
- Amount of exercise and "restless" movement
- Use of laxatives, diuretics, and diet pills

Unbearable Lightness: Portia de Rossi

At age fifteen, Australia's Amanda Lee Rogers took the name Portia de Rossi, anticipating a glamorous acting career. She could never have imagined how she would almost lose it all to an eating disorder that took root during her crash dieting days as a child model. "Ever since I was twelve years old, I would starve myself daily and then binge after the job was over. And that was just the diet I returned to every single time I needed to lose weight," she told Robin Roberts on *Good Morning America*. "From that age I learned that what I looked like was more important than what I thought, what I did and who I was. I think when your self-esteem is based on how you look, you're always going to be insecure. There's always a fresher face, a thinner girl."[b]

Privately wrestling with food and sexual orientation, de Rossi moved to the United States to pursue her Hollywood dream. She got her first big break in 1998 on the set of *Ally McBeal*, playing lawyer Nelle Porter for four seasons. In an especially moving and intimate memoir, she details her growing obsession with weight loss and her fears of being outed as a lesbian. After a year and a half run with anorexia, she collapsed on a film set in 2000. In the hospital, de Rossi was diagnosed with cirrhosis, lupus, osteoporosis, and imminent organ failure. Having hit the proverbial rock bottom, she then began a slow and often-times painful ascent to well-being, taking advantage of outpatient treatment at Monte Nido Treatment Center in Malibu. "Now I look in the mirror and I think I'm exactly where I'm supposed to be," she said. "I think that it's important to not be so concerned about how you look. As women, it's really important to be focused on things other than what is on the plate in front of you and get on with your life and develop your mind and career and not be so obsessed with how you look and what you weigh."[c] De Rossi's trip from beginning to end lasted over fifteen years. She considers herself fully recovered. "My struggle with anorexia, coming to terms with my sexuality, I realized I had struggled with self-acceptance my whole life," she said in a *People* interview in 2010. "To be able to get to a point where you're just happy with who you are, I think that's when you know what real peace feels like."[d]

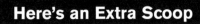

Here's an Extra Scoop

Ipecac syrup, a longstanding remedy to ingested poison, is no longer dispensed as an over-the-counter item, per requests by the American Academy of Pediatrics to get pharmacists to take it off the shelf. Clinicians see far less abuse of the toxic substance in their practices than in years past.[10]

- Use of other stimulant and depressive sorts of drugs (caffeine, nicotine, alcohol, narcotics, etc.)
- Sleep habits and motivation in daily activities

In addition, the clinician should take a comprehensive patient and family history, noting former eating patterns, attitudes and beliefs about body image and eating, incidence of obesity and other weight issues, and the presence of psychological and substance use disorders among all family members. A history helps establish a timeline for when behavioral and physical abnormalities took place. Occurrences such as loss of a menstrual cycle, periods of constipation, even refusal to go to school are helpful for establishing contributing factors and triggers for eating disorders. Time points like these also give the doctor an idea of a patient's healthy weight range and physical status.

Such interviews are not easy for anybody. A good specialist is tactful and non-accusatory, creating a safe environment for every family member involved in the interview. Dr. Jahraus has sat across from many glaring patients, who are quite unhappy about being compelled to talk to him:

> The way I'll [get them to open up] is I'll . . . acknowledge their discomfort and say, "You don't look very happy to be here today," and they'll say, "I'm not," . . . and I'll say, "Tell me what the issue is." [The patient will say,] "They think I have an eating disorder, and I don't." [Then I'll say,] "I'll tell you what, I'll be honest with you, we'll talk about this and try to figure this out. I'll let you know if I think you have an eating disorder, and if you don't, I'll let the others know that you don't have an eating disorder as well." So I'm . . . trying to work on [building] that relationship, that therapeutic relationship, from the very first minute.[10]

Specialists are also on the lookout for physical signs and symptoms that suggest how critical the health impact of disordered eating might be, regardless of what the patient or family is telling them. They observe and question

- rapid or remarkable weight change, unrelated to another medical condition
- fine hair growth (*lanugo*) and the body and thinning hair on the head
- hypotension/dizziness (low blood pressure)
- menstrual cycle interruptions (in female patients)
- hyperactivity (fidgeting/rocking) with complaints of fatigue
- hypothermia (low body temperature)
- edema (swelling in feet and hands)
- slow (bradycardia) or irregular heartbeat
- chronic sore throat and reflux
- ongoing constipation or diarrhea
- calluses on middle/index fingers ("Russell's sign")
- hemorrhages in the eyes

"I remember when my mom brought me in to our pediatrician who had known me since I was seven years old and had seen me grow up healthy and happy," said Ruth.

At seventeen, I was beyond skinny, and though I didn't let on to anyone, I was frightened that my brain might really be out to lunch. "Look at her eyes," my mom kept saying. "There's something wrong with her eyes." The extreme weight loss might have happened from any of a number of life-threatening illnesses, cancer, maybe, or some foreign bacteria or viral infection. Anorexia had opened a window in my pupils and gave itself away. My doctor saw me on a Friday. On Monday morning, he admitted me to the ED ward at University Hospital in Madison, Wisconsin, ninety miles from home.[11]

Every initial evaluation should take into account a full plate of lab tests. Lab work is also an ongoing part of any treatment program. After a physical exam notes a patient's age, height, weight, body mass, blood pressure, pulse, and general physical description, a medical doctor will recommend a standard work-up that includes a complete blood count with urinalysis to look for blood and urine abnormalities. Other tests check for liver and thyroid dysfunction; altered electrolyte, blood sugar, and hormone levels; and nutrition deficiencies. A drug screen, pregnancy test, and electrocardiogram for heart function might also be called for. A DEXA scan, to check bone mass, need not be done at the initial assessment of underweight patients—although a doctor might use it to convince a reluctant patient of her dire situation. As treatment progresses and weight is restored, clinicians can get a fuller picture of bones' current density and determine whether any actual bone loss has occurred.

The Dentist in Your Corner

For many people with eating problems, the first medical professional who is alerted to early signs of anorexic and bulimic behavior is a dental practitioner. Because young people are likely to visit a dentist or dental hygienist more often than their regular doctor, an oral exam can pick out subtle clues to an eating disorder before it can advance. Patients may be less intimidated at a dental office and be more willing to volunteer details when concern is expressed. Dental practitioners can check for shrunken or swollen salivary, parotid, and submandibular glands; gum disease; tooth decay and eroding enamel; dry mouth (xerostomia); and soft palate damage. All are signs of nutritional deficiencies, dehydration, and effects of regurgitated stomach acid and trauma due to techniques of vomiting. Although not an early indicator, another dental complication associated with EDs is degenerative arthritis within the tempero-mandibular joint (TMJ), where the lower jaw attaches to the skull.[e] Drs. Robert Schlossberg and Deborah Klotz, dentists from Bethesda, Maryland, advise those struggling with disordered eating behaviors to take special care to practice good oral hygiene.

1. Brush and floss regularly after eating, and always rinse with water only after a binge-purge cycle.
2. Avoid brushing immediately after vomiting to keep from scrubbing acids into tooth enamel.
3. See a hygienist for thorough cleaning as often as recommended.

Where Angels Fear to Tread—Methods of Therapy

Once upon a time, physicians drilled holes in patients' skulls in order to let the demons out. Less than 100 years ago, patients in psychiatric hospitals might undergo lobotomies (brain removal operations) to calm severe paranoia, rage, and depression. The therapies for mental illness today are less violent, but success takes tremendous effort on the part of the patient and dogged dedication by the treatment team. Recovery can make sufferers feel worse, at least for a while,

Down to the Bone

The teen years and early twenties is the prime time for the body to fully develop the strength of its bones. If bone-building amounts of calcium, magnesium, phosphorus, and Vitamin D aren't available, bones can't develop their full density, and they can become further depleted by the rest of the body's need for these nutrients. Severe malnutrition with any ED can lead within a year to various degrees of bone loss that are not readily reversible. It's been estimated that about half of teens and young adults with anorexia nervosa will have to deal with the chronic effects of osteopenia or osteoporosis, such as increased risk of fractures, for the rest of their lives. This often permanently impacts the duration and type of physical activity that they are able to do. Only about 4 percent of depleted bone is able to be restored in some individuals with proper attention to nutrition and exercise—most are unable to restore bone at all.[f]

because the brain fights to hang onto familiar and comfortable coping strategies. Specialists treating any form of ED know it's important to stabilize a patient's medical condition first, so the individual can better benefit from psychotherapy. Just as low or excessive body weight by itself cannot indicate an eating disorder, neither does weight restoration signify a cure. Even as bodies recover from starvation, malnutrition, or obesity, sufferers are highly vulnerable to relapse after initial treatment programs end. Regular medical monitoring should continue along with whichever kind of psychotherapeutic approach is utilized.

Recovery can feel worse than the disease for everyone in the family. Parents and siblings are pressured to learn new ways to relate to each other. They must deal with thoughtless slings and arrows coming from the insensitivity and ignorance of others. They realize that after months, years, and thousands of dollars, their loved one may still be lost in the woods. By age twenty-one, Mary Polan of Westhampton, New York, had been fighting anorexia for ten years. Her father, Mike, recalled multiple day and evening treatment programs with three hospital stays. "We tried everything we could as parents," he said. "You put the blame on yourself."[12] Even he was shaken by the trauma when Mary had to have a PEG (feeding tube) inserted. The sense of sadness, hopelessness, and helplessness was overwhelming.[13] At last, Mary entered a longer-term, step-down program in

(Re)Feeding a Hungry Heart

An ongoing debate appears to be over how much underweight patients should be fed and how quickly they should be expected to gain. Starving a growing body causes it to rev its metabolism into overdrive, once it starts feeding adequately again. It can take a lot of daily calories, many more than normal teenagers eat, to bring someone with anorexia to a healthy weight. Too much food, too fast, can cause fluid and electrolyte levels to shift dangerously in the body. Medical directors of treatment centers are concerned about *refeeding syndrome*, a potentially lethal situation that can develop if a patient is fed too aggressively. Clinicians must look out for edema, arrhythmia, gastrointestinal distress, hepatitis symptoms, and central nervous system depression, while increasing anoretic patients' daily calorie allowance. Even patients who are not low in weight but have been extremely malnourished (and especially when alcohol or laxative use is involved) must be monitored for refeeding syndrome.

Underfeeding, however, because of the traditional mantra "start low, advance slow" can set weight restoration back a week or more. "There is a body of evidence that our older, more cautious feeding strategies are older and more cautious than they need to be," said Dr. David S. Rosen, a professor of pediatrics, internal medicine, and psychiatry at the University of Michigan Medical School, who leads the American Academy of Pediatrics Committee on Adolescence.[9] Newer feeding regimens start patients at almost 2,000 calories per day, increasing to 3,000 or more within a week if a patient remains metabolically sound. This can feel really uncomfortable for those used to surviving on only a few hundred daily calories. A digestive system, forced to wake up and push through three or four times as much food as usual, complains. Patients may experience painful stomach cramps, constipation, diarrhea, reflux, and a bloated "buddha belly." Some must deal with drug and alcohol withdrawal at the same time. It's also psychologically traumatic to see such quick changes taking place in a body that's been under personal control for so long. Marjorie Nolan, a spokeswoman for the Academy of Nutrition and Dietetics, is a registered dietitian in New York

City who specializes in eating disorders. She recalled one of her patients whose hospitalization at age fifteen set her recovery back in the long term. "They got the weight back on her," she said, "and medically stabilized her to a degree, which was necessary, but it was so aggressive that now, several years later, she's still traumatized by it."[h]

California, where she did well. She has moved into her own apartment, is a shift manager at her job, and is taking classes at a local community college, her father reported in an essay for NEDA. His advice? "Realize when the disease takes over they [sic] are not thinking clearly" and "Be there to support, not fix."

For people with anorexia, the idea, let alone the reality, of weight gain is traumatic. Many with bulimia go to counseling to stop binging, with no intention of ending compulsive exercise or food control practices. Overweight binge eaters, too, are often only seeking the "perfect diet." Although many therapists insist eating disorders are not about the food, eating does symbolize the struggle with underlying psychological issues. Continuing unhealthful patterns directly influence the ability to recover well. Therefore, it's essential to directly address disordered eating and compulsive behaviors in the early stages of therapy. Several psychotherapy approaches have been evaluated for their effectiveness in treating EDs. According to F.E.A.S.T., two have shown excellent results under rigorous and controlled test studies and are thus defined as evidence based:

- Cognitive behavioral therapy (CBT)—Method that teaches individuals to recognize their distorted thoughts and feelings about food, eating, and body image, and replace them with alternatives that lead to healthier behaviors. CBT helps sufferers readjust all-or-nothing thinking, exaggerating and minimizing, overgeneralizing and personalizing, assuming, and fantasizing. Therapists often have clients utilize proactive techniques such as workbooks, journaling, and various homework challenges. The method has a long track record in treating young adults with bulimia and binge eating. New enhancements (CBT-E) have been shown to be effective in treating anorexia and unclassified EDs, as well as co-occurring substance use disorders.[14]
- Family-based (or Maudsley) treatment (FBT)—Chosen mainly by families whose ill child is still living at home, the Maudsley approach is named for Maudsley Hospital in London, England, where the protocol was first designed in the eating disorders unit by Christopher Dare, MD, and his colleagues during the early 1980s. It has a remarkably high success rate

for treating youngsters with anorexia. A modified version for bulimia is also in use. Supported by their treatment team, parents are empowered to make regular eating possible for their child. Follow-up studies show 60–90 percent will have fully recovered within four to five years. Only 10–15 percent will remain seriously ill.[15] In 2012, psychiatrist James Lock and psychologist Daniel le Grange, who together had written the original FBT training manual for the United States, published results from a four-year study. Maudsley was superior to individual therapy for adolescents in keeping them symptom free from anorexia six to twelve months after the end of treatment.[16]

Other promising psychotherapeutic approaches include the following:

- Interpersonal therapy (IPT)—The IPT approach attempts to improve how ED sufferers relate to both themselves and others. The techniques help to identify and express emotions, and bolster communication skills. IPT is not designed to address eating behaviors per se, but rather the depressive and anxious symptoms that accompany most disordered eating behavior. For patients who binge, or binge and purge, studies examining the long-term results of IPT have shown they improve about as well as with behavioral therapies. The American Psychiatric Association treatment guidelines recommend it for patients who do not respond well to CBT.
- Dialectical behavior therapy (DBT)—Originally developed to treat borderline personality disorder, DBT views the inability to regulate emotions as the core problem of eating disorders. It has been adapted by therapists to help people overcome bulimia and binge eating. DBT focuses on building mindfulness skills to handle distress and reinterpret emotions so that patients feel free to choose other behaviors that manage food cravings and related urges and preoccupations. One 2011 study ended when early results showed outpatients counseled with DBT improved so much more than those counseled with other approaches.[17]
- Acceptance and commitment therapy (ACT)—ACT helps patients to accept that inner turmoil is part of life, yet we can still get on with it in a positive way. Although few studies have looked at ACT's effectiveness in treating eating disorders, research has noted it works well at addressing the urges to avoid or control difficult feelings, thoughts, and sensations. Many ED therapists are utilizing ACT techniques to good effect in their practices. One 2013 study of patients in residential treatment for anorexia and bulimia showed both groups decreased their symptoms more by undergoing ACT than similar patients in the traditional program. The

Triggering Debate: Behavior Mod

Getting people to change their behavior through reward (positive reinforcement) and punishment (negative—or, rather, lack of—reinforcement) is the oldest trick in the book. Is this a valid means to get someone with anorexia to reach a goal weight? Or someone who binges to quit? Is it wrong to reward, or deny, yourself using food? What other strategies could we use to lower our fears about eating, and treat food more normally again?

ACT patients also showed lower rates of re-hospitalization during the six months after discharge.[18]

Harriet Brown, an award-winning journalist whose fourteen-year-old daughter was diagnosed with anorexia in 2005, strongly favors choosing a therapist who uses evidence-based therapy, or one who is at least aware of the latest research findings. A number of mental health practitioners view their practice as more of an art than a science, she reported in 2013.[19] But data clearly shows that certain therapeutic techniques have a greater impact than others on a patient's recovery no matter the strength of relationship between the people involved. She and her husband chose the Maudsley (or FBT) method rather than send their daughter, "Kitty," to a residential treatment center. "She needed us, it was really clear to me, and we needed to be part of it," she told Diane Rehm in 2010. "There were no FBT therapists in our town, but we had a great pediatrician and a great therapist who both said, okay, we're on board with you. We're going to educate ourselves about this and we're going to be your support team. So we did [it]."[20] When choosing therapists, Brown advises you interview to find out what kind of training and certifications they have, how they keep up with the latest research, and how many of their clients get well.

Lynn Grefe, CEO of NEDA, agrees with her. People diagnosed with eating disorders should see a specialist, she advised on *The Diane Rehm Show.* "I would want to know that they're members of the Academy for Eating Disorders. . . . Or they've been trained and received some training from IAEDP, which is the International Association of Eating Disorder Professionals. . . . I'd want to know, if it's a treatment center, what's the age population? As good as that program could be, it probably will not be effective unless that person's in a population that's similar to that individual."[21] Age and gender similarities are important, she thinks, because men have different life issues than women, and teenagers have concerns that differ from older people.

Starving for Two: Pregorexia

Health complications that result from a full-blown eating disorder can cause a person serious short- and long-term problems. If a patient is pregnant with an ED, the problems double. Although not a medical term, *pregorexia* refers to females who worry about their changing body shape during pregnancy and limit fat and calories to avoid gaining weight. Without sufficient energy and nutrition, the bodies of mothers and their unborn child fight each other for survival. A developing fetus demands what it needs to grow, plundering stored resources, and worsening the physical complications of an ED. Young mothers, those in their teens and early twenties who significantly restrict food, are at much higher risk for all possible pregnancy complications, including diabetes, stroke, and organ failure. Pregnancy plus an ED accelerates the aging process, especially in bones.

A malnourished fetus can suffer all kinds of mental and physical repercussions. Babies who haven't gotten enough to eat—or enough oxygen due to mom's excessive exercise—may be premature and low birth weight, or be diagnosed with autism or attention-deficit/hyperactivity disorder. Research on the resulting effects of starvation suggests more about the long-term effects. In 1944, the Germans occupying Holland forced starvation on the Dutch for months, now known as the Dutch Hunger Winter. The children born during or just after the famine have been the subject of many health studies since 1976. As Stanford neurobiology professor Robert Sapolsky explained in a 2011 documentary, starving fetuses in the second and third trimesters are already learning that the environment is menacing, resources are not plentiful, and getting what is needed to survive is not easy.[i] Their cells adjust physiologically to slow metabolism and raise their capacity to store fat.

Professor Tessa Roseboom of the University of Amsterdam has interviewed and examined 2,400 Dutch citizens since 2000 and found the ones born to women who had starved in the occupation were at a higher risk for psychological disorders, cardiovascular disease, and metabolic syndrome than children born before or after the famine. "You could say that these babies were exposed to stress in fetal life, and they're still suffering the consequences of that now, sixty years later,"[j] she reported in a National Geographic documentary.

Pregorexia is unusual, even for those with a long history of eating restriction. According to Dr. Paula Deakins of the Melrose Institute in St. Louis Park, Minnesota, 60–70 percent of eating disorder patients get relief from anorexia symptoms when they become pregnant.[k] Binging and bulimic behavior is much more likely—regular binge eating during a first pregnancy is as high as 25–44 percent.[l] Obstetricians need to recognize when a new mom is caring about her baby more than herself, says Dr. Deakins. It gives an excellent window of opportunity to effectively treat her ED.[m]

"One woman I knew lost all her teeth by the time she was twenty-three. She had battled her eating disorder through three pregnancies, one of which was twins. When I met her, she was pretty much recovered, but at age thirty-five she had a complete set of dentures, a heart murmur, and had to be extra careful about falling and breaking a bone."

—Ruth[n]

Put It All Together—Integrated Medicine

Each therapeutic method has its limitations. A balanced, or integrated, approach can offer patients and their families the best of all worlds, but it can take trial and error (and money!) to locate the specialists who practice just the mix of conventional and alternative therapy that works. Integrated medicine (IM) refers not only to the contributions of multiple care practitioners, but also to the blend of healing disciplines each one provides.

Health care professionals who practice IM often call themselves *holistic* practitioners. Holistic philosophy is to heal the whole person—mind, body, and spirit—and not just eliminate disease symptoms. *Integrated approaches* are well-designed to treat EDs because of the complexity of biological, psychological, and sociocultural forces that contribute to them. There is plenty of evidence that

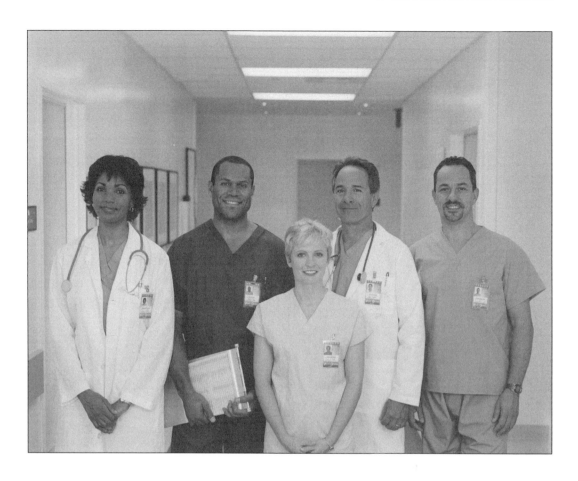

people benefit most when they are cared for by at least three health professionals, a primary care physician, a mental health practitioner, and a nutritionist (dietician). Although some therapeutic methods may seem to come from outer space, it's wise to choose professionals with open minds about the causes and cures for illness and who recognize the value not only of "evidence-based treatment" but also "treatment-based evidence."

The first step after an evaluation is to assemble a team of health care providers. For those entering an inpatient setting, this is standard operating procedure in eating disorder hospital units and residential facilities. For those entering or continuing with outpatient programs, the three-pronged approach to follow-up care supports ongoing recovery and helps prevent relapse. "In my years of working in the field, I have learned there is not one, true, cookie-cutter way to treat patients with eating disorders," says Kourtney Gordon, a certified eating disorders registered dietician in Largo, Florida. "I am mindful to where they are in their motivation to recover. I often find myself in the role of just listening one session and setting goals in another, being a coach one week and a confronter the next. The care team is always in the background, helping to lay a foundation that the family can use to foster support."[22]

> **Here's an Extra Scoop**
>
> People with EDs benefit especially from integrated treatment programs when they suffer from co-occurring disorders. Over half of all those with an ED have a *dual diagnosis* of another mental illness, such as depression, anxiety, or substance use disorder. Effective treatment of this second condition is critically important for proper treatment of an ED.° The Substance and Mental Health Services Administration recommends evidence-based, integrated treatment, from either the same practitioner or treatment team, for those suffering from multiple mental health issues.

Conventional Western medical practices monitor patients' vital signs and take care of emergencies and side effects that may occur as patients' eating and physical activity are stabilized. Whole food-based nutrition and rehydration can usually improve an individual's status in a matter of days. Cornerstones of integrated medicine that could be added as patient's health becomes less critical include

- individual, group, and family therapies
- art and movement therapies
- eye movement desensitization and reprocessing (EMDR)
- nutritional counseling
- wilderness adventure program
- equine/animal-assisted therapies
- mind-body therapies
- herbal and botanical therapies
- neurofeedback
- bright light therapy
- pharmacotherapy (medication)

Many types of treatment have not had enough studies done to show evidence that they work. But they could still be effective for somebody. Treatment decisions are usually made by both doctors and families based on considerations other than conclusive research.

At the Eating Recovery Center (ERC), a fully comprehensive, integrated treatment facility in Denver, Colorado, the medical staff has pulled out all the stops, using computerized technology to treat the toughest cases. Body motion sensors keep track of every calorie patients burn, and biofeedback measures the physical benefit they get from stress-relief exercises. "Flexibility training," originally developed to help traumatic brain injury victims, teaches patients to lose rigid thought processes by having them take different seats in group sessions, or using the less-dominant hand to brush their teeth, Sophie Maura reported in *Marie Claire* in 2011. The changing routine builds new neuropathways, relieving obsessive thinking.[23] Families are involved in every level of treatment and in whichever type of therapy program their loved one enters. "We have drifted away from shaming and blaming of families and have moved toward an understanding that families are an integral part of eating disorders treatment, not only in helping an individual respond well to treatment, but also go[ing] on to lasting recovery,"[24] said Dr. Ovidio Bermudez, medical director of Child and Adolescent Services at ERC.

Prescription for Recovery

Psychiatric disorders today are readily treated with medication. People suffering symptoms of depression, anxiety, bipolar disorder, ADD (attention deficit disorder), or ADHD (attention-deficit/hyperactivity disorder) might be given Zoloft, Paxil, Seroquel, Adderal, Ritalin, or combinations of these and other drugs. Drug companies developed *selective serotonin reuptake inhibitors* (SSRIs) to combat mood and anxiety disorders, which are common to many ED sufferers. They are thought to work by interfering with serotonin receptors and transporters, so that the neurotransmitter stays longer in the synapse between neurons. A newer class of antidepression medications, *selective norepinephrine reuptake inhibitors* (SNRIs), is believed to target norepinephrine in the same way. *Neurologists don't have a crystal-clear explanation for how most psychiatric drugs actually work in the brain.* Rather than increasing low amounts of neurotransmitters, researchers now think both types of reuptake inhibitors might be stimulating the growth of new neurons. More brain cells could give patients better ability to respond to other therapies, which in turn helps lift the symptoms of depression and anxiety.

Two Food and Drug Administration–approved SSRIs for young people under eighteen are *fluoxetine* (Prozac) and escitalopram (Lexapro). SNRIs, such as duloxetine (Cymbalta) and venlafaxine (Effexor), are available for licensed child psychiatrists to treat children and adolescents. No psychotropic (mind-altering) medication cures an eating disorder, but medical doctors prescribe them to further the course of therapy in cases with co-occurring conditions.

SSRIs and SNRIs do not automatically give full relief to everyone, and resolving EDs is more complex than simply raising levels of brain chemicals. Besides, antidepressants take a while to kick in and can have annoying side effects. It can be quite complicated, especially for teenagers, to get a dosage right. Even though patients might be handed a pharmacy of medication by a doctor, there is remarkably little evidence that drugs alone work well on ED symptoms. Nevertheless, fluoxetine (Prozac) has been shown to be more effective than a *placebo* in clinical trials for treating people with bulimia or binge eating disorder.[25] Although many people with eating disorders are under psychiatric care and receive medication for anxiety and depression, no other drug appears to be as consistently effective for binging and purging behaviors. Anorexia has a particularly poor track record of improvement with pharmacotherapy, although a few studies support the use of *olanzapine* (Zyprexa) for weight gain, and the use of olanzapine, quetiapine (Seroquel), and risperidone (Risperdal) for depression, anxiety, and core eating pathology.[26]

Fear No More: Special K

A new, faster acting class of antidepression/antianxiety drugs might be right around the corner. For years ketamine (brand-name, Ketalar), which is similar to Valium and PCP, has been used as a general anesthetic for surgical procedures in children and adults. On the street, it's a recreational club drug known as Special K. The drug dissociates perceptions from cognition, sending the brain into a calm, relaxed state. For those suffering from symptoms of major depression, bipolar disorder, and types of anxiety, ketamine may not only provide relief when traditional antidepressants have failed; it's also proving to work much faster.

Researchers at the National Institute of Mental Health and at Yale University believe ketamine restores and increases connections in the brain's glutamate system, another neurotransmitter. "A healthy neuron looks like a tree in spring, with lots of branches and leaves extending toward synaptic connections with other neurons," said Carlos Zarate of the Mood and Anxiety Disorders Program at NIMH. "What happens in depression is there's a shriveling of these branches and these leaves and it looks like a tree in winter. And a drug like ketamine does make the tree look like one back in spring."[p]

A few significant studies have indicated that some of the thinking processes prevalent in people with EDs, could potentially improve with a drug like ketamine. The goal of experiments with ketamine and other drugs that affect glutamate is to show pharmaceutical companies how they could design drugs that'll take away the hopelessness that comes from mood disorders and the panic that comes from anxiety, and at the same time reduce side effects.

The trouble is that eating disorder patients face a diversity of mental and physical health challenges. They may be dangerously under- or overweight and malnourished. They may be clinically depressed and anxious, unable to control compulsions or eliminate racing thoughts. They may be addicted to other substances and behaviors. *Nutritional rehabilitation* and weight restoration reduce symptoms of companion disorders for most patients, but some aspects of intense moods and thinking processes prevent full recovery from disordered eating, and can even lead to relapse. Psychiatrists work with patients' unique circumstances to find tolerable medications that help them make the most of additional therapies.

The types of psychotropic medications doctors commonly prescribe to people with EDs include antidepressants, antipsychotics, mood stabilizers, ADD/ADHD medications, and antianxiety and antiobesity agents. Table 9.1 has a few brand-name recommendations from the American Academy of Child and Adolescent Psychiatry.[27]

An Expert Weighs In: Dr. James Greenblatt—Start with the Food

Besides developing better psychotherapies to help people recover, nutritional rehabilitation is one of the newest frontiers in the treatment of EDs. Among mental health specialists that practice integrated approaches, anorexia, in particular, is being recognized as a disease mainly of malnutrition, rather than disturbed psychology. Dr. James M. Greenblatt is the chief medical officer of Walden Behavioral Care in Massachusetts. A licensed psychiatrist, Dr. Greenblatt has counseled thousands of children, teens, and adults with EDs and companion disorders. Resolving nutritional deficiencies should be the number one goal of every stage of recovery, he says, and every treatment plan should be uniquely tailored, taking into account patients' individual biochemistry, specific behaviors, and surrounding circumstances. Patients can progress in therapy when a body gets what it's missing, because brain functions improve. They are better able to handle the stress that disordered their eating in the first place.

"I cannot overstate the importance of a sound nutritional program in the treatment of EDs, particularly in anorexia nervosa,"[28] he writes in *Answers to Anorexia*.

> A nutritionally optimal environment makes recovery easier and plays a major role in the prevention of relapse. When the brain is receiving proper nourishment, symptoms may be relieved, and patients will feel more motivated to participate in psychotherapy.[29]
>
> I am not suggesting that a vitamin pill can erase psychological stresses or negative emotions, nor that nutritional supplement[s] alone will cure

Table 9.1. Prescription Meds

Anti depressants	Anti psychotics	Mood stabilizers	ADD/ADHD medications	Antianxiety agents	Antiobesity agents*
SSRIs:	Clozaril	Lithium (not for	Dexedrine	(not typically	Topamax
Prozac	Seroquel	patients with	Ritalin	prescribed for	Xenical
Lexapro	Invega	bulimia nervosa)	Strattera	underage patients)	Belviq
Zoloft	Risperdal	Depakote		Xanax	Qsymia
Paxil	Abilify	Lamictil		Ativan	
Luvox				Valium	
Celexa				Klonopin	
SNRIs:				Vistaril	
Effexor					
Pristiq					
Cymbalta					

* With the exception of Topamax (topiramate), weight-loss drugs have not been found effective in reducing binging behavior, unless combined with psychotherapy.

the disease. I am well aware that long standing relationship struggles and dysfunctional family dynamics need to be addressed for successful recovery . . . supplements are safe and cost-effective strategies that can dramatically affect outcomes.[30]

Dr. Greenblatt points out by the time problem eating conditions are diagnosed as an eating disorder, they are nutritional diseases that have nutritional solutions. He has coined the term "malorexia," to refer to the major deficiencies present in a majority of patients with anorexia—and perhaps in bulimics and bingers, too. Low levels of zinc, vitamin B_{12}, and the amino acid tryptophan have all been implicated in symptoms of anxiety, depression, and poor sleep habits. In fact, the striking similarity between physical and psychological signs of anorexia and zinc deficiency, led doctors over a century ago to feed anorexic patients foods that were rich in zinc. Numerous reports in medical journals show that at least half of those who suffer from anorexia are measurably deficient in zinc, probably because they aren't getting enough of it in their diet, but also because they can't readily absorb it.[31]

Many young people experience deficits in these three essential nutrients when they choose to become vegetarian as a means of dietary restriction. Although you can surely get enough calories in a vegetarian diet, if protein, carbohydrates, and fats are unbalanced or insufficient, your brain is not getting what it needs to fully develop. Dr. Greenblatt proposes a five-point nutritional solution for those suffering from anorexia, which is also a logical plan for anyone malnourished through extreme eating practices:

1. Optimize zinc levels.
2. Evaluate deficient digestive enzymes and the flora in the gut.

By the Numbers: The Harris Benedict Formula

The Harris Benedict Equation was developed in 1919 to calculate a body's basal metabolic rate—the energy you need just to maintain basic body function. By computing numbers for height, body weight, and age according to gender, you can figure out how many calories are needed to maintain your current weight at a certain activity level. Unfortunately, the formula doesn't account for weight composition, so it can be way off for people whose body fat–to–muscle ratio is skewed. A 2007 study discovered that weight fluctuations and ethnicity also affect the accuracy of the formula's prediction.[9] For people with disordered eating history, therefore, it's advisable to work with a registered dietician to determine caloric and nutritional needs.

3. Correct underlying nutritional deficiencies, especially B vitamins and essential fatty acids.
4. Look for celiac disease (wheat gluten allergy) and other food allergies.
5. Take a brain scan to identify which medications might be effective.

For the last point, Dr. Greenblatt highly recommends using a referenced-electroencephalogram (rEEG) to measure brainwaves. The diagnostic tool gives clinicians a readout that can be compared to the profiles of other similar-aged patients. This takes the guesswork out of prescribing a particular drug or drug combination.

One Is Never Enough

Getting rid of an ED is never quick and easy. As much as everyone would like for ninety days of treatment to fix the problem, rehab is not like taking a vehicle into

Spotlight on Timberline Knolls, Residential Treatment Center

Located west and slightly south of Chicago on a pristine campus in Lemont, Illinois, Timberline Knolls Residential Treatment Center (TK) opened its doors in 2005 to treat women and girls age twelve and up with all forms of EDs, as well as other types of substance and behavioral addictions. The center, known for its success with patients who have co-occurring disorders and histories of trauma, has earned the Joint Commission Gold Seal of Approval, a distinction of excellence for health care organizations. The staff practices an integrated, holistic approach to care through an individualized treatment plan for every resident. This may include a variety of talk therapies (dialectical behavioral and family) and expressive therapies (art, dance/movement, yoga, and equine), along with a full complement of therapeutic group activities. Medical staff is on site 24/7. "I believe one of the most important changes I have made . . . was learning to love myself," said a former TK resident from Florida. "Self-worth is so crucial to your recovery because the self-destruction will slowly stop if you believe your life is worth living/saving."[r] Find Timberline Knolls on Facebook and YouTube and at www.timberlineknolls.com.

the shop. It's more like a cancer operation. When you go in to have it removed, you want doctors to find all the tentacles that are hiding. They hold tight to body tissue and can look very different in different places. You can't help but lose some blood and healthy parts as well. After getting stitched up and sent home, that's when the real work of recovery begins.

Initial treatments for eating disorders are directed at and are effective in relieving symptoms, but symptom-free does not mean cured. This makes it tough to evaluate the success of courses of treatment. ED mentality can stick around a long time—your brain, after all, has taken years to train itself to handle thoughts and emotions in specific ways. Relapse is common, and so is shifting to other compulsive, compensating behaviors, especially when motivation or support is inadequate. The American Psychiatric Association has observed that patients with co-occurring substance abuse and anorexia or bulimia nervosa appear to have more severe problems with impulsivity in general, including greater risk of shoplifting, self-injurious and suicidal behaviors, and laxative abuse.[32] Integrated medicine continues to draw on the latest scientific understanding of how the brain works, the way the body and brain influence each other, and what they both require in terms of energy and nutrition. It's turning out to be the most effective method to treat all varieties of EDs for the majority of patients whose eating disorder becomes evident in the teen years.

Staying Strong: Demi Lovato

Timberline Knolls's most recognizable alumna is pop singer and Disney starlet Demi Lovato. The multitalented Demi, at her parents' insistence, arrived reluctantly in October 2010 to deal with bulimia, alcohol abuse, and self-injury. While there, she was diagnosed with bipolar disorder. On March 6, 2012, MTV premiered a news video, *Demi Lovato: Stay Strong*, in which Demi details her road to recovery through rehab, in the genuine hope that her story will help others. "I thought that when I was in there that that was the end of my life," Demi said in a clip. "I thought there's no way I was going to get better, I'm in here for good. . . . I didn't want to get better when I was in there, I thought, this is how I'm supposed to be."[s]

But Demi did get better, and she visited TK a year later to encourage new residents. "I came here to tell you guys that it gets easier. I needed someone to tell me that when I was here. . . . I wish that every single person here could live in freedom . . . 'cause it's so worth it. Utilize your time here 'cause this place will change your life. It changed mine."[t]

Although it might be possible to outgrow symptoms of EDs through means of self-help—the use of books, online materials, and supportive friends and family—for those diagnosed with full-blown disorders, ongoing professional help is almost always necessary for recovery. So is fresh, wholesome, nutrient-rich food—seemingly an enemy for so long, it's exactly the friend needed to get well. It's essential to make peace with it and be vigilant about potential health issues. Complete recovery is possible. Let's see how some folks are making that happen.

More Food for Thought

Read

Cynthia M. Bulik. *Crave: Why You Binge Eat and How to Stop*. New York: Walker & Company, 2009.

Lindsey Hall and Leigh Cohn. *Bulimia: A Guide to Recovery*. 25th anniversary edition. Carlsbad, Calif.: Gürze Books, 2011.

Cheryl Kerrigan. *Telling ED No! and Other Practical Tools to Conquer Your Eating Disorder and Find Freedom*. Carlsbad, Calif.: Gürze Books, 2011.

Jenni Schaefer, with Thom Rutledge. *Life without Ed: How One Woman Declared Independence from Her Eating Disorder, and How You Can, Too*. New York: McGraw-Hill, 2004. www.jennischaefer.com/books/life-without-ed.

Listen

Geneen Roth. *When Food Is Food and Love Is Love: A Step-by-Step Spiritual Program to Break Free from Emotional Eating*. Louisville, CO: Sounds True, Inc., 2005 (6 CD audio program). www.soundstrue.com.

Watch

Thin (documentary, 102 minutes). Lee Kazin and Lauren Greenfield for HBO Independent Productions. Premiered Nov. 14, 2006. Released to DVD in 2012. www.laurengreenfield.com.

Learn

Academy for Eating Disorders. Eating disorders information, conferences and education, and resources for professionals, the public, and the press. www.aedweb.org.

The Johns Hopkins Eating Disorders Program. Johns Hopkins Medical Center, Baltimore, Maryland. Inpatient treatment for the most severe cases of eating disorders. www.hopkinsmedicine.org/psychiatry/specialty_areas/eating_disorders.

Maudsley Parents: A Site for Parents of Eating Disordered Children. www.maudsleyparents.org.

UCSD Eating Disorders Center for Treatment and Research. University of California, San Diego, School of Medicine. Day treatment for adolescents and adults; intensive multi-family therapy. eatingdisorders.ucsd.edu.

FINDING BALANCE: THE HEALTHY WEIGH TO RECOVERY

···

You don't have to control your thoughts, you just have to stop letting them control you.

—Dan Millman

Way of the Peaceful Warrior: A Book That Changes Lives, 1980

Is full recovery possible? What are some of the stumbling blocks? Explore tips and techniques for healthful eating, weight management, and spiritual renewal that help improve self-image and restore zest for living.

Regain, Reclaim, Recover

There are millions of ways to suffer from eating problems, and millions of ways to recover from EDs or stop disordered eating. No two are the same; every sufferer is different. Each person must figure out what methods, tools, and strategies work best, and put them into long-term practice. No symptoms are too insignificant to require help. The nature of behavioral disorders is to deny a problem exists, resist change, and retreat into isolation and hopelessness. Treatment gives the best hope of surviving the worst consequences of the illness, and gives sufferers the chance to establish patterns that will keep them well. Recovery is rarely a straight road. For most, it's about as difficult and complex as the disorder.

The first key to recovery, according to therapists Carolyn Costin and Gwen Schubert Grabb, is motivation. Finding the desire to get better is necessary to keep the work of recovery on track. Once you believe there is a better way to live, and that it's possible to achieve it, you'll be open to learning new ways to think

"The last thing I wanted to do was let go of the eating disorder. It was my best friend and yet my worst enemy; it was what I knew and what I could count on. It was safe and although very dangerous, very comfortable. I knew what it was like to have an eating disorder; I didn't know what it was like to recover."

—Johanna S. Kandel, survivor, www.facebook.com/johanna.kandel
Founder of the Alliance for Eating Disorders Awareness
Author of *Life beyond Your Eating Disorder* [a]

about yourself. You'll develop patience in the struggle to accept healthful eating behaviors and physical activity. The urge to control feelings through food will gradually seem less and less intense. Over time, the reasons why people want to get better change as thinking processes improve. Good treatment programs and therapists try to find additional motivators so they can direct clients to advanced stages of recovery and prevent relapse.

Motivation saved Bailey Monarch of Tarpon Springs, Florida, whose family committed 100 percent to eradicate the grip of anorexia. In the spring of 2009, the high school sophomore honors student decided to get serious about healthy eating and drop a few pounds. Already fit and trim from years of ballet classes, Bailey lost over a third of her body weight in less than five months. "I started noticing she wasn't eating what I was leaving for her," said her mom, Cherié, who told the story on the website for F.E.A.S.T. (Families Empowered and Supporting Treatment for Eating Disorders) at www.feast-ed.org. "Gradually I came to realize she was trying not to eat at all."[1] The Monarchs discussed the concern with their family doctor, but did not become alarmed immediately, thinking Bailey would turn around on her own.

Numbness in Bailey's right foot and increasing difficulties with concentration sent her to the Internet to research her symptoms. Realizing that she probably had anorexia, she nevertheless assured her parents she was okay. "I didn't want to miss school so I said I'd eat. I thought I could take care of it myself," Bailey later recalled for a local news reporter. She agreed to see a therapist and build herself back up. As she entered her junior year, it was clear she couldn't do it alone. "My foot became paralyzed," she said. "I couldn't dance, couldn't do what I loved."[2] Her hair fell out, lack of blood circulation turned her toes and fingers blue, and eventually her entire right side became numb. "Eating was the one thing I could control," she said, "[but it] became my ultimate fear. My eating disorder took control of me—and no matter how bad I wanted to get better, it would tell me, 'no, don't even think about it.'"[3]

Because the family's doctor didn't have much direct experience, Cherié had begun to call around and read everything she could to learn more. "It did not take very much reading for me to realize that things in the eating disorder treatment world were changing rapidly and no one that we talked to was up to date."[4] When her doctor advised hospitalization, Bailey feared missing her high school graduation. Her parents quickly decided to enroll in an intensive Maudsley training program at the University of California, San Diego. Treatment therapists educated the Monarchs how to supervise Bailey's meals, and showed Bailey how

Medicate, Regulate, Alleviate

Science has made nutritional rehabilitation the big name of the recovery game, but it's also making strides to find better medications that may be equally important to treating eating disorders. Researchers at the Endocrine Society knew estrogen replacement therapy had been successful in treating anxious female rats that had had their ovaries removed. Because anxiety disorder symptoms are particularly common in girls with anorexia (most of whom fail to ovulate), they wondered whether using estrogen to reduce anxiety would also show a change in anorexic eating attitudes or body image concerns. In a *placebo-controlled* study, the investigators used standardized questionnaires to survey seventy-two teenage girls in treatment for anorexia. Like the animal studies, anxiety scores correlated with estrogen levels. After the replacement therapy, the girls with high anxiety/low estrogen showed a measurable improvement. As long as they also gained weight, their attitudes toward body image and food did not worsen. "Identification of therapies that reduce the tendency to experience anxiety and reduce body dissatisfaction with weight gain may have a major impact in reducing relapse," said the study's lead author, Dr. Madhusmita Misra. "These findings have the potential to impact therapy in anorexia nervosa with early implementation of estrogen replacement in girls who are estrogen-deficient."[b]

to deal more effectively with stressful feelings and the urge to restrict. Back at home, everyone, including Bailey's two sisters, was determined to make Bailey well. Weight restoration took eleven months, but her psychological symptoms had been so severe that the Monarchs continued meal supervision, and closely monitored her weight, for another six months. "We added another layer of treatment," added Cherié. "We took her to a specialty clinic that treats behavioral problems nutritionally. They put her on some personally tailored supplementation, [so] we also saw further help from that."[5]

Bailey's recovery was so positive, she found extra energy and motivation to lobby the Florida legislature for insurance coverage for mental disorders, support the Federal Response to Eliminate Eating Disorders (the FREED Act) on Capitol

Demi's Daily Battle

Shortly after checking out of treatment, teen recording artist Demi Lovato moved into a sober living house in Los Angeles to stay on track. Bulimia, self-mutilation, and depression still rattled her cage. "I check in with many, many people every single day," she told the Associated Press in 2011. "I have a very strong treatment team and it's actually kind of overwhelming sometimes to have that many people just focused on you and your problems."[c] A year later, when SuChin Pak of MTV News asked how she was doing at the premiere of her hour-long documentary *Stay Strong* (2012), she replied, "I'm doing awesome right now. I am living a really healthy lifestyle and I have the support that I need. You know, it's not easy, like I said it's a daily battle—I struggle every single day, but each day gets easier and I'm in a really good place today."[d]

Demi continues to strengthen her recovery through her commitment to various social and environmental causes. Together with the Substance Abuse and Mental Health Services Administration, she focuses on the importance of social connectedness for young adults who are at risk for psychological disorders and substance abuse and advocates for their access to health care services. On May 7, 2013, Children's Mental Health Awareness Day, Demi appeared at a press briefing with Kathleen Sebelius, secretary of the U.S. Department of Health and Human Services. She accepted an award for her work as a mentor to young adults challenged with mental health and substance use.[e]

Hill, and coordinate with the National Eating Disorders Association (NEDA) for the first NEDA Walk in the Tampa Bay area in 2011. She graduated high school in 2012 and entered Vanderbilt University. Her family has remained watchful. Cherié highly recommends that parents seek out specialists and educate themselves thoroughly. The quality of care is variable, she said, which can make the difference between lifelong problems and complete recovery.

An ongoing support system is absolutely necessary following any initial course of treatment. Eating disorder symptoms reassert themselves, even as a survivor continues therapy sessions and stabilizes nutrition with a healthful meal plan. In the early stages of recovery, the side that craves normalcy and freedom from illness—what many therapists refer to as "the healthy self"—needs new options to counteract old behaviors. Having opportunities to develop steady, supportive relationships helps to build self-esteem, self-confidence, and self-worth. Group therapy, moderated by licensed counselors, is excellent for this, but self-help options can be beneficial, too. Self-help is any method that lets recovering sufferers practice healthy coping skills that strengthen their self-image. For instance, when survivors get in touch with other survivors who are further along the road to full recovery, it decreases the sense of isolation and makes them feel worthy of care. By developing satisfying human relationships, issues of bad body image and self-hatred start to ease. Eating and exercise compulsions become less necessary.

Seeds of Change

Just as eating disorders develop at different rates and to different levels of intensity in each individual, recovery is a process that takes place in stages. Various specialists describe as many as ten, but the well-known—though hotly debated—Stages of Change model has five—Precontemplation, Contemplation, Preparation, Action, and Maintenance. The schema breaks down the process of recovery from all compulsive and addictive behaviors, from sufferer's first awareness of the problem to being able to sustain new and better ways of dealing with it. Originated in the late 1970s by psychology professors James Prochaska and Carlo DiClemente at the University of Rhode Island, Stages of Change, also known as the Transtheoretical Model, has evolved through multiple versions with contributions from other researchers. It has been used to tailor interventions and therapy programs for addictive disorders and for anyone adapting to life challenges.

Here's an example of how the model might represent the shifting attitudes of people in the midst of an ED recovery.

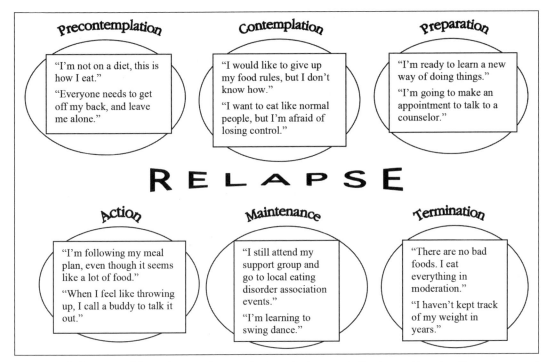

Stages of change. Although not always designated as a sixth stage, Termination appeared in the 1992 version to represent the end of the road. Relapse is not a stage, rather a process of transition back to an earlier stage. *Schema created by the author in accordance with Prochaska and DiClemente models, 1983 to present.*

Basically, recovery starts once positive change begins. But rather than a step-ladder, you might picture recovery stages as a roller coaster at an amusement park. The climb up may be steep or more gently sloped. The ride through it is sometimes fast, sometimes slow, and filled with unexpected twists and turns, tunnels and water landings—maybe even flipping you upside down. Some people happily reach solid ground after one experience and never look back. Others go around again (and again), or look for another midway ride to leap on. How far along the recovery path someone gets and how quickly it happens is due to many factors, but perhaps the biggest one is how well supported the intention is to change the mind and behavior. The more support you receive from others who are equipped to walk with you, and the better you can teach them how to help you, the better you'll be able to sustain your progress. It may take years to put all the puzzle pieces together, but full return to normal is possible—and worth it. Never give up because of setbacks. "Stick with it," says Ruth, "stick with it. Recovery is an opportunity to learn to handle any adversity you'll encounter in life. You'll become calmer and more sure of yourself. You'll be a better friend. People who overcome eating disorders, and other addictions, are kinder, more compassionate human beings. The world needs more people like that."[6]

Watch Your Self-Talk

Have you ever heard the statement "What you think about, you bring about"? The saying comes from a biblical quote, Proverbs (23:7): "For as one thinketh in his soul, so is he." Maybe the writers of the Old Testament understood how our mind is influenced by the nature of our thoughts. Our subconscious mind is primed to agree with what it hears. That's why words matter. The positive affirmations and the negative putdowns we tell ourselves affect us as much as those we hear from others—perhaps more so, because we tell ourselves the same things over and over again. Negative self-talk is not characteristic of being humble, says Michael Cartwright, founder of American Addiction Centers. "Besides being disingenuous, this sort of talk is counterproductive. Honest humility acknowledges our strengths as well as our weaknesses, our failures as well as our successes. We don't need to get puffed up over our successes; nor do we need to flagellate ourselves for our failures."[f]

Self-talk can be either a stumbling block or a useful tool to recovery. Berating yourself for mistakes you make, reminding yourself of your shortcomings and telling yourself your efforts are hopeless, tears down self-esteem. Conversely, by consistently practicing positive self-talk and visualizing the kind of life you want to live, you create the belief that you are the kind of person you want to be; that you deserve to be happy, healthy, and successful; and that you have the power to get anything you desire. "I was used to hiding my body," wrote ED survivor and author Cheryl Kerrigan about a clothes shopping trip she took soon after she had reached her goal weight. "As I looked at myself [in the mirror], negative thoughts jumped into my mind, but so did positive ones. I liked the way the outfit fit my new body and was happy with what I saw. So I said to myself, 'Damn, I look good.'"[g]

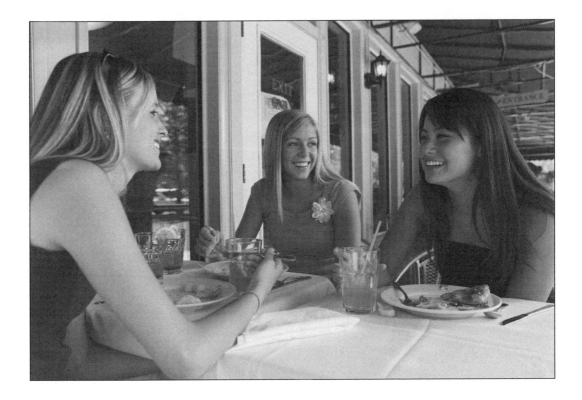

Lots of people compare recovery work to planting a garden. The seeds you sow are the new strategies you learn to outsmart your disorder. There are alternative techniques for identifying and expressing feelings, and you can learn recovery tools—healthy behaviors that effectively deal with stressful situations. Some of these might be daily breathing and meditation exercises, creating a recovery scrapbook, following a predetermined meal plan. Once you commit to practicing these tools, they take root and grow. Before you know it, you have a life garden full of color. Along the way, you harness the traits that perpetuated disorder to strengthen your recovery. Carolyn Costin and Gwen Schubert Grabb call this "using a healthy self to heal an ED self." "We teach people, this isn't a battle that somebody else is going to step in and take away your eating disorder," Costin explains. She gives an example of how a patient would feel unable to stop an urge to purge, but would know just what to say to discourage someone else with the same feelings. "Usually someone has a healthy self inside for somebody else. They know what to say, but they don't use it for themselves."[7] Sufferers can learn to use their intuitive knowledge of healthy attitudes, a voice that had been muted by their illness, to heal.

Twelve Steps to Wellness

Twelve-step programs attempt to repair psychological problems by transforming the spirit. The twelve-step approach to treat addictive behaviors began with Alcoholics Anonymous (AA) in 1935, when two men, Bill Wilson and Dr. Bob Smith (a.k.a. Bill W. and Dr. Bob), discovered they could help each other stay sober, and that other alcoholics could stay sober, when they gathered together to guide one another through a course of action for recovery. Founded on principles of Christian fellowship, the model developed to support people in crisis with addictive and compulsive behaviors or other emotional problems. No religious affiliation is necessary or expected. Groups function through members' commitment to sharing their experiences and observations at fellowship meetings, working together to practice directives intended to bring them closer to a spiritual awakening.

In 1953, Bill W. explained the principles that had guided AA's objectives during the first four years and that became the foundation for the curriculum.[8] When adapted for all twelve-step recovery programs, they can be summarized in six steps:

1. Admitting the inability (powerlessness) to control one's behavior
2. Facing the truth about the seriousness of one's affliction
3. Being honest with an experienced member-sponsor
4. Making amends for the harm done to others
5. Working with others in the same circumstances
6. Acknowledging the power of a greater entity that assists the recovery process

The American Psychiatric Association (APA) endorses twelve-stepping as a source of community support for people with EDs, but does not recommend it as the sole form of treatment for those diagnosed with an eating condition. Too much variation exists between patients and in the knowledge, attitudes, beliefs, and practices of fellowship chapters and sponsors. Also, no systematic studies of the long-term results are available.[9] Certain treatment centers do incorporate the twelve-step model into their programs, but the APA cautions against using it as a substitute for appropriate medical, psychological, and nutritional therapies. If patients wish to include twelve-stepping as part of their overall choice of therapeutic approaches, their experience should be closely monitored by at least one member of the treatment team. The best time to incorporate a twelve-step approach is probably after disordered eating behaviors have eased, and the focus shifts to relapse prevention.

A goal of the twelve-step curriculum is to banish problem behaviors (i.e., maintain sobriety) by completely eliminating use of (i.e., abstinence from) the substance that triggers the loss of control. In the case of alcohol or drug addiction, the approach is straightforward—give up drinking, inhaling, shooting up, and so on. The idea is to remain free from disease, so to work the program effectively, you must avoid the behavior that triggers the illness. For a few compulsive

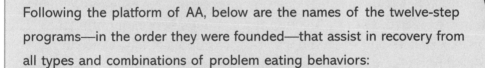

The Food Fellowships

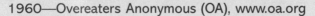

Following the platform of AA, below are the names of the twelve-step programs—in the order they were founded—that assist in recovery from all types and combinations of problem eating behaviors:

1960—Overeaters Anonymous (OA), www.oa.org

1979—Compulsive Eaters Anonymous—H.O.W. (CEA-HOW), www.ceahow.org

1984—Recoveries Anonymous (RA), www.r-a.org

1987—Food Addicts Anonymous (FAA), www.foodaddictsanonymous.org

1989—Dual Recovery Anonymous (DRA), www.draonline.org

1993—Anorexics and Bulimics Anonymous (ABA), aba12steps.org

1994—Recovery from Food Addiction (RFA), www.recoveryfromfoodaddiction .org

1995—Eating Addictions Anonymous (EAA), www.eatingaddictionsanonymous .org

1998—Food Addicts in Recovery Anonymous (FA), www.foodaddicts.org

1998—GreySheeters Anonymous (GSA), www.greysheet.org

2000—Eating Disorders Anonymous (EDA), www.eatingdisordersanonymous .org

RA and DRA are not food fellowships, per se. They were each formed to apply the twelve step approach to cope with emotional problems in someone's life. DRA, specifically, is for people experiencing both a psychological disorder and chemical dependency.

behaviors, gambling, gaming, and self-harm, the abstinence model can be applied pretty well. With eating disorders, though, the concept is murky, because recovery means being able to deal with food in a normal, healthy way. The original food fellowship, OA was designed to help anyone with compulsive eating problems control hunger and change the emotional relationship to food. Although the first step of OA is admitting powerlessness over food, the objective is not to abstain from eating, but rather from eating compulsively. To work the program effectively, members identify "trigger foods" and define a food plan that normalizes eating routines and enables them to reach and maintain a healthy weight. Other food fellowships adhere to specific food rules, such as weighing and measuring everything eaten, not eating between meals, or eliminating certain binge-worthy foods, such as sugar and flour. Strict rules such as these may not be helpful for overcoming an ED, especially if a sufferer has a lengthy history of dieting and purging.

The essence of the twelve steps enables sufferers to build stable relationships so that the hyperfocus on food and eating can transform into positive engagement with the inner self and the rest of the world. Steps two through eleven are about the methods to effect that change. The twelfth step entails service work—the intent to use newfound skills and wisdom to assist with the recovery of other sufferers. Letting go of eating problems allows the development of a new sense of purpose, a major step in discovering a true self. All of the food fellowships feature a set of tools for recovery that members can use to stay on track. Many are similar to what a therapist might suggest, whether or not he or she adheres to twelve-step principles in counseling sessions. Tools include keeping in touch with a sponsor, reaching out to connect with other members, reading twelve-step literature, recording thoughts and feelings, volunteering for duties within the chapter, and, of course, attending and speaking up at meetings regularly.

Chart Your Progress: Journaling for Self-Discovery

Writing is an extraordinarily powerful tool to use on the journey through recovery. Putting pen to paper provides an outlet for galloping thoughts and intense emotions, diffusing the urges that fire disordered eating. Carolyn Jennings is the author of *Hunger Speaks: A Memoir Told in Poetry*. "Shaping my experiences from disease and recovery into poetry was therapeutic and empowering," she wrote in a recovery essay for NEDA. "The process clarified details and connections, as well as switched me from [being a] victim of something into being an observer and a creator."[h]

Long before she wrote poetry, journaling became a key to her recovery from binge eating. Inspired by personal experience, Jennings became a Journal to the Self certified instructor and workshop coordinator. Writing practice builds self-awareness, she says, which is essential for recovery. Once you distinguish between the voice of illness and the voice of health, you can disentangle from the disease.

To support your recovery, Jennings recommends a technique called Topics du Jour. Originally conceived by writer Kathleen Adams, founder of the Center for Journal Therapy (www.journaltherapy.com), the practice begins by creating a list of topics that are major concerns in your life. "I listed areas that I relate to my recovery and that I wanted to check on regularly," Jennings said. "My list totals seventeen and includes the categories *body, mind, emotions, spirit, food and drink, anxiety, sexuality, cooking, self-expression, play*, and *relationships/isolation/ intimacy*. I love being able to track each of these topics easily over time to see what's developing, changing, staying stuck, needing attention or deserving praise. Over time, Topics du Jour reveal growth and change, good habits of health and self-care or slips back toward disease and despair. I am more aware of wholeness and fullness. Important areas don't go neglected and forgotten."[i]

Want to try it? Here are the instructions:

Jot down a list of topics you'd like to track in your life or your recovery. If you'd like to write daily, aim to list 30 topics. This way, on the first day of every month, you'll write about a certain relationship or school, on the second day about your food plan or exercise, etc. If writing daily doesn't appeal, let the length of the list arise naturally, but do write as often as you can; simply start at the top of the list, focus on the next topic each time you write, and then start at the top of the list again. Set up a computer file or select a small notebook. Play with Topics du Jour just five to fifteen minutes at a time. You can set a timer and try it for a few months. Occasionally read your postings over time on a specific topic and take note of progress or stuck points that can be brought to your therapist or recovery support team. See if you find this technique helpful and easy for you.[j]

Jennings contributes the *Writing for Recovery Blog Series* for NEDA (www .nationaleatingdisorders.org/blog), where she shares tips and techniques for developing a therapeutic writing practice. Contact her through her website, www .writingourwings.com.

Get Your Motor Running

Psychotherapy not only helps sufferers resolve the underlying feelings of emptiness, unworthiness, and disconnectedness that they usually have, but also the ego inflation and distorted thinking that goes along with disordered eating and weight loss and obsessive exercise. Twelve-step study can help sufferers rediscover themselves or create a new identity in the company of others with similar struggles. "When I hear some morning news nutritionist say, 'Diets don't work,' I laugh," says Kelly. "For some of us, they work *way too well*." Kelly joined OA after she became pregnant. "There's a nationwide war on obesity—here I was proving to be the best soldier. I thought I knew everything about fat percentages, carbohydrate grams and calorie counts. I did cardio-conditioning and strength training, drank lots of water. I thought I was being healthy as 'Bully' took over my life. It validates the powerful side of you. That's one reason why it's so hard to give up."[10] With good prenatal counseling, Kelly's bulimia went underground, but resurfaced soon after she gave birth. With the support of her mother and husband, she contacted a treatment center that offered nutrition services. She continues to attend twelve-step meetings and has discovered her storytelling voice. She's now a published author of murder mysteries.

Any kind of compulsive disorder becomes an incredibly powerful way of taking care of the stress that painful emotions cause. This is why many therapists remind patients that "fat" is not a feeling and insist that eating disorders are not about food. Try to tell that to someone who panics over everyday food decisions—What? When? How much?—and constantly evaluates the consequences of eating—Will this make me fat? How will I make up for it this time? Fat is a feeling, and EDs are about food for many in treatment. Addressing strategies to manage food choices is a vital part of recovery. *Meal support*, a concept that originated in the food fellowships, is the method utilized in the family-based treatment (FBT), or Maudsley approach, and in many residential treatment centers. Having someone else take charge of food decisions is very scary for someone who has been tightly controlling eating behaviors. The terror of eating, an effect of the illness itself, can provoke a lot of explosive words, tears, even violence, and cause parents to worry whether they are traumatizing their child. Before choosing the Maudsley program, Harriet Brown and her husband had been trying to get their child to eat the foods she had formerly loved without success. It was adversarial, difficult, and complicated, she told radio interviewer Diane Rehm in 2010. After thoroughly reviewing the FBT approach, she found she could cajole her daughter to eat by sitting with her at meals as long as it took her to eat them and by setting simple consequences—no TV, books, showers, phone or sleep, until she finished what was in front of her. "I sort of developed things I would just say over and over again, like a politician staying on message," she said. "And I would tell my daughter, 'I love you and I'm not going to let you starve.' And that kind of became our mantra. So when we sat at the table and she was terrified about eating, you know, 'I love you, I'm not going to let you starve. You can do it. You can't go to school until you do it.' We kind of used a whole toolbox of strategies to help with that."[11] Studies have found no evidence that the bonds between children and their parents are destroyed—in fact, the opposite is true. Reports from families indicate that they grow closer to each other as a result of working through FBT and the process of nutritional recovery from either anorexia or bulimia.[12]

Meal support also helps people who are no longer dependent on their parents. "I know someone who arranged Meals on Wheels deliveries," said Christina, twenty-nine, of Tampa, Florida. "I took my meals at a local convent one summer. Having someone else make my food choices was a great relief. You just have to be at a point where you are strong enough to trust the spirit of recovery and believe your Higher Power is working through other people to make you well."[13] When you're healed, you'll be able to take on the responsibility for caring for yourself again, this time in a healthy way. Twelve-step programs call this "being restored to sanity."

Another way to regain control is through *intuitive eating*, a method for getting in touch with your body's true need for nourishment. Intuitive eating is choosing to eat what you feel like eating when you feel like eating it, as much as you feel is right for you. It is not carte blanche to go whole hog. It's the anti-diet approach to eating, and many have used it successfully to reprogram their attitudes about food and eating, body size, and shape. Learning to eat intuitively takes time and practice. It requires a lot of trust and patience in the process (attunement) as you develop a positive sense of self. Those in recovery should be sure to line up plenty of good emotional support and guidance from treatment professionals. A 2012 study published in the journal *Appetite* showed strong support for intuitive eating as a measure of health. Young men and women who reported trusting their body to tell them how much to eat had better physical and mental health indicators than those who did not have such trust. Females who stopped eating when they were full had lower odds of chronic dieting and binge eating than those who did not stop eating when full.[14] Intuitive eaters were less likely to be disordered eaters and more likely to have normal body mass.

Nutrition therapist, author, and speaker Evelyn Tribole strongly advises those who are still fighting to gain weight in recovery to follow the meal plan laid out by their dietician, at least until they are restored and stable, before exploring intuitive eating. Sticking to a structured schedule and meal plan assures consistent nutrition with sufficient calories.[15] You learn what a normal, balanced diet is. As weight is restored, you can start to pay attention to what it feels like to be hungry and full, and learn to distinguish false signals from what is true. When your

Healthy Wealthy and Wise: Health at Every Size®

A new body peace movement is taking root "on the simple premise that the best way to improve health is to honor your body."[k] Health at Every Size (HAES®) promotes a health-centered rather than a number-oriented approach to health and wellness, and advocates for greater acceptance of the diversity of body types in society. HAES operates on the principles of intuitive eating—focus on pleasurable eating and exercise habits and on the natural cues for hunger, satiety, and appetite to establish optimal and stable health for body and mind. Research findings indicate that when treated with an HAES, or similar, non-diet approach, subjects show significant medical improvement in terms of biological measures (e.g., blood pressure, blood lipids), eating behaviors, and concerns about self-esteem and body image.[l] HAES achieves these results more successfully than conventional weight-loss programs and without the potential dangers associated with traditional weight-control attempts.

Shifting our actions to trust our own body's wisdom also saves us money. "I started following HAES a couple years ago after a lifetime of dieting," reads a comment on a *New York Times* blog. "My weight has become relatively steady instead of bouncing up and down, which is better for my heart (yo-yo dieting is worse for you than staying fat) and better for my wallet (I'm not constantly having to buy clothes in different sizes). . . . I actually get *more* exercise because I do what I enjoy and I do it because I want to, not because I feel like I have to. I eat better because I listen to what my body wants. And I am mentally better because I'm not constantly agonizing over calorie counts and pounds."[m]

All major advocacy groups in the eating disorders field support HAES and encourage health practitioners to adopt the guidelines presented by the Association for Size Diversity and Health. To show your support and commitment, sign the pledge at www.haescommunity.org.

"It's well documented that overweight people can lead long, disease-free lives. In fact, BMI [body mass index] is almost irrelevant, according to a study by the renowned Cooper Institute in Dallas. If you're fat but fit—meaning you can be active for twenty to thirty minutes—you can live longer than people who are thin and out of shape! Putting all the emphasis on weight, regardless of diet or fitness, is harmful to everyone. It can lead thin people to believe it's okay to eat junk and be unhealthy, and it implies that the best thing you can do if you're overweight is diet. The truth is, the vast majority of dieters regain their lost weight, with some ending up heavier—a pattern that's a big risk factor for many diseases that are too quickly blamed on weight. If you eat a good diet and exercise, you're likely to be healthy, no matter what the scale says."

—Linda Bacon, PhD, @LindaBaconHAES
Professor of Nutrition, City College, San Francisco
Author of *Health at Every Size: The Surprising Truth about Your Weight*[n]

meters are repaired, you can rely on those biological cues. You'll eat for physical rather than emotional reasons and give yourself unconditional permission to eat. Over time, you calmly (maybe joyfully?) choose the types of foods in the amounts that reenergize you. Your body gravitates to its natural proportions, and you'll be able to keep your weight stable. Trusting intuition lets you make all life's decisions with confidence.

Psychology professor emeritus Jean Kristeller of Indiana State University developed a ten-week course that successfully treats symptoms of binge and compulsive eating using mindfulness meditation and guided mindfulness practices. Mindfulness is paying attention to what's going on around you and inside you. Designed to address the core issues of binge eating disorder, Mindfulness-Based Eating Awareness Training helps with all degrees of compulsive eating by teaching how to control responses to various emotions, make conscious food choices, develop an awareness of hunger and satiety cues, and cultivate self-acceptance.[16]

Leaders of eating support groups might be able to teach techniques of *mindful eating* to help those in recovery find their intuition. The exercises use deliberate thought to increase awareness of eating behaviors. Mindful eating encourages you to identify the sensations of eating—the sight, smell, texture, even the sound of food. It forces you to slow down and consider your true emotions when

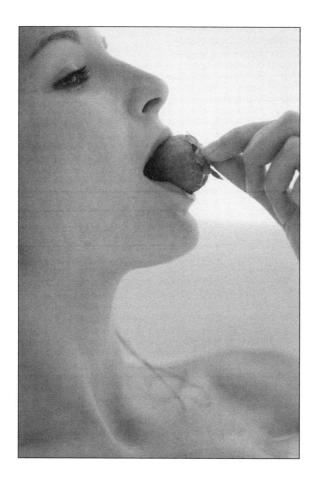

Meditation for Mindfulness

Meditation and breath work are mindful practices that have been used by spiritual seekers—particularly Buddhist and Christian monks—throughout human history. The techniques focus attention, teaching how to be at ease with thoughts and sensations in the mind and body. They are self-soothing activities that can be used as part of therapy for any type of compulsive, stress-related behaviors, no matter how severe. Mindfulness-Based Stress Reduction (MBSR), developed by Jon Kabat-Zinn at the University of Massachusetts Medical Center, brings together guided meditation, yoga stretches, and group discussion. The eight-session program is offered in medical centers and by private psychotherapists around the country who integrate behavior modification approaches with mindfulness training. MBSR is especially useful in

ED recovery—it's a tool to calm a yammering mind, reduce impulsivity, and encourage a safe exploration of troublesome feelings through simple observation. Meditative practices commonly utilized include

- belly breathing
- alternate nostril breathing
- walking meditation
- listening meditation
- chanting

The thought of trying to sit quietly and do nothing sounded almost impossible to Cheryl Kerrigan. "How could I try to just 'be' when inside my head Ed was screaming the entire time? *How could that be helpful?*" she asked. "Nevertheless, I wanted the things that meditation could provide . . . so one day I went to a Zen meditation class."° Cheryl's ED voice was pretty loud that first day, protesting and telling her how stupid and selfish she was. Yet, by the end of class, "he backed down just enough for me to have a few minutes of peace." That's when Cheryl knew she was onto something. She took more classes and sat at home, becoming more invigorated, yet peaceful. "[Whenever] Ed speaks, push his voice from your thoughts and concentrate on your breath," she counsels. "Be patient and kind with yourself and don't give up." Afterward, she continues, you can deepen the experience by writing about the feelings you discover before, during, and after the meditation.

confronted with food. You learn to notice your impressions, letting them pass through your mind without passing judgment, or responding immediately to your first impulses. You simply breathe, chew slowly, savor the flavor, and swallow, one bite at a time.

Cleveland Clinic psychologist Susan Albers, PsyD (@DrSusanAlbers, www .facebook.com/eatdrinkmindful), works one-on-one and with groups of people struggling with eating and body image concerns. She is also is a prolific author on the subject of mindful eating. Changing behavior is a marathon, not a sprint, she says. She suggests 26.2 tips (26, plus a final written reminder) as you build a new relationship with food and train yourself to eat well. Here are a few of her recommendations:[17]

11. Rate Your Hunger before You Eat (helps you to honestly evaluate your need)
15. Don't Multi-Task (put down the book, leave the computer, never eat in front of the TV)
17. Don't Fight Cravings (give yourself permission to eat what you want, when you're hungry for it)
23. Try New Foods (even a "fear" food)
25. Put Even More Effort into What You Do Well, Instead of Trying to Change What You Struggle With (emphasizing strengths instead of weaknesses will always put you ahead in the game)

Dr. Albers believes anyone troubled by food can put mindful eating into practice, no matter how chaotic their eating behaviors have become. Read her books and find more of Dr. Albers's tips in at www.eatingmindfully.com/mindful-eating-tools.

No Guarantees—Setbacks, Slip-ups, and Stumbling Blocks

Dropping habits that have taken months and years to evolve is a tremendously difficult task—especially when they have worked so effectively in relieving stress. Replacing compulsive weight and body controlling behaviors with better, and

Yoga for Body Wisdom

Yoga practice can open you up to a totally new relationship to your body. It quickly becomes a favorite activity for many ED survivors, particularly those who have been compulsive exercisers. Learning a few basic poses (*asanas*), either through an instructor-led class or a well-presented DVD, will immediately improve circulation, balance, and your ability to relax. Every movement, no matter the style or school you choose, is done to breathe, which focuses energy. "I had thought yoga was the lazy person's exercise, or for people that needed physical therapy because of injury," says Ruth. "I didn't come to it until very late in my recovery, when I was experiencing some leg pain, different from any body complaint I had had before. It resolved within weeks and I knew I had found the solution to all my obsessive exercise. Yoga changes your mind and body in incalculable ways. Fifteen years later, it continues to open up my inner world and keep me whole."[P]

"It is so easy to get addicted to our tension, and it's our tension that blocks our ability to feel. For us to be able to do the work we need to do in the world, to be able to hold that light for spirit, what is required is great empathy. If we're not feeling us, how can we feel the world around us? So by doing yoga and by breathing deep, by meditating and chanting and by expressing yourself in all sorts of positive ways, allows us to remember who we truly are. We're not these bodies, we're not the job that we do, not the money that we make, not the relationship we think we're in control of. We're none of these things. We're beautifully and infinitely a child of spirit. And truly adored."

—Seane Corn, yoga instructor and activist[q]

more healthful, life-appropriate strategies takes conscious commitment, time, and practice. Slip-ups and setbacks, whether long or short, are an expected part of the struggle to reeducate disordered thought processes. Some psychotherapists consider them necessary to sustaining recovery because of the opportunity they offer for problem solving. Up to two-thirds of those struggling with anorexia and bulimia succumb to relapse. The riskiest period of time, according to studies reported by F.E.A.S.T., is in the six to seven months after eating behaviors have improved and symptoms have dissipated.[18]

A true relapse is more intense and severe than skipping one meal, or chowing down extra birthday cake. It signals the return of the "food as relief" mind-set and usually entails a significant change in weight or reengaging in binging or binge-purge cycles. While an outsider cannot know for sure when a series of setbacks becomes a full relapse, the sufferer surely does. At twenty-two, after five years of bulimic symptoms, Ruth's college roommate, "Liza," was questioned by her dental hygienist. She admitted her problem and agreed to be evaluated. Her hygienist referred her to community mental health services, and she saw a counselor there for a while. Then she quit therapy, thinking she'd gotten everything she needed out of the sessions. She did well on her own for about five months, keeping her bulimia under control until her boyfriend, a newly commissioned Marine Corps officer, left for training. Within just a few weeks, she was triggered after a family dinner, went home, and had, as she put it, "a saxophone colossus."[19] Ruth and Liza agreed, if they never had to eat again, recovery would be much easier. The trouble with eating disorders is, unlike alcohol and drugs, food isn't all or nothing.

The problem is the cure.

Before the healthy self gets good at using recovery tools, old coping mechanisms are bound to assert themselves. This is the reason for a relapse prevention plan—a set of predetermined possibilities for action rather than relying on disordered eating and exercise in triggering situations. Plans such as eating prescribed meals at standard times, bringing certain foods along when eating outside home, and keeping a contact list close at hand for calling or texting a buddy when troublesome feelings arise. People with eating disorders are usually pretty good at following self-imposed rules. Establishing alternative rescue methods may not only interrupt a potential relapse; it's actually making use of one's natural temperament and abilities that contributed to the illness. Relapse prevention techniques are meant to resolve problems before they come up, helping to steadily integrate a healthy mind and body.

Switching Sides: Junkie Weight Control

Substance abuse is common in roughly half of all cases of people with eating disorders, and over a third of people who abuse drugs or alcohol also experience an ED.[r] A 1998 survey of cocaine abusers found 72 percent of the women who also qualified as eating disordered had chosen to use the drug specifically as a method of weight control. Eighty-five percent claimed they also used alcohol as an appetite suppressant.[s] In addition to amphetamines like cocaine, teens and young adults use an array of substances to lose or keep from gaining weight, or to maintain a fit physique: benzodiazepines, opiates and opioid narcotics, steroids, caffeine, tobacco, diuretics, laxatives, and both over- and under-the-counter appetite suppressants, metabolism boosters, and weight-loss drugs. All can be habit forming when used excessively by those susceptible to addiction.

Substance abuse may occur before, during, or after ED symptoms become apparent. When people qualify for a dual diagnosis of chemical dependency and an ED, an integrated treatment program is the best option to address both issues and develop a comprehensive relapse prevention plan. If alternative strategies to reduce emotional stress aren't put in place, relapse is practically guaranteed. Substituting one form of addictive behavior for another is all too common in the struggle for full recovery. Amy Winehouse, the soulful singer-songwriter whose defiant anthem "Rehab" was a hit in 2006, became a British tabloid sensation because of her troubles with alcohol and drug dependency. But she had also filled her plate with bulimia and self-injury before she was seventeen. She lost the battle with all of them in 2011 at the age of twenty-seven. "She would have died eventually, the way she was going," her older brother, Alex, told a British news source in 2013, "but what really killed her was the bulimia . . . it left her weaker and more susceptible. Had she not had an eating disorder, she would have been physically stronger."[t]

One of the pitfalls of the recovery road is the danger of crossing over into a second eating disorder diagnosis. The state of starvation, for example, is extraordinarily difficult for a body to maintain over a lifetime—which is why chronic anoretics are dead within twenty years. With normal access to food, the desire to survive typically foils a mind's competing attempt to diet into the grave. The APA has indicated that 50–64 percent of those diagnosed with anorexia turn to bulimia and binge eating.[20] People who initially binge have been known to develop anorexic symptoms as they pursue a diet. Others cross over into a subthreshold ED diagnosis, or slip into new disordered eating and exercise behaviors while recovering from others.

One of the interesting findings from the National Comorbidity Survey—Replication study was the reported average length of time that "recovered" anoretics had been ill—a year and a half, versus a bit over eight years for either bulimia or binge eating respondents.[21] This evidence suggests the majority of anoretics who do not become chronic sufferers—roughly two-thirds, that is—have a "dip in, dip out" period that is rather short, much shorter than has been generally understood. For such a serious, life-threatening illness, this is good news, but it's important to realize that body weight is not a marker of normal psychology. Although it's rare for prior anoretics to become obese, it's not unusual for them to be plagued with eating and body image issues long after their physiological health has stabilized. If initial treatment hasn't been thorough for any ED, relapses can occur years later due to a major life stressor—marriage or divorce, job change, the birth of a child, or death of a family member. Swift intervention, close monitoring with an appropriate treatment program, and long-term vigilance is the best insurance for sticking to the recovery road without slipping into the chasm forever.

Cut to the Chase, Quick: Self-Injury

Eating disorders and self-injurious behavior (SIB) serve up together like PB&J. Self-injury, self-harm, self-mutilation, all better known as "cutting," is a release for extreme emotional distress, and is not unusual among those with ED symptoms who regularly purge. Over sixteen kinds of self-harming methods have been documented among teenagers and children even younger than seven. Slicing, burning, punching, scratching, even hair pulling (trichotillomania) are directed to any part of the body, but most often on lower legs and forearms, ankles and wrists, stomach, and thighs.[u] The cuts, bruising, and scarring may be superficial or they may need medical attention and cause lasting disfigurement. Forty percent of 1,432 eating disordered adolescents between the ages of ten and twenty-one reported SIB. This was most common in female patients with a history of bulimic symptoms, a co-occurring mood disorder, and substance abuse.[v]

Mary, from Atlanta, Georgia, was treated at the Renfrew Center in Coconut Creek, Florida. "The easiest thing to do was roll up my sleeve and cut my arm," she explained in the documentary, *Thin*. "Then I got obsessed with having all of the scars in one place and having them all the same length and depth and looking the same. I have hundreds of cuts. It got to where the only way I could feel good was if I broke through the skin enough to where I exposed muscle or bone and I would have to get stitches."[w] Mary, twenty-four, started restricting food when she was fourteen. The cutting began when she was seventeen. "Talking has always been hard for me," she told producer Lauren Greenfield. "Showing my emotions through my body was an easy way to get them out. It was about looking on the outside the way I felt on the inside. To show people I hurt this much." Dialectical behavior therapy, the counseling approach that teaches interpersonal skills, emotional regulation, distress tolerance, and problem solving combined with mindfulness training, has shown promise for many who punish themselves with food and knives.

An Expert Weighs In: *You*

The real recovery experts are not psychotherapists, medical doctors, nutritionists, or scientific researchers, but the ones who go through it. Even though having an eating disorder doesn't make you the disease's expert, it does make you an expert in your own disorder. An ED has a lot to teach anyone—the sufferers, their families, and all observers who are willing to grow from the experience. Here are some real voices from the trenches to tell us what they've learned:

Now that I approach my meals and my exercise with the attitude "what makes me healthy" instead of "what makes me thinner," I have been able to keep a weight that is natural for my body type and age, enjoy real meals and enjoy exercising, instead of living in fear of food, or punishing myself with extreme workouts.—sztt[22]

I still feel part of me is too concerned about what I look like or how I eat. My goal is that someday I'll be like I was in high school where I could eat a chocolate chip cookie as big as your face and not think for two seconds about whether that was healthy or how much I would need to run to counteract that. It does seem like I'm getting better at that all the time.—Margaret M.[23]

I felt recovery itself was much harder than actually being in the eating disorder in the midst of it all, 'cause that didn't take any energy—I knew exactly what I needed to do, I knew exactly what I was supposed to eat, exactly what exercise I was supposed to be doing. In recovery, it was like, well, if I work out is that obsessive? I know I'm supposed to eat this but should I really be eating this?—Emily H.[24]

I knew I could never be the wife and life partner to my wonderful husband or truly follow my dreams of performing until I let go of my destructive behaviors. I spent half of my life a prisoner of my eating disorder but I never gave up hope. That hope gave me the courage to keep fighting and it gave me the courage to finally reach out for help.—Asha B.[25]

Having an ED, that temptation is always gonna be there, no matter what. I have an addiction. I'll have it all my life. But now I have weapons to battle the war. I'm gonna keep doing it. It's been life changing, life saving.—Rickywayne M.[26]

I have made more room in my life for things that bring me joy; things that I never had time for when I was busy with my eating disorder . . . things like singing in a choir, having "Pinterest" dates, trying out new recipes with friends, and learning to play the piano!—Ericka C.[27]

I'm doing great now. It's no coincidence that this is the first time in 8 years that I've been experiencing full nutrition in a non-chaotic, sustained way. I truly believe that full nutrition for an extended period of time has really been the turning point for me.—L.[28]

One of the most helpful things for me in my recovery is to talk with others in the same situation. In my opinion, this is done best in group therapy. I have had a wonderful group leader that helps us to maintain the goal of getting healthy, rather than just giving each other negative tips.—Becky[29]

I decided that I was going to let my family support me, as they had wanted to do from the beginning. Allowing my family to help me to maintain this healthy body [weight] until I was healthy enough in my mind to do it for myself . . . I have been nine months symptom free.—Hannah[30]

One of the most important things that I've learned about my recovery is that nothing changes overnight, and it is far from perfect. I would be lying to you if I said I hadn't had any of the thoughts I had previously, or if I told you I have never done some of the actions I used to do since I entered recovery but every day is another step away from that life, and the missteps become smaller and [it gets] easier to get back on track.—Justin S.[31]

I didn't want to be hurt anymore. So I started to believe that nothing could prevent me from becoming totally healthy and "normal" as a grown woman. I made up my mind to no longer define myself based on my past.—Holly A.[32]

Sharing Stories Responsibly

Once people get into treatment, they can start to find out what their ED is really all about. Recovery is a time for learning what makes you tick, what satisfies your soul, and how to live an authentic life. The discoveries and newfound understanding could offer a beacon for others, and you might feel that you'd like to share your experience to help families in crisis, or as a means of ED prevention.

? Triggering Debate: Wellness at Work

Can we all learn to live healthy, wealthy, and wise in the world today? How might someone in recovery use qualities like perfectionism, compulsiveness, and willpower as weapons against an ED? How would you advise a friend to avoid temptation when triggers arise?

Speaking about personal experience can be rewarding, but also stressful—care must be taken to tell the story responsibly. Our culture places a high value on self-control, and it's easy to send the wrong message to middle and high school students who wish for "just a touch of anorexia." Even elementary school children see losing weight—or eating vast quantities without gaining—as a great accomplishment. Audiences should be made aware of the serious health problems that come from eating disorders. People should be encouraged to talk to a parent, trusted adult, or health professional if feelings ever become overwhelming.

Various eating disorder organizations offer guidelines for sharing recovery stories. Here are a few recommendations:

- Protect yourself from overexposure and inappropriate responses. Be sure you are comfortable opening up to others who may not be understanding. Set limits on what you divulge.
- Practice fielding common questions and addressing the false assumptions your audience may have. Be ready to direct people to organizations with professional resources for specific guidance.
- Stay away from "triggering" content. Leave out play-by-play details having to do with pounds lost, foods eaten or avoided, or any methods used to hide or perpetuate the illness.
- Focus on medical complications and the negative mental and social consequences you and your family experienced, but always end by instilling hope that recovery is attainable.
- Emphasize the importance of early intervention, finding qualified treatment professionals, and staying calm in the face of the storm.

Beyond the ups and downs of setbacks and relapses, does the recovery road have an end? Can anyone who has struggled with an eating disorder find a peaceful relationship with food? What does the future look like? Living life free from disordered eating and compulsive activity means something different to every former sufferer. Let's consider a few final thoughts.

More Food for Thought

Read

Jennifer Ashton with Christine Larson. *The Body Scoop for Girls: A Straight-Talk Guide to a Healthy, Beautiful You.* New York: Avery, 2009.

Gina M. Biegel. *The Stress Reduction Workbook for Teens: Mindfulness Skills to Help You Deal with Stress.* Oakland, Calif.: New Harbinger Publications, 2010.

Robin F. Brancato. *Food Choices.* Lanham, Md.: Scarecrow Press, 2010.

Carolyn Costin and Gwen Schubert Grabb. *8 Keys to Recovery from an Eating Disorder: Effective Strategies from Therapeutic Practice and Personal Experience.* New York: W. W. Norton, 2011.

Jenni Schaefer. *Goodbye Ed, Hello Me: Recover from Your Eating Disorder and Fall in Love with Life.* New York: McGraw-Hill, 2009. www.jennischaefer.com/books/goodbye-ed-hello-me.

Evelyn Tribole and Elyse Resch. *Intuitive Eating: A Revolutionary Program That Works.* 3rd ed. New York: St Martin's Griffin, 2012. www.intuitiveeating.com.

Watch

Fat: What No One Is Telling You (documentary, 85 minutes). A production of Twin Cities Public Television and WGBH Educational Foundation, 2007. www.pbs.org/wbgh/takeonestep/fat/index.html.

Happy :) (documentary, 75 minutes). Shady Acres Productions/Wadi Rum Films, 2011. www.thehappymovie.com.

How to Cook Your Life: Find Nirvana in the Kitchen (documentary, 94 minutes). Roadside Attractions/Megahertz TV Fernsehproduktion GmBH, 2007.

Shiva Rae, Fluid Power Vinyasa Flow Yoga (exercise video/two-DVD set, 243 minutes). Acacia and Yoga Tribe Culture Production for Acorn Media, 2006.

Learn

The Alliance for Eating Disorders Awareness. Volunteer-run community education, professional training programs, and advocacy work. www.allianceforeatingdisorders.com. For info: 866-662-1235.

Association for Size Diversity and Health. Advocates for Health at Every Size®, the movement to promote a health-centered approach to weight management. www.sizediversityandhealth.org.

The Center for Mindful Eating. Teleconferences, training, newsletter, events. www.thecenterformindfuleating.org.

Take Action

MentorCONNECT. A match-up service providing one-on-one and group support for ED survivors, ages fourteen and up, in any stage of recovery. www .mentorconnect-ed.org.

SMITHTeens: A home for personal storytelling. Publish your six-word memoir and connect with the community. www.smithteens.com.

Epilogue:
What Recovery Looks Like

"Self-improvement can have temporary results, but lasting transformation occurs only when we honor ourselves as the source of wisdom and compassion."

—Pema Chöndrön
The Places That Scare Us: A Guide to Fearlessness in Difficult Times, 2001

Can we tell when an ED is gone? Does anyone fully recover? What is the real cure for EDs? Let's take one last swig before the journey's end.

Making Peace

Eating disorders mess up minds, ruin friendships, and keep people from living life to the fullest. Having an ED is like being in a bad relationship that will ultimately kill. Still, extreme and bizarre eating and exercise habits shield many of us from the pain of emotions that seem too big to deal with. They put us in control of our image and our appetites in an intense, fast-paced world that values idealism and ambition. For a while. Eating disorders are not choices, but recovery is. When sufferers decide to call a truce with their inner demons, nourish their body and spirit in ways that build true confidence and self-worth, they often feel better than ever before. "I feel like I'm becoming the person I really am," wrote L. to Laura Collins, who posted her letter on www.feast-ed.org. "The better I eat, the better I feel, the clearer I think. Sometimes, when I'm struggling to eat, I wonder to myself: What do I want more—no weight gain at all costs or the recovered life? And the answer is simple. I want the recovered life."[1]

Anyone treated for an eating disorder gets a glimpse of what wellness looks like. When the desire to be well exceeds the dependence on disordered eating and exercise, courage can overcome the fear of making the lifestyle changes necessary to recuperate. Everyone faces obstacles as they let go of old thinking patterns and practice new stress relievers. Sticking to the wellness path, living life with true self-reliance, is challenging for most former sufferers. Many often wonder what "normal" actually means.

What is full recovery? Let's consider three final questions.

How Do We Tell When an ED Is Gone?

Therapists Carolyn Costin and Gwen Schubert Grabb, both survivors of severe eating disorders, insist recovery is more than no longer showing diagnosable signs. Recovery is feeling free from disordered behaviors and thoughts without reacting to former triggers. Full recovery means you completely accept your body's natural size and shape. "When you are recovered, food and weight take a proper perspective in your life," says Costin. "What you weigh is not more important than who you are; in fact, numbers are of little importance at all. . . . When you are recovered, you do not use eating disorder behaviors to deal with, distract from, or cope with other problems."[2]

In many cases, particularly among very young patients with anorexia, solving the biochemical problems with a weight restorative meal plan and appropriate medication may be enough to drive an ED away for good. "When I got into my weight range, it was amazing," Bailey Monarch said in a 2010 interview. "I felt like myself again, healthy and happy. My schedule and stress hasn't changed, but the way I dealt with it has."[3]

Some former sufferers may feel as if they are in remission. Even though they neither show outward signs, nor feel triggered to act out, they sense the potential for disordered eating remains underground. The precise contributing factors, the overall consequences, and the challenges of getting well are unique to each person who has ever struggled with eating and body issues. The "recovered life" is something every former sufferer discovers and defines over time.

Can Anyone Truly Fully Recover?

Absolutely! You may have heard full recovery is impossible, partly because of a dirty little secret among treatment professionals. "A reasonably high percentage of people who treat eating disorders have had them themselves, and a lot of them never really fully recovered," Harriet Brown pointed out in *Jezabel*. "And so I think that if you got sick, you were sick for 10 years, or 15 years or whatever, and then you got better, but maybe not all the way better, . . . you are used to thinking about your illness in terms of psychodynamics. You know, 'I had a wretched mother, and an absent father, and this happened to me when I was a child.'"[4] It's natural to project that view on the rest of the world, she said. The attitude could hold other sufferers back from believing in their potential to be free from their disorder.

   The state-of-the-art perspective among the best-informed treatment professionals is to focus on treating eating disorders with good nutrition and create a circle of healing that reduces stress. Therapy opens new opportunities for strengthening family relationships and increases self-development and social skills. With conscious attention to self-care, permanent change takes place. "I didn't just want to maintain my weight, suppress the urge to purge, and still have a list of foods that were 'safe' to eat," Portia de Rossi wrote in her memoir. "I never wanted to think about food and weight ever again."[5] Her journey took her from an anorexic low to a bulimic high, as she stumbled toward a recovery that gradually brought her to sanity and self-acceptance. In 2008, de Rossi married comedienne and talk show host Ellen DeGeneres, legally changing her name to Portia Lee James DeGeneres in 2010.

Spotlight on Gürze Books,
Eating Disorders Resource Publisher

The only clearing house for resources exclusive to eating disorders, Gürze Books (@GurzeBooks) publishes titles and distributes an expanded catalogue of books for family members and treatment professionals, those in recovery, and anyone who wants to discover more about the complex world of disordered eating and body issues. The bookstore has over 300 specialty titles (memoirs, treatment guides, healthy eating, self-image, etc.), while the website, www.edcatalogue.com, offers educational articles, links to national organizations, conferences and events, a directory of support groups, and contact information for therapists and treatment centers. Two companion sites, www.eatingdisordersblogs.com and www.eatingdisordersrecoverytoday.com, incorporate writing from professional experts and hold space for stories of personal recovery. Founded by Leigh and Lindsey Cohn in Carlsbad, California, the couple established the company in 1980 as Lindsey was recovering from bulimia.[a] *Bulimia: A Guide to Recovery* details Lindsey's battle and was one of the first practical self-help guides for people with EDs. Find it and read more online at www.gurzebooks.com.

People with eating disorders can go on to lead fully actualized and authentic lives. The challenge is to generate access to supportive resources for all sufferers, and to counteract the triggering pressures in our society.

What's the Real Cure?

The solution to remedy any disordered eating is deceptively simple: Normalize eating and body weight with full nutrition and balanced activity. Seek the help of knowledgeable professionals. Keep caring family members involved. Learn to relax. Simple, far from easy, and feels like crap. Perhaps the distance between "recovering" and "recovered" is how much sufferers practice new skills for dealing with stress, despite how uncomfortable it may feel in the beginning. In the process of getting well they discover who they are without an ED. Here are some thoughts that may be helpful to those still working their way through recovery:

Eating disorders fight to stay alive, so never give up on yourself, your friend, or family member.
Breathe through the difficult moments.
Choose a daily practice that feels centering, grounding, and mindful.
Maintain a low-stress lifestyle. Don't take on more than you can handle at one time.

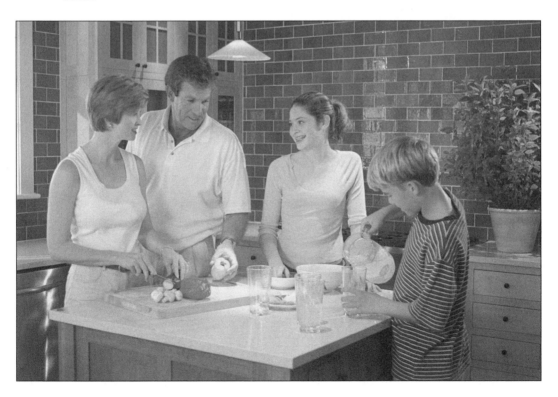

Never lose hope.

There will never be enough peanut butter, cinnamon buns, or chocolate shakes to fill the emptiness you feel inside. So don't try.

Pay attention to good nutrition, not numbers. Never diet. Find fitness activities that you enjoy and can switch into as your life progresses.

Don't let yourself get too isolated, overscheduled, or hungry.

Do something really nice and helpful for someone else. Participate in community works projects.

Let's hear one last commentary from survivor Jenni Schaefer (@JenniSchaefer; www.facebook.com/LifeWithoutEd), author, speaker, singer-songwriter, and champion of ED recovery for all. In the course of her treatment, Jenni chose to divorce her illness, as she would a guy that was no good for her. Like any breakup, it was painful and healing took a long time. It's very possible to say goodbye to Ed forever, she says in her books and on her website (www.jennischaefer.com), and find complete freedom:

I wondered if recovery was going to be worth it. Finally, fully recovered, I now know the answers to those questions. Yes, recovery is worth all the hard work. No, I'm not fat and miserable. In fact I'm happier than ever before, and I love my body. No, I'm not as thin as I used to be, but here's the miracle—I don't want to be. Don't quit before the miracle of full recovery happens to you.[6]

Glossary

Explore more at glossary.feast-ed.org.

adaptive function: a method by which we seek to satisfy our human needs and desires or cope with circumstances we can't control. If the technique brings negative consequences, it's considered a maladaptive function. Example: healthy eating and exercise are adaptive functions for weight control; fasting or extreme exercise would be maladaptive for the same purpose.

addiction: unrelenting cravings, resulting from changes in the brain, that push us into compulsive behavior, despite negative outcome.

amenorrhea: absence of the menstrual cycle

amygdala/amygdalae: two almond-shaped neural bundles located in the medial temporal lobe with direct connections to the hypothalamus, thalamus, hippocampus, septum, sensory and prefrontal cortex, and brainstem. They are essential for the emotional interpretation of stress, the retention of emotional memory, and reading emotion in others. Also important in the formation of sexual orientation.

analgesic: a substance that causes relaxation and freedom from pain.

anemia: lack of iron in the blood.

anorexia mirabilis: an illness of self-starvation afflicting young (almost exclusively Catholic) women of the Middle Ages who fasted and practiced other religious austerities to prove piety.

anorexia nervosa (AN): an eating disorder characterized by a relentless drive to maintain an abnormally low body weight.

asceticism: the practice of extreme restraint in regular human activity in order to gain greater spiritual awareness and religious sanctity. Most organized religions incorporate a degree of abstinence or self-discipline into normal, traditional practices, such as dietary laws, the observance of fast days, or by placing restrictions on types of clothing worn or sexual activity engaged in.

atypical eating disorder: eating disorder symptoms that feature unusual behavior, for example, chewing and spitting out food without swallowing, or that fall short of the classically defined eating disorder types by one or two criteria. See *(Feeding and) Eating Disorders Not Elsewhere Classified.*

avoidant/restrictive food intake disorder (ARFID): refusing food or avoiding eating to the extent of causing significant nutritional deficiency and either weight loss (in adults) or failure to grow normally (in children and teens).

axon: the long "tail" segment of a neuron.

bigorexia: a form of *body dysmorphic disorder*, almost exclusive to males, also called reverse anorexia. The syndrome causes sufferers to perceive their musculature as smaller and weaker than it actually is.

binge: consuming huge portion(s) of food in one sitting.

binge eating disorder (BED): an eating disorder characterized by recurrent episodes of massive food consumption, which doesn't involve purging, followed by feelings of distress, guilt, and self-chastising. *Deprivation-sensitive* BED follows periods of calorie restriction. *Dissociative-addictive* BED develops as a coping response to painful emotions, usually quite early in life.

binge priming: period of caloric or food restriction that makes a person more prone to overeat or abuse a drug.

body dysmorphic disorder: a distortion of body image in which sufferers perceive imagined defects, or are unable to accurately assess the size and shape of their body or body parts. They can, however, properly see other bodies realistically.

brainstem: our "reptilian" brain (evolutionarily, the oldest part) that manages basic organ functions, reflexes, sleep-wake cycles, and attention. Centers include the medulla oblongata, the reticular formation, the pons, and the midbrain.

bulimia nervosa (BN): an eating disorder characterized by recurring episodes of eating binges followed by a form of compensation, usually vomiting.

bulimirexia/bulimarexia: nonmedical term for someone who shows symptoms of both anorexia and bulimia, such as an anorexic who uses purging behavior, that is, vomiting or laxatives to restrict calories, or a bulimic who undergoes periods of fasting and excessive exercise. See *exercise (or "aerobic") bulimia.*

calorie: the energy needed to raise one gram of water one degree centigrade. Food calories are actually kilocalorie (1,000 calorie) measurements.

central nervous system: comprised of the brain and spinal cord.

cerebral cortex: layer of outermost brain tissue, divided into four lobes that process sensory information (parietal lobe), motor movements and cognition (frontal lobe), vision (occipital lobe), and hearing (temporal lobe). Although the limbic lobe lies inside the brain and underneath the other lobes, it's considered the fifth lobe of the cortex as its connection to them is so profound.

comorbidity: two or more illnesses (diseases, disorders, syndromes) occurring at the same time in the same person. Does not assume that either is the cause of the other.

compulsive eating: enhanced drive to eat, normally outside ordinary biological cues for nourishment. Used interchangeably with *binge eating* and is often a response to a prolonged period of calorie restriction.

diabulimia: unofficial medical condition where a type 1 diabetic controls her caloric intake by manipulating the amount of prescribed insulin.

disordered eating: any chronic restrictive and ritualistic compulsive eating problem leading to nutritional imbalance. First coined by the Women's Task Force of the American College of Sports Medicine.

dopamine: neurotransmitter produced in the ventral tegmental area of the midbrain, responsible for the experience of pleasure and pain relief. Essential for motor coordination, motivation, and impulse control.

dual diagnosis: having enough disease symptoms that qualify a patient for two separate medical disorders, for example, bulimia and alcohol dependence.

eating disorder (ED): deviant patterns of compulsive eating behavior marked by pathological self-preoccupation and body concerns.

emetic: substance used to induce vomiting, for example, ipecac syrup.

endocrine system: the highway of hormones secreted by glands in organs throughout the body.

endogenous: natively produced, such as specific proteins, hormones, cells, and so on, manufactured by the body.

endorphin: naturally occurring, opioid hormones produced by neurons that soothe pain.

enzyme: specialized proteins that assist (catalyze) biochemical reactions.

epidemic: the accelerated spread of a disease through a population. Epidemics occur when the number of disease cases exceeds what would normally be expected.

epidemiology: study of the occurrence of a particular disease or disorder.

etiology: cause of a physical disease or psychological disorder.

exercise (or "aerobic") bulimia: obsessive exercise performed solely as a reason to burn fat and calories, rather than as a means to stay active and healthy. Associated with symptoms of agitation and depression if the sufferer is forced to cease.

(Feeding and) Eating Disorders Not Elsewhere Classified (EDNEC): encompasses atypical eating behavior and physical symptoms of malnutrition that don't match the classic definitions for anorexia, bulimia, and binge eating disorder. Introduced in 2013 with the *DSM-5* (*Diagnostic and Statistical Manual of Mental Disorders*, fifth edition), it replaced EDNOS (Eating Disorders Not Otherwise Specified) with two subcategories, OSFED (Other Specified Feeding or Eating Disorder) and UFED (Unspecified Feeding or Eating Disorder).

female athlete triad: a form of atypical eating disorder, identified by the Women's Task Force of the American College of Sports Medicine, consisting of three intersecting health problems in young women who exercise prodigiously: (1) insufficient nutrition, (2) menstrual irregularities, and (3) weakened bones.

fluoxetine: antidepressant drug (Prozac) approved for the treatment of bulimia.

food insecurity/security: access to sufficient, safe, nutritious food to maintain a healthy active life.

ghrelin: hormone responsible for feelings of hunger.

heritable: passed along from generation to generation. Eating disorders themselves are not heritable diseases. Neurological, physical, and behavioral traits have characteristics that are due to gene influence inherited from parents and to the context (the surrounding culture and biochemical environment) that forms them.

holistic: a balanced, mind-body approach to the practice of medicine that seeks to address the underlying causes of physical and psychological disease to remedy symptoms.

hormones: specialized protein molecules produced by glands that signal the need for chemical reactions to take place in the body. Examples include insulin/glucagon (digestion), estrogen/testosterone (sexual arousal), melatonin (sleep), leptin/ghrelin (hunger), adrenal corticoids (stress), endorphins (pain control), and oxytocin (love bonding).

hypothalamus: the control station for many autonomic body and brain functions, including hunger, thirst, body temperature, sleepiness/wakefulness. It also commands the pituitary gland, which is essential in producing human growth hormone. The lateral hypothalamus makes us want to eat. The ventromedial hypothalamus lets us know when to stop.

incidence: the actual number or percentage of individuals annually diagnosed with an illness, that is, the number of new cases in a given year.

insulin: hormone secreted by the pancreas when blood sugar levels rise.

integrated approach: practice of medicine and wellness care that involves diverse disciplines, incorporating the health of mind, body, and spirit.

ketones: chemical compound by-product produced in the body as it utilizes fat and protein for energy.

lanugo: fine, soft body hair that develops as a body attempts to conserve heat.

leptin: hormone responsible for feelings of satiety.

limbic system: structures of the brain that deal with emotions, olfaction, learning, and memory. Centers include the amygdale, hypothalamus, hippocampus, corpus callosum, and others.

malnutrition: health condition resulting from a diet that is deficient in nutrients and energy required by the body.

manorexia: misnomer referring to anorexia symptoms in males.

meal support: placing the responsibility for food decisions on someone other than the one eating. Not a method of force feeding, it reduces the trauma of eating for someone afflicted with an eating disorder.

mindful eating: tuning into the body's natural signals to eat when hungry and stop when satisfied.

mood disorder: defective brain activity that upsets our ability to effectively process emotion and modulate feelings. Examples include major depressive disorder, dysthymia, bipolar disorder, and cyclothymia.

neuromodulation: the hormonal activity of certain neurotransmitters, such as dopamine, serotonin, norepinephrine, and acetylcholine, that subtly control feeling phenomena and various mood states of the brain.

neuron: nerve cell. Over 200 different kinds exist throughout our nervous system.

neuroplasticity: the phenomenon of how "practice makes perfect." Specific behavior shapes the brain's chemical response, building neural pathways that are resistant to alteration. Young brains are especially adaptive in this respect, which explains why adolescents are more readily able to learn another language or play an instrument than adults.

neurotransmitters: specialized brain hormones produced by neurons that stimulate or inhibit communication between nerve cells. Common ones include serotonin, dopamine, GABA, acetylcholine, glutamate, aspartate, and norepinephrine.

night eating syndrome: eating condition that compels the sufferer to consume at least half a normal day's calories after dinner and into the night. Many victims also suffer from insomnia, rising in the middle of the night to binge. Some never actually wake, preparing and eating food in their sleep. Also referred to as sleep-eating disorder.

norepinephrine: a substance that is both produced in the brain (the locus coeruleus of the brainstem) as a neurotransmitter and in the body as a hormone (manufactured in the adrenal gland). Helps to regulate mood and stress levels and functions in sleep and learning. Also known as noradrenaline.

normative discontent: the concept that unhappiness and dissatisfaction is so common, the feelings can be considered normal.

nutritional rehabilitation: the process of returning an ED sufferer to a healthful diet that provides energy and nutrients necessary for ongoing recovery. Expert treatment professionals encourage that this take place as quickly as possible.

obesity: ingestion of excess food energy relative to activity level, causing the body to store unused calories as fat.

olanzapine: drug used to treat anorexia because of its effectiveness as an appetite stimulant and inducement for the body to store fat.

opioid: behaving like an opiate, an analgesic compound derived from the opium poppy plant. The substance can cause feelings of intense pleasure because of the cascade effect on dopaminergic neurons. The human brain produces protein compounds (for example, endorphins/enkephalins, dynorphins), which, even though they are shorter lived and less intense than narcotic drugs, might still cause addictive behavior.

orthorexia: disordered eating resulting from compulsions to eat as healthfully as possible, eventually causing overly restrictive eating habits, malnutrition, and usually significant weight loss.

osteopenia: the initial stage of osteoporosis.

osteoporosis: the leaching of calcium from bone when the body needs it for cell use elsewhere. Results in weakening the bones to the point of breakage.

partial syndrome eating disorder: disordered eating patterns that can be considered pathological behavior, but don't meet the full diagnostic criteria for an eating disorder named in the *DSM*.

pathology: signs and symptoms of illness that identify a particular disease, disorder, or syndrome. *Psychopathology* refers to brain chemistry and behavioral aspects that reflect a psychological illness.

peripheral nervous system: nerves of the body, outside the central nervous system, that are able to respond to stimuli in both the internal and external environment.

placebo: a "sugar pill" or "dummy" medication given to some of the subjects in clinical research drug experiments. Because the act of taking medication can have a measurable effect in lessening disease symptoms, placebo-controlled studies are necessary to prove the effectiveness of a new drug therapy.

prevalence: the actual number or percentage of individuals affected by an illness in a given population, that is, how many are suffering at a particular point in time. *Lifetime prevalence* refers to the number of people who are affected at some point in their life.

pro-ana/pro-mia: encouragement of disordered eating and exercise habits as a bona fide lifestyle. Many ED social media sites masquerade as support groups for people with ED behaviors, but are particularly triggering and tend to keep participants from seeking recovery. See *thinspiration ("thinspo")*.

process addiction: addiction to a behavior or activity.

protective factor: specific biological markers and environmental cues that limit vulnerability to developing a disease or disorder.

purge: a means of forcing one's body to eliminate food energy consumed, for the sake of weight control

purging disorder: behavioral condition that compels the sufferer to expel or expend calories through vomiting, the use of laxatives, fasting, extensive exercise, or other extreme behavior. May be identified as a companion syndrome in anorexia; it is devoid of binging behavior.

receptor molecule: protein "locks" that occupy sites along a cell membrane, awaiting stimulation from its special type of hormone.

refeeding: the process of introducing essential and sufficient nutrition to patients who have been starving.

refeeding syndrome: a radical shift in blood mineral levels that leads to heart, liver, and kidney complications during a patient's shift from starvation to normal diet.

relapse: a return of eating disorder symptoms, after a period of improvement.

reuptake: process by which transporter molecules physically pump neurotransmitter from a synapse back into the presynaptic neuron.

risk factors: specific biological markers and environmental pressures that increase the chance that one will develop physical or mental illness. *Protective factors*, conversely, help to prevent the onset of disease or disorder.

selective serotonin reuptake inhibitors (SSRIs): drugs for depression that delay or block transport of serotonin back into the presynaptic nerve cell. Examples are Prozac, Paxil, Zoloft, and Luvox.

serotonin: neurotransmitter produced in the rafae nuclei of the brainstem. Essential for balancing moods, regulating body temperature, sleep, appetite, and pain control.

serotonin norepinephrine reuptake inhibitors (SNRIs): drugs for depression that delay or block transport of serotonin *and* norepinephrine back into the presynaptic nerve cell. Examples are Cymbalta and Effexor.

starvation: the physical state of extreme undernourishment and lack of food energy.

subthreshold binge eating disorder: binge eating disorder that varies from the classically defined categorical symptoms by one or two features; a sufferer, having had bariatric (stomach stapling) surgey, binges on seemingly normal amounts of food.

subthreshold bulimia nervosa: bulimia nervosa that varies from the classically defined categorical symptoms by one or two features; for example, a sufferer whose binge-purge cycles occur less often than once per week.

synapse: intercellular space between the axon of one neuron and the cell body (or dendrite) of another.

thinspiration ("thinspo"): social media content, through both imagery and words, meant to inspire the drive to be thin.

transporter molecule: protein "pack mules" that remove excess transmitter hormone from intercellular space and bring it back to the originating neuron.

trigger/triggering: environmental factor that sets off an eating disorder in someone who is specifically vulnerable to it. Triggers are different for everyone. Something such as looking at pictures of perfected body images can be triggering for some, but not others.

wannarexia: disordered eating that develops in dieting individuals who know some things about anorexia and bulimia and want to acquire an eating disorder by imitating the behaviors.

Notes

Prologue

1. Carolyn Costin, *The Eating Disorder Sourcebook*, 3rd ed. (New York: McGraw Hill, 2007), 2.

---

a. "Weight Loss Market Sheds Some Dollars in 2013" (press release), PRWeb, February 5, 2014, www.prweb.com/releases/2014/02/prweb11554790.htm.

Chapter 1

1. Renfrew Center Foundation for Eating Disorders, *Eating Disorders 101 Guide: A Summary of Issues, Statistics and Resources*, September 2002 (revised October 2003), 2.
2. National Eating Disorders Association (NEDA), "What Are Eating Disorders?" (handout), 2012, 4. Available at www.nationaleatingdisorders.org/sites/default/files/ResourceHandouts/GeneralStatistics.pdf.
3. Cheryl Alkon, "What Is an Eating Disorder?" *Teen Voices Magazine* 3, no. 4 (1994), www.feminist.com/resources/artspeech/body/voices.htm (accessed May 2012).
4. Courtney E. Martin, *Perfect Girls, Starving Daughters: How the Quest for Perfection Is Harming Young Women* (New York: Berkley Books, 2007), 2.
5. According to the American Psychiatric Association (APA) treatment guidelines from 2006 (reconfirmed in 2012), the prognosis for anorexia does not appear to have improved since the 1993 publication. Anorexia is infamous for the rule of thirds—one-third die, one-third recover, and one-third continue to struggle with eating- and weight-related issues, as well as other health conditions, for the rest of their lives.
6. APA, "Practice Guidelines for Eating Disorders," *American Journal of Psychiatry* 150, no. 2 (1993): 212–228. As reported by the Alliance for Eating Disorder Awareness in "Eating Disorder Statistics," 2. Available at www.ndsu.edu/fileadmin/counseling/Eating_Disorder_Statistics.pdf (accessed March 26, 2012).
7. NEDA, "What Are Eating Disorders?" 1.
8. Walter Kaye and Danyale McCurdy, "Prevalence and Correlates of Eating Disorders in Adolescents," *Archives of General Psychiatry* (presently, *JAMA Psychiatry*), 2011: E1–E10. As reported to NEDA, "Prevalence and Correlates of Eating Disorders in Adolescents" (handout), 2012. Available at www.nationaleatingdisorders.org/sites/default/files/ResourceHandouts/PrevalenceAndCorrelatesofEatingDisordersinAdolescents.pdf.
9. Renfrew Center Foundation, *Eating Disorders 101 Guide*, 1.
10. National Association of Anorexia Nervosa and Associated Disorders (ANAD), "Eating Disorders Statistics," www.anad.org/get-information/about-eating-disorders/eating-disorders-statistics/ (accessed May 2012).

11. S. Bryn Austin, Najat J. Ziyadeh, Sara Forman, Lisa A. Prokop, Anne Keliher, and Douglas Jacobs, "Screening High School Students for Eating Disorders: Results of a National Initiative," *Preventing Chronic Disease* 5, no. 4 (October 2008): 1, www.cdc.gov/pcd/issues/2008/oct/pdf/07_0164.pdf (accessed June 2012).

12. Mirasol Eating Disorder Recovery Centers, "Eating Disorder Statistics for Children and Adolescents," www.mirasol.net/eating-disorders/information/eating-disorder-statistics.php (accessed June 2012).

13. Claire Bates, "Half of Anorexia Sufferers 'Develop Eating Disorder by Age of 10,'" *Mail Online*, Health, October 7, 2010, www.dailymail.co.uk/health/article-1318429/Half-anorexia -sufferers-develop-eating-disorder-age-10.html (accessed June 2012).

14. Frédérique R. E. Smink, Daphne van Hoeken, and Hans W. Hoek, "Epidemiology of Eating Disorders: Incidence, Prevalence and Mortality Rates," *Current Psychiatry Reports* 14, no. 1 (May 2012): 412. doi: 10.1007/s11920-012-0282-y.

15. Walter Kaye, "Mortality and Eating Disorders" (handout), NEDA, 2012. Available at www .nationaleatingdisorders.org/sites/default/files/ResourceHandouts/MortalityandEatingDisor- ders.pdf

16. Kathleen Ries Merikangas, Jian-ping He, Marcy Burstein, Sonja A. Swanson, Shelli Ave- nevoli, Lihong Cui, Corina Benjet, Katholiki Georgiades, and Joel Swendsen, "Lifetime Prevalence of Mental Disorders in U.S. Adolescents: Results from the National Comorbid- ity Study-Adolescent Supplement (NCS-A)," *Journal of the American Academy of Child and Adolescent Psychiatry* 49, no. 10 (October 2010): 980–989. doi: 10.1016/j.jaac.2010.05.017.

17. Centers for Disease Control and Prevention (CDC), "Youth Risk Behavior Surveillance— United States, 2011," *Morbidity and Mortality Weekly Report (MMWR)* 61, no. 4 (June 8, 2012): 39. Available at www.cdc.gov/mmwr/pdf/ss/ss6104.pdf.

18. Dianne Neumark-Sztainer, *I'm, Like, SO Fat! Helping Your Teen Make Healthy Choices about Eating and Exercise in a Weight-Obsessed World* (New York: Guilford Press, 2005), as noted in NEDA, "What Are Eating Disorders?"

19. Daniel Eisenberg, Emily Nicklett, Kathryn Roeder, and Nina Kirz, "Eating Disorder Symp- toms among College Students: Prevalence, Persistence, Correlates, and Treatment-Seeking," *Journal of American College Health* 59, no. 8 (September 2011): 700–707. dx.doi.org/10.1080 /07448481.2010.546461.

20. NEDA, "National Eating Disorders Association Announces Results of College Survey" (press release), February 25, 2013, www.nationaleatingdisorders.org/national-eating-disorders -association-announces-results-college-survey (accessed September 2013).

21. ANAD, "Eating Disorders Statistics (Students)," National Association of Anorexia Nervosa and Associated Disorders 10-Year Study, 2000. www.anad.org/get-information/about-eating -disorders/eating-disorders-statistics/ (accessed May 2012).

22. Eisenberg et al., "Eating Disorder Symptoms," 705.

23. NEDA Parent, Family and Friends Network, "Eating Disorders in the *DSM-5*: Implications of Changes in the Diagnostics Categories and Criteria" (webinar). Conducted by B. Timothy Walsh, MD, Evelyn Attia, MD, Stephen Wonderlich, PhD, for PFN, Network of the National Eating Disorders Association, May 30, 2013.

24. Ruth (the author), June 5, 2012.

25. B. Timothy Walsh, "Eating Disorders in Adolescents: Strategies for the Primary Care Pro- vider—Focus on Anorexia Nervosa and *DSM-5*" (webinar). TeenScreen National Center for Mental Health Checkups at Columbia University, January 12, 2012.

26. APA, *Diagnostic and Statistical Manual of Mental Disorders*, 5th ed. (Washington, D.C.: Author, 2013), as presented in NEDA Parent, Family and Friends Network, "Eating Disorders in the *DSM-5*."

27. Robert Frederich, Shousheng Hu, Nancy Raymond, and Claire Pomeroy, "Leptin in Anorexia Nervosa and Bulimia Nervosa: Importance of Assay Technique and Method of Interpretation," *Journal of Laboratory and Clinical Medicine (Translational Research)* 139, no. 2 (February 2002): 72. doi:10.1067/mlc.2002.121014.

28. Andrew J. Brown, "Low-Carb Diets, Fasting and Euphoria: Is There a Link between Ketosis and γ-hydroxybutyrate (GHB)?" *Medical Hypotheses* 68, no. 2 (October 2007): 269. doi:10.1016/j.mehy.2006.07.043.

29. APA, *"DSM-5" Development*. Previously available at www.dsm5.org/ProposedRevision/Pages/proposedrevision.aspx?rid=25 (accessed June 2012).

30. Jordana, "Jordana," in *Thin*, by Lauren Greenfield (San Francisco: Chronicle Books with Melcher Media, 2006), 130.

31. Frederich et al., "Leptin in Anorexia Nervosa," 72.

32. Michael Strober, Roberta Freeman, Carlyn Lampert, Jane Diamond, and Walter Kaye, "Controlled Family Study of Anorexia Nervosa and Bulimia Nervosa: Evidence of Shared Liability and Transmission of Partial Syndromes," *American Journal of Psychiatry* 157, no. 3 (March 1, 2000): 393–401. doi:10.1176/appi.ajp.157.3.393.

33. Juvenile Diabetes Research Foundation, "Diabulimia: Skipping Insulin to Lose Weight," *Countdown*, December 18, 2008, jdrf.org/blog/2008/diabulimia-skipping-insulin-to-lose-weight/ (accessed July 2012).

34. Weight Information Network, "Binge Eating Disorder," NIH Publication No. 04–3589, National Institutes of Health (Washington, D.C.: U.S. Department of Health and Human Services, June 2008 [updated December 2012]). Available at win.niddk.nih.gov/publications/PDFs/bingedis10.04.pdf.

35. "Ben and Josh." *Intervention*, season 4, episode 55, January 21, 2008, GRB Entertainment for A&E TV Networks, www.aetv.com/intervention/episode-guide/season-4.

36. Carolyn Costin, *The Eating Disorder Sourcebook*, 3rd ed. (New York: McGraw-Hill, 2007), 14.

37. APA, *"DSM-5" Development*.

38. Cheryl D. Fryar, Margaret D. Carroll, and Cynthia L. Ogden, "Prevalence of Obesity among Children and Adolescents: United States, Trends 1963–1965 through 2009–2010," NCHS Health E-Stat (Hyattsville, Md.: National Center for Health Statistics, September 2012), 3. Available at www.cdc.gov nchs/data/hestat/obesity_child_09_10/obesity_child_09_10.pdf.

39. Standard labels for *overweight*, *obese*, and *morbidly obese* depend on the scale of measurement. For this book, consider *overweight* to refer to any amount of pounds or body fat over one's ideal weight. Consider *obese* to mean extra body fat 20 percent or more above normal, and *morbidly obese* as having 50 percent extra body fat, or one hundred plus pounds over ideal weight.

40. Sara Selis, "Binge Eating Disorder: Surprisingly Common, Seriously Under-treated," *Psychiatric Times*, April 3, 2007. Available at www.psychiatrictimes.com/articles/binge-eating-disorder-surprisingly-common-seriously-under-treated.

41. James I. Hudson, Eva Hiripi, Harrison G. Pope Jr., and Ronald C. Kessler, "The Prevalence and Correlates of Eating Disorders in the National Comorbidity Survey Replication," *Biological Psychiatry* 61, no. 3 (February 2007): 348–358. doi: 10.1016/j.biopsych.2006.03.040.

42. Peter Lewinsohn, Ruth Striegel-Moore, and John Seeley, "Epidemiology and Natural Course of Eating Disorders in Young Women from Adolescence to Young Adulthood," *Journal of the*

American Academy of Child & Adolescent Psychiatry 39, no. 10 (October 2000): 1284–1292. doi:10.1097/00004583-200010000-00016.

43. Ruth Striegel-Moore, John Seeley, and Peter Lewinsohn, "Psychosocial Adjustment in Young Adulthood of Women Who Experienced an Eating Disorder During Adolescence," *Journal of the American Academy of Child and Adolescent Psychiatry* 42, no. 5 (May 2003): 587–593. doi:10.1097/01.CHI.0000046838.90931.44.

44. Austin et al., "Screening High School Students," 2.

45. Renfrew Center Foundation, *Eating Disorders 101 Guide*, 1.

a. Mark Moran, "Binge Eating Disorder May Be Added to *DSM-5*," *Psychiatric News*, Clinical and Research News 47, no.1 (January 6, 2012), psychnews.psychiatryonline.org/newsarticle.aspx?articleid=181255 (accessed May 2012).

b. Carol L. Otis, Barbara Drinkwater, Mimi Johnson, Anne Loucks, and Jack Wilmore, "ACSM Position Stand: The Female Athlete Triad," *Medicine & Science in Sports & Exercise* 29, no. 5 (May 1997): i–ix, cscca.org/document/acsmposition (accessed July 2012).

c. Ruth (the author), May 15, 2012.

d. National Institute on Drug Abuse, "DrugFacts: Club Drugs (GHB, Ketamine, and Rohypnol)," Publications, DrugFacts Series, National Institutes of Health, revised July 2010, (Washington, D.C.: U.S. Department of Health and Human Services, 2013). Available at www.drugabuse.gov/sites/default/files/clubdrugs10.pdf.

e. National Heart, Lung and Blood Institute, "Sleep Apnea Linked to Increased Risk of Death," News and Reports, Press Releases, National Institutes of Health (Washington, D.C.: U.S. Department of Health and Human Services, August 2008). Available at www.nhlbi.nih.gov/news/press-releases/2008/nhlbi-media-availability-sleep-apnea-linked-to-increased-risk-of-death.html.

f. American Academy of Sleep Medicine, "Sleep Apnea Increases Your Risk of Death," August 2008, yoursleep.aasmnet.org/article.aspx?id=1017 (accessed June 2012).

g. Alkon, "What Is an Eating Disorder?"

h. "Rickywayne / Jessica (Texas)," *Heavy*, season 1, episode 2, January 24, 2011, A&E TV Networks, www.aetv.com/heavy/episode-guide.

i. Katherine McNeil, reader comment to Shirley S. Wang, "Parental Role Aids Anorexia Recovery," *Wall Street Journal*, Business, October 5, 2010, online.wsj.com/community/33f33fd4-9125-40c4-8bc1-63ba36dd7800/activity (accessed July 2012).

Chapter 2

1. G. Terence Wilson, "Eating Disorder, Obesity and Addiction," *European Eating Disorders Review* 18, no. 5 (September–October 2010): 341–351. doi: 10.1002/erv.1048. (With grateful appreciation to Michael P. Levine, PhD.)

2. Gabor Maté, *In the Realm of Hungry Ghosts: Close Encounters with Addiction* (Berkeley, Calif.: North Atlantic Books, 2010), 154.

3. Bruno Dubuc, "Anxiety Neurotransmitters," The Brain from Top to Bottom, Emotions and the Brain, Fear, Anxiety and Anguish (Intermediate Level), thebrain.mcgill.ca (accessed August 2012).

4. John Heminway, *Stress: Portrait of a Killer*, a co-production of National Geographic Television and Stanford University, 2008, killerstress.stanford.edu and www.pbs.org/programs/killer-stress.

5. "Understanding Stress" (supporting video clip), *This Emotional Life*, a production of NOVA and Vulcan Productions with Kunhardt McGee Productions, 2009, video.pbs.org/video/1218735872 (accessed August 2012).

6. National Institute of Mental Health, "Anxiety Disorders," NIH Publication No. 09-3879, *National Institutes of Health* (Washington, D.C.: U.S. Department of Health and Human Services, 2009), 1. Available at www.nimh.nih.gov/health/publications/anxiety-disorders/nimhanxiety.pdf.

7. American Psychiatric Association Practice Guidelines, "Treatment of Patients with Eating Disorders, Third Edition, Part B," *American Journal of Psychiatry* 163 (supplement) (May 2006; AHRQ panel reviewed and revalidated, 2011). doi: 10.1176/appi.books .9780890423363.138660.

8. Marilyn Arce, Vasiliki Michopoulos, Kathryn N. Shepard, Quynh-Chau Ha, and Mark E. Wilson, "Diet Choice, Cortisol Reactivity, and Emotional Feeding in Socially Housed Rhesus Monkeys," *Physiology & Behavior* 101, no. 4 (November 2, 2010): 446–455. doi: 10.1016/j.physbeh.2010.07.010.

9. Maté, *In the Realm of Hungry Ghosts*, 167.

10. Carlo Colantuoni, Pedro Rada, Joseph McCarthy, Caroline Patten, Nicole M. Avena, Andrew Chadeayne, and Bartley G. Hoebel, "Evidence That Intermittent, Excessive Sugar Intake Causes Endogenous Opioid Dependence," *Obesity Research* 10, no. 6 (June 2002): 478–488. doi: 10.1038/oby.2002.66.

11. "Jill/Johnny (South Carolina)," *Heavy*, season 1, episode 7, February 28, 2011, A&E TV Networks, www.aetv.com/heavy/episode-guide.

12. "Jill/Johnny (South Carolina)."

13. "Jill/Johnny (South Carolina)."

14. "Jill/Johnny (South Carolina)."

15. Maté, *In the Realm of Hungry Ghosts*, 224.

16. Maté, *In the Realm of Hungry Ghosts*, 137, 158, 224.

17. Maté, *In the Realm of Hungry Ghosts*, 147.

18. Carolyn Costin, *The Eating Disorder Sourcebook: A Comprehensive Guide to the Causes, Treatments and Prevention of Eating Disorders*, 3rd ed. (New York: McGraw-Hill, 2007), 4.

---

a. "Ben and Josh," *Intervention*, season 4, episode 55, January 21, 2008, GRB Entertainment for A&E TV Networks, www.aetv.com/intervention/episode-guide/season-4.

b. Josh, "Josh's Story" (video clip), Turning Point of Tampa, Inc., www.tpoftampa.com/programs/eating-disorders.html (accessed August 2012).

c. "Ben and Josh."

d. Josh, "Josh's Story."

e. "Ben and Josh."

f. Kelly M., personal communication, May 30, 2012.

g. Paul Johnson and Paul J. Kenny, "Dopamine D2 Receptors in Addiction-Like Reward Dysfunction and Compulsive Eating in Obese Rats," *Nature Neuroscience* 13, no. 5 (May 2010): 635–641. doi:10.1038/nn.2519.

h. U.S. Department of Energy, Brookhaven National Laboratory, "Binge Eaters' Dopamine Levels Spike at Sight, Smell of Food," *ScienceDaily*, Science News, February 28, 2011, www.sciencedaily.com/releases/2011/02/110228104308.htm (accessed August 2012).

i. Ashley N. Gearhardt, Sonja Yokum, Patrick T. Orr, Eric Stice, William R. Corbin, and Kelly D. Brownell, "Neural Correlates of Food Addiction," *Archives of General Psychiatry* (presently *JAMA Psychiatry*) 68, no. 8 (August 2011): 808–816. doi:10.1001/archgenpsychiatry.2011.32.

j. Joan Arehart-Treichel, "Overeating Is an Addiction, Brain Imaging Shows," *Psychiatric News*, Clinical and Research News, 46, no. 18 (September 16, 2011), psychnews.psychiatry online.org/newsarticle.aspx?articleid=116627 (accessed August 2012).

k. "Laurie and Jessie," *Intervention*, season 2, episode 33, December 10, 2006, GRB Entertainment for A&E TV Networks, www.aetv.com/intervention/episode-guide/season-2. All quotes in this sidebar come from this episode.

l. Bruno Dubuc, "Molecules That Reduce Pain," The Brain from Top to Bottom, Pleasure and Pain, Avoiding Pain (Beginner Level), thebrain.mcgill.ca (accessed August 2012).

m. Ellen Kuwana, "Discovering the Sweet Mysteries of Chocolate," *Neuroscience for Kids*, October 1, 2010, faculty.washington.edu/chudler/choco.html (accessed August 2012).

n. National Public Radio, "Getting Old Is Hard, Even (and Especially) for Models," *Fresh Air*, WHYY-FM, July 30, 2012. Transcript available at www.npr.org/2012/07/30/157590245/getting-old-is-hard-even-and-especially-for-models.

o. Kelly M., personal communication, May 30, 2012.

Chapter 3

1. Larkin McPhee, *Dying to Be Thin*, a NOVA Production by Twin Cities Public Television, Inc., for WGBH/Boston, 2000. Transcript available at www.pbs.org/wgbh/nova/body/dying-to-be-thin.html.

2. Katherine A. Halmi, Suzanne R. Sunday, Michael Strober, Alan Kaplan, D. Blake Woodside, Manfred Fichter, Janet Treasure, Wade H. Berrettini, and Walter H. Kaye, "Perfectionism in Anorexia Nervosa: Variation by Clinical Subtype, Obsessionality, and Pathological Eating Behavior," *American Journal of Psychiatry* 157, no. 11 (November 1, 2000): 1799–1805. doi:10.1176/appi.ajp.157.11.1799.

3. Cynthia M. Bulik, Federica Tozzi, Charles Anderson, Suzanne E. Mazzeo, Steve Aggen, and Patrick F. Sullivan, "The Relation between Eating Disorders and Components of Perfectionism," *American Journal of Psychiatry* 160, no. 2 (February 1, 2003): 366–368. doi:10.1176/appi.ajp.160.2.366.

4. "VCU Study Links Perfectionist Trait and Eating Disorders," VCU News Services, Virginia Commonwealth University, February 1, 2003, www.govrel.vcu.edu/news/Releases/2003/jan/013103.html (accessed September 2012).

5. "VCU Study."

6. Catherine M. Shisslak, Marjorie Crago, and Linda S. Estes, "The Spectrum of Eating Disturbances," *International Journal of Eating Disorders* 18, no. 3 (November 1995): 209–219. doi: 10.1002/1098-108X(199511)18:3<209::AID-EAT2260180303>3.0.CO;2-E.

7. Ruth (the author), September 8, 2012.

8. "Photographer Records Women Dying to Be Thin" (video clip), Meredith Viera interview with Lauren Greenfield and Nancy Etkoff, *Today: Books*, Wednesday, November 8, 2006, today.msnbc.msn.com/id/15613726 (accessed September 2012).

9. CASAColumbia®, *Food for Thought: Substance Abuse and Eating Disorders* (New York: National Center on Addiction and Substance Abuse at Columbia University, 2003), ii.

10. Sara Dingle, "Eating Disorder Genes Triggered by Dieting," *World Today* (ABC News), August 21, 2012, www.abc.net.au/worldtoday/content/2012/s3572329.htm (accessed September 2012).

11. "Laurie and Jessie," *Intervention*, season 2, episode 33, December 10, 2006, GRB Entertainment for A&E TV Networks, www.aetv.com/intervention/episode-guide/season-2.
12. "Amy P.," *Intervention*, season 7, episode 115, April 19, 2010, GRB Entertainment for A&E TV Networks, www.aetv.com/intervention/episode-guide/season-7.
13. "Laurie and Jessie."
14. "Amy P."
15. Tami Roblek and Guido K. W. Frank, "Intolerance of Uncertainty: A Risk Factor in the Development of Anxiety and Eating Disorders," *Eating Disorders Review* 23, no. 1 (January–February 2012). Available at eatingdisordersreview.com/nl/nl_edr_23_1_1.html.
16. Ronald C. Kessler, Patricia A. Berglund, Olga Demler, Robert Jin, Kathleen R. Merikangas, and Ellen E. Walters, "Lifetime Prevalence and Age-of-Onset Distributions of *DSM-IV* Disorders in the National Comorbidity Survey Replication (NCS-R)," *Archives of General Psychiatry* (presently, *JAMA Psychiatry*) 62, no. 6 (June 2005): 593–602. doi:10.1001/archpsyc.62.6.593.
17. National Institute of Mental Health, "National Survey Confirms That Youth Are Disproportionately Affected by Mental Disorders," *Science News*, September 27, 2010, www.nimh.nih.gov/news/science-news/2010/national-survey-confirms-that-youth-are-disproportionately-affected-by-mental-disorders.shtml (accessed September 2012).
18. National Institutes of Health, "Mood Disorders," *Research Portfolio Online Reporting Tools (RePORT)*, Fact Sheet (Washington, D.C.: U.S. Department of Health and Human Services, updated October 2010). Available at report.nih.gov/NIHfactsheets/Pdfs/MoodDisorders(NIMH).pdf.
19. World Health Organization, "Global Burden of Disease, 2004 Update," WHO Department of Health Statistics and Informatics, 2008, 51. Available at www.who.int/healthinfo/global_burden_disease/GBD_report_2004update_full.pdf.
20. Colette Boucher, "Serotonin: 9 Questions and Answers," WebMD, 2008 (reviewed October 12, 2011), www.webmd.com/depression/features/serotonin (accessed September, 2012).
21. McPhee, *Dying to Be Thin*.
22. Walter Kaye and Michael Strober, "Serotonin: Implications for the Etiology & Treatment of Eating Disorders," *Eating Disorders Review* 10, no. 3 (May–June 1999). Available at eatingdisordersreview.com/nl/nl_edr_10_3_1.html.
23. McPhee, *Dying to Be Thin*.
24. "Photographer Records Women."
25. "Amy P."
26. McPhee, *Dying to Be Thin*.
27. Timothy Brewerton, MD, DFAPA, FAED, DFAACAP, personal communication, July 14, 2013.

---

a. McPhee, *Dying to Be Thin*.
b. American Medical Association, "EPoCH CME: Screening and Managing Eating Disorders in Primary Practice" (online training manual), *Resources*, released April 9, 2012, expires April 9, 2014, www.ama-cmeonline.com/eating_disorders (accessed May 18, 2013).
c. CASAColumbia, *Food for Thought*, i.
d. Substance Abuse and Mental Health Services Administration, "Clients with Substance Use and Eating Disorders," *SAMHSA Advisory* 10, no. 1 (Washington, D.C.: U.S. Department of Health and Human Services, February 2011), 4. Available at store.samhsa.gov/shin/content/SMA10-4617/SMA10-4617.pdf.

e. Emily M. Pisetsky, Y. May Chao, Lisa C. Dierker, Alexis M. May, and Ruth H. Striegel-Moore, "Disordered Eating and Substance Use in High-School Students: Results from the Youth Risk Behavior Surveillance System," *International Journal of Eating Disorders* 41, no. 5 (July 2008): 464. doi: 10.1002/eat.20520.

f. Prader-Willi Syndrome Association, "What Is Prader-Willi Syndrome?" *Be Informed*, 2012, www.pwsausa.org/syndrome/index.htm (accessed November 12, 2012).

g. The Committee on Genetics, "Clinical Report: Health Supervision for Children with Prader-Willi Syndrome," *Journal of the American Academy of Pediatrics* 127, no. 1 (January 1, 2011): 199. doi: 10.1542/peds.2010-2820.

h. The Committee on Genetics, "Clinical Report," 203.

i. Barton J. Blinder, Edward J. Cumella, and Visant A. Sanathara, "Psychiatric Comorbidities of Female Inpatients with Eating Disorders," *Psychosomatic Medicine, Journal of Biobehavioral Medicine* 68, no. 3 (May 2006): 454–462. doi: 10.1097/01.psy.0000221254.77675.f5.

j. Walter H. Kaye, Cynthia M. Bulik, Laura Thornton, Nicole Barbarich, Kim Masters, and the Price Foundation Collaborative Group, "Comorbidity of Anxiety Disorders with Anorexia and Bulimia Nervosa," *American Journal of Psychiatry* 161, no. 12 (December 2004): 2215–2221. doi: 10.1176/appi.ajp.161.12.2215.

Chapter 4

1. David Grubin, *The Buddha: The Story of Siddhartha*, David Grubin Productions for PBS in conjunction with the exhibition, Pilgrimage and Buddhist Art, Asia Society Museum, New York, 2010, www.pbs.org/thebuddha.

2. Henri Chabrol, Stacey Callahan, and Sean O'Halloran, "The Pressure to Be Thin on Adolescent Girls in Ancient Rome," *Journal of the American Academy of Child & Adolescent Psychiatry* 39, no. 11 (November 2000): 1345. doi:10.1097/00004583-200011000-00007. As reviewed in vaughanbell, "Size Zero Culture in Ancient Rome," *Mind Hacks* (blog), October 22, 2009, mindhacks.com/~/size-zero-culture-in-ancient-rome (accessed November 2012).

3. Harriet Brown, *Brave Girl Eating: A Family's Struggle with Anorexia* (New York: William Morrow, 2010), 98.

4. Barton J. Blinder and Karin H. Chao, "Bulimia Nervosa/Obesity: A Historical Overview," in *Understanding Eating Disorders: Anorexia Nervosa, Bulimia Nervosa, and Obesity*, ed. LeeAnn Alexander-Mott and D. Barry Lumsden (Washington, D.C.: Taylor & Francis, 1994), 17. Available at www.ltspeed.com/bjblinder/publications/bulimiahistory.htm.

5. Mario Redo and Giuseppe Sacco, "Anorexia and the Holiness of Saint Catherine of Siena," trans. Graeme Newman, *Journal of Criminal Justice and Popular Culture* 8, no. 1 (2001): 44, www.albany.edu/scj/jcjpc/vol8is1/reda.html (accessed November 2012).

6. Hyder E. Rollins, "Notes on Some English Accounts of Miraculous Fasts," *Journal of American Folklore* 34 (Champaign: University of Illinois Press, 1921), 361. Available at www.jstor.org/stable/534924.

7. Rollins, "Notes on Some English Accounts," 357.

8. Rollins, "Notes on Some English Accounts," 367.

9. Rollins, "Notes on Some English Accounts," 372.

10. Richard Morton, *Phthisiologia: Or a Treatise of Consumptions, Wherein the Difference, Nature, Causes, Signs and Cure of All Sorts of Consumptions Are Explained*, Book I, 2nd. ed. (London:

Printed for W. and J. Inneys at the Prince's Arms, the West end of St Paul's Churchyard, 1694), 8–9. Available at www.collegeofphysicians.org/hmdlsubweb/catalogue.htm.

11. Morton, *Phthisiologia*, 10.
12. Morton, *Phthisiologia*, 4.
13. Sir William Withey Gull, *A Collection of the Published Writings of William Withey Gull, M.D.*, volume CXLVII, ed. Theodore Dyke Acland (London: New Sydenham Society, 1874), 310. Available at archive.org/details/collectionofpubl01gulluoft.
14. Gull, *Collection*, 310.
15. "Succi's Long Fast—the Italian Says That He Will Go without Food for 45 Days," *New York Times*, November 6, 1890.
16. "Succi Breaks His Fast—Forty-five Long Days He Has Lived on Air and Water," *New York Times*, December 21, 1890.
17. M. K. Gandhi, *An Autobiography: The Story of My Experiments with Truth*, trans. Mahadev Desai (Boston: Beacon Press, 1957), 418–420.
18. Sharman Apt Russell, *Hunger: An Unnatural History* (New York: Basic Books, 2005), 86.
19. Hillel Schwartz, *Never Satisfied: A Cultural History of Diets, Fantasies, and Fat* (New York: Free Press, 1986), 183, as cited in Leigh Ann Love, "The Diet Culture Phenomenon and Its Effect on the United States Orange Juice Industry" (unpublished thesis, University of Florida, 2005), 6.
20. Michele Leight, "The Model as Muse: Embodying Fashion, Metropolitan Museum of Art, May 6 to August 9, 2009," *City Review*, Style, June 29, 2009, www.thecityreview.com/modelmuse.html (accessed November 2012).
21. Martin Beckford, "Sister of Tragic 'Size Zero' Model Found Dead," *Telegraph*, UK News, February 15, 2007, www.telegraph.co.uk/news/uknews/1542707/Sister-of-tragic-size-zero-model-found-dead.html (accessed November 2012).
22. Louisa Barnett, "Twiggy Lashes Out at 'Size Zero' Actresses," *Mail Online*, News, November 19, 2006, www.dailymail.co.uk/news/article-417254/Twiggy-lashes-size-zero-actresses.html (accessed November 2012).
23. Kent Demaret, "Psychiatrist Hilde Bruch Saves Anorexia Nervosa Patients from Starving Themselves to Death" (archived article), *People* 9, no. 25 (June 26, 1978), www.people.com/people/archive/article/0,,20071146,00.html (accessed November 2012).
24. National Association of Anorexia Nervosa and Associated Disorders (ANAD), "ANAD's Beginnings," www.anad.org/get-information/about-anad/history (accessed November 2012).
25. Terence M. O'Keefe, "Suicide and Self-Starvation," *Philosophy* 59, no. 229 (New York: Cambridge University Press, 1984), 349. Available at www.jstor.org/stable/3750951.
26. Russell, *Hunger*, 164, 251.
27. Richard Carpenter (with Suzanne Adelson), "A Brother Remembers: An Account of Karen Carpenter's Brave Battle over the Years against Anorexia Nervosa" (archived article), *People* 20, no. 21 (November 21, 1983), www.people.com/people/archive/article/0,,20198418,00.html (accessed November 2012).
28. Randy L. Schmidt, *Little Girl Blue: The Life of Karen Carpenter* (Chicago: Chicago Review Press, 2010), 283.
29. Schmidt, *Little Girl Blue*, 285.
30. "Among the Beautiful People," *People*, Celebrity Central, Kate Moss: Biography, May 1993, www.people.com/people/kate_moss/biography (accessed November 2012).
31. James Fox, "The Riddle of Kate Moss," *Vanity Fair*, no. 628 (December 2012), 168.

32. Fox, "The Riddle of Kate Moss," 168.

33. Jesse McKinley, "A Magician Seeking Simplicity in a Cage," *New York Times*, Arts, August 19, 2003, www.nytimes.com/2003/08/19/arts/a-magician-seeking-simplicity-in-a-cage.html (accessed November 2012).

34. "World Record Set with 49-Day Fast," *Epoch Times*, May 18, 2004, www.theepochtimes .com/news/4-5-18/21492.html (accessed November 2012).

35. Binge Eating Disorder Association, "New Association Serves Binge Eating Disorder Community" (press release), bedaonline.com, September 11, 2008 (accessed November 2012).

36. Karen Kersting, "An Evolutionary Explanation for Anorexia?" *Monitor on Psychology* 35, no. 4 (April 2004): 22, www.apa.org/monitor/apr04/anorexia.aspx (accessed November 2012).

37. Kersting, "An Evolutionary Explanation for Anorexia?" 22.

38. Kersting, "An Evolutionary Explanation for Anorexia?" 22.

---

a. Carol Lawson, "Anorexia: It's Not A New Disease," *New York Times*, Style, December 8, 1985, www.nytimes.com/1985/12/08/style/anorexia-it-s-not-a-new-disease.html (accessed November 2012).

b. Joan Jacobs Brumberg, "Chlorotic Girls, 1870–1920: A Historical Perspective on Female Adolescence," *Child Development* 53 (December 1982): 1469.

c. W. K. Stewart and Laura W. Fleming, "Features of a Successful Therapeutic Fast of 382 Days Duration," *Postgraduate Medical Journal* 49 (March 1973): 203. doi:10.1136/pgmj.49.569.203.

d. National Eating Disorder Information Centre, "Adults," Statistics Archive, 2012. nedic.ca/ statistics-archive (accessed November 2012).

e. Ann M. Gustafson-Larson and Rhonda D. Terry, "Weight-Related Behaviors and Concerns of Fourth-Grade Children," *Journal of the American Dietetic Association* (presently, *Journal of the Academy of Nutrition and Dietetics*) 92, no. 7 (July 1992): 818–822. PMID:1624650.

f. Laurel M. Mellin, Charles E. Irwin, and Sarah Scully, "Disordered Eating Characteristics in Girls: A Survey of Middle Class Children," *Journal of the American Dietetic Association* (presently, *Journal of the Academy of Nutrition and Dietetics*) 92, no. 7 (July 1992): 851–853. PMID:1624655.

g. Adolescent Medicine Committee, Canadian Paediatric Society, "Eating Disorders in Adolescents: Principles of Diagnosis and Treatment," *Paediatrics and Child Health* 3, no. 3 (May–June 1998): 189–192. PMID:20401245.

h. Julie K. I. Dam, "How Do I Look?"(archived article) *People* 54, no. 10 (September 4, 2000), www.people.com/people/archive/article/0,,20132200,00.html (accessed November 2012).

i. Mike Adams, "U.S. Weight Loss Market Worth $46.3 Billion in 2004—Forecast to Reach $61 Billion by 2008," *NaturalNews.com*, March 30, 2005, www.naturalnews.com/006133.html (accessed November 2012).

j. Yafu Zhao and William Encinosa, "Hospitalizations for Eating Disorders from 1999 to 2006," *HCUP Statistical Brief #70* (Rockville, Md.: U.S. Department of Health and Human Services, April 2009), 1. Available at www.hcup-us.ahrq.gov/reports/statbriefs/sb70.pdf.

k. Yafu Zhao and William Encinosa, "An Update on Hospitalizations for Eating Disorders, 1999 to 2009," *HCUP Statistical Brief #120* (Rockville, Md.: U.S. Department of Health and Human Services, September 2011), 1. Available at www.hcup-us.ahrq.gov/reports/statbriefs/ sb120.pdf.

l. World Health Organization, "Obesity and Overweight." Media Centre Fact Sheet No.311, May 2012 (updated March 2013), www.who.int/mediacentre/factsheets/fs311/en (accessed November 2012).

Chapter 5

1. National Eating Disorders Association (NEDA), "Males and Eating Disorders: Research" (handout), 2012, 1. Available at www.nationaleatingdisorders.org/sites/default/files/ResourceHandouts/ResearchonMalesandEatingDisorders.pdf.

2. NEDA Parent, Family and Friends Network, "Males with Eating Disorders: An Update" (webinar), conducted by Theodore Weltzin, MD, with panelists Troy Roness, Ron Saxen, and Chris Skarinka, July 31, 2012.

3. "Men and Binge Eating Disorder" (video clip), Tanya Rivero interview with Ron Saxen, *ABC News: Healthy Living*, November 1, 2011, abcnews.go.com/Health/video/binge-eating-disorder-14861041 (accessed December 2012).

4. Ruth Striegel-Moore, Richard Bedrosian, Chun Wang, and Steven Schwartz, "Why Men Should Be Included in Research on Binge-Eating," *International Journal of Eating Disorders* 45, no. 2 (March 2012), 233. doi: 10.1002eat.20962.

5. The Alliance for Eating Disorder Awareness, "Males and Eating Disorders," www.allianceforeatingdisorders.com/portal/males-and-eating-disorders (accessed December 2012).

6. Tracey D. Wade, Anna Keski-Rahkonen, and James Hudson, "Epidemiology of Eating Disorders," in *Textbook in Psychiatric Epidemiology*, 3rd ed., ed. M. Tsuang and M. Tohen (New York: Wiley, 2011), 343, as noted in NEDA, "What Are Eating Disorders?" (handout), 2012. Available at www.nationaleatingdisorders.org/sites/default/files/ResourceHandouts/GeneralStatistics.pdf.

7. Renfrew Center Foundation for Eating Disorders, *Eating Disorders 101 Guide: A Summary of Issues, Statistics and Resources*, September 2002 (revised October 2003), 3.

8. Columbia University Mailman School of Public Health, "According to Study, Gay and Bisexual Men Have Significantly Higher Prevalence of Eating Disorders than Heterosexual Men," *At The Frontline* 2, no. 2, May 2007, www.mailmanschool.org/e-newsletter/AtTheFrontline-vol2no2/Pdf/Re-GBLeatingdisorders.pdf (accessed December 2012).

9. NEDA, "Males and Eating Disorders: Research," 3.

10. Christopher Hines, *The Adonis Factor*, Rogue Culture Productions, 2010, www.theadonisfactor.com.

11. Hines, *The Adonis Factor*.

12. Hines, *The Adonis Factor*.

13. Hines, *The Adonis Factor*.

14. Hines, *The Adonis Factor*.

15. Amy Norton, "Gay, Bisexual Teens at Risk for Eating Disorders," *Reuters Health*, September 19, 2009, www.reuters.com/article/2009/09/17/us-eating-disorders-idUSTRE58G68G20090917 (accessed December 2012).

16. S. Bryn Austin, Najat J. Ziyadeh, Heather L. Corliss, Margaret Rosario, David Wypij, Jess Haines, Carlos A. Camargo Jr., and Alison E. Field, "Sexual Orientation Disparities in Purging and Binge Eating from Early to Late Adolescence," *Journal of Adolescent Health* 45, no. 3 (September 2009): 238. doi: 10.1016/j.jadohealth.2009.02.001.

17. Eric Stice, C. Nathan Marti, and Shelley Durant, "Risk Factors for Onset of Eating Disorders: Evidence of Multiple Risk Pathways from an 8-Year Prospective Study," *Behavior Research and Therapy* 49, no. 10 (October 2011): 622–627. doi: 10.1016/j.brat2011.06.009 9. (With grateful appreciation to Carolyn Costin.)

18. Daniel Clay, Vivian L. Vignoles, and Helga Dittmar, "Body Image and Self-Esteem among Adolescent Girls: Testing the Influence of Sociocultural Factors," *Journal of Research on Adolescence* 15, no. 4 (November 2005): 452. doi: 10.1111/j.1532-7795.2005.00107.x.

19. Connect with Kids, *Mirror, Mirror: Topic—Body Image* (educational DVD), CWK Network, Inc., 2004, connectwithkids.com.

20. American Society of Plastic Surgeons, "2011 Plastic Surgery Procedural Statistics," 2012, www.plasticsurgery.org/Documents/news-resources/statistics/2011-statistics/2011_Stats_Full_Report.pdf (accessed January 2013).

21. Connect with Kids, *Mirror, Mirror.*

22. Laurel M. Mellin, Charles E. Irwin, and Sarah Scully, "Prevalence of Disordered Eating Characteristics in Girls: A Survey of Middle Class Children," *Journal of the American Dietetic Association* 92, no. 7 (July 1992): 851–853.

23. Marya Hornbacher, *Wasted: A Memoir of Anorexia and Bulimia* (New York: HarperCollins, 1998), 13.

24. Jennifer A. O'Dea and Suzanne Abraham, "Eating and Exercise Disorders in Young College Men," *Journal of American College Health* 50, no. 6 (May 2002): 275. doi: 10.1080/07448480209603445.

25. NEDA Parents, Friends and Family Network, "Males with Eating Disorders."

26. "Amy P.," *Intervention*, season 7, episode 115, April 19, 2010, GRB Entertainment for A&E TV Networks, www.aetv.com/intervention/episode-guide/season-7.

27. Darryl Roberts, *America the Beautiful 2: The Thin Commandments*, Harley Boy Entertainment, 2010, www.americathebeautifuldoc.com.

28. Roberts, *America the Beautiful 2.*

29. Roberts, *America the Beautiful 2.*

30. Adrian Furnham, Nicolla Badmin, and Ian Sneade. "Body Image Dissatisfaction: Gender Differences in Eating Attitudes, Self-Esteem, and Reasons for Exercise," *Journal of Psychology* 136, no. 6 (November 2002): 593. doi: 10.1080/00223980209604820.

31. Connect with Kids, *Mirror, Mirror.*

32. Hines, *The Adonis Factor.*

33. Dale L. Cusumano and J. Kevin Thompson, "Body Image and Body Shape Ideals in Magazines: Exposure, Awareness, and Internalization," *Sex Roles* 37, nos. 9–10 (November 1997): 702. doi: 10.1007/BF02936336.

34. Hines, *The Adonis Factor.*

35. Kjerstin Gruys, "Day 365: An Interview with Cynthia Bulik, PhD, Author of *Woman in the Mirror*," *Mirror, Mirror, Off the Wall* (blog), March 24, 2012, www.ayearwithoutmirrors.com/2012/03/day-365-interview-with-cynthia-bulik.html. (With grateful appreciation to Kjerstin Gruys and Cynthia Bulik.)

36. Discovery Channel School, *Reality Matters: Extreme Measure, Body Image* (educational DVD), 2004, www.cosmeo.com.

37. Discovery Channel School, *Reality Matters.*

a. "Jill/Johnny (South Carolina)," *Heavy*, season 1, episode 7, February 28, 2011, A&E TV Networks, www.aetv.com/heavy/episode-guide.

b. "Transgender Research Sees Body Dissatisfaction, Eating Disorders," *WSU News* (Washington State University), May 14, 2012, news.wsu.edu/~/transgender-research-sees-body-dissatisfaction-eating-disorders (accessed October 13, 2013).

c. Troy Roness, "My Journey Back," NEDA—Stories of Hope, www.nationaleatingdisorders.org/stories-of-hope/my-journey-back-troy-roness (accessed December 2012).

d. YWCA, *Beauty at Any Cost—the Consequences of America's Beauty Obsession on Women & Girls* (Washington, D.C.: Author, August 2008). Available at www.docstoc.com/docs/150918014.

e. Carolyn Costin, *The Eating Disorder Sourcebook: A Comprehensive Guide to the Causes, Treatments, and Prevention of Eating Disorders*, 3rd ed. (New York: McGraw-Hill, 2007), 82.

f. "Inside the Episode" (video clip), *Girls*, season 1, 01 Pilot, April 15, 2012, HBO Series TV, www.hbo.com/girls/index.html (accessed January 2013).

g. Hines, *The Adonis Factor.*

h. Hines, *The Adonis Factor.*

i. Ryan K. Sallans, "Finding Me: Looking Past the Surface to Discover My Transgender Identity," NEDA, 2012, www.nationaleatingdisorders.org/finding-me-looking-past-surface-discover-my-transgender-identity. (With grateful appreciation to Ryan Sallans.)

j. Eve Ensler, *The Good Body* [Acting edition] (New York: Villard, 2005), 68.

k. Ensler, *The Good Body*, 69.

l. Darryl Roberts, *America the Beautiful: Is America Obsessed with Beauty?* Darryl Roberts and Sensory Overload Entertainment, 2007, www.americathebeautifuldoc.com.

Chapter 6

1. Shelley Levitt, "The Disordered Eating Epidemic," *More*, October 2010, www.more.com/health/wellness/disordered-eating-epidemic (accessed February 2013).

2. Federica Tozzi, Laura M. Thornton, Kelly L. Klump, Manfred M. Fichter, Katherine A. Halmi, Allan S. Kaplan, Michael Strober, D. Blake Woodside, Scott Crow, James Mitchell, Alessandro Rotondo, Mauro Mauri, Giovanni Cassano, Pamela Keel, Katherine H. Plotnicov, Christine Pollice, Lisa R. Lilenfeld, Wade H. Berrettini, Cynthia M. Bulik, and Walter H. Kaye, "Symptom Fluctuation in Eating Disorders: Correlates of Diagnostic Crossover," *American Journal of Psychiatry* 162, no.4 (April 2005): 732. doi:10.1176/appi.ajp.162.4.732.

3. Christopher G. Fairburn and Kristin Bohn, "Eating Disorder NOS (EDNOS): An Example of the Troublesome 'Not Otherwise Specified (NOS)' Category in *DSM-IV*," *Behavior Research and Therapy* 43 no. 6 (June 2005): 691–701. doi: 10.1016/j.brat.2004.06.011.

4. Jordana, "Jordana," in *Thin*, by Lauren Greenfield (San Francisco: Chronicle Books with Melcher Media, 2006), 130.

5. American Psychiatric Association Practice Guidelines, "Treatment of Patients with Eating Disorders, Third Edition, Part A," *American Journal of Psychiatry* 163 (supplement) (May 2006; AHRQ Panel reviewed and re-validated, 2011). doi: 10.1176/appi.books.9780890423363.138660.

6. Darryl Roberts, *America the Beautiful: Is America Obsessed with Beauty?* a film by Darryl Roberts and Sensory Overload Entertainment, 2007, www.americathebeautifuldoc.com.

7. Carolyn Costin, "From Diet to Disorder—How a Diet Can Progress to an Eating Disorder" (video clip), Monte Nido Video Gallery, March 14, 2012, www.montenido.com/media_events/video_gallery (accessed July 2013).

8. Michael Strober, "The Path from Illness to Recovery," in Greenfield, *Thin*, 160.

9. Nina, "Nina," in Greenfield, *Thin*, 129.

10. National Public Radio, "Research News—Study: Depression, Autism And Schizophrenia Share Genetic Links," *All Things Considered*, Audie Cornish interview with Jordan Smoller, MD, March 1, 2013. Transcript available at www.npr.org/2013/03/01/173271247/-study-depression-autism-and-schizophrenia-share-genetic-links.

11. Larkin McPhee, *Dying to Be Thin*, NOVA Production by Twin Cities Public Television, Inc., for WGBH/Boston, 2000, www.pbs.org/wgbh/nova/body/dying-to-be-thin.html (accessed September 2012).

12. National Institute of Mental Health, "Director's Blog: Spotlight on Eating Disorders," *My Blog: Tom Insel, MD*, February 24, 2012, www.nimh.nih.gov/about/director/2012/spotlight -on-eating-disorders.shtml (accessed February 2013).

13. Yafu Zhao and William Encinosa, "Hospitalizations for Eating Disorders from 1999 to 2006," *HCUP Statistical Brief #70* (Rockville, Md.: U.S. Department of Health and Human Services, April 2009), 1. Available at www.hcup-us.ahrq.gov/reports/statbriefs/sb70.pdf.

14. Walter Kaye and Danyale McCurdy, "Prevalence and Correlates of Eating Disorders in Adolescents," *Archives of General Psychiatry* (presently, *JAMA Psychiatry*), 2011: E1–E10, as reported to the National Eating Disorders Association (NEDA), "Prevalence and Correlates of Eating Disorders in Adolescents" (handout), 2012. Available at www.nationaleatingdisorders .org/sites/default/files/ResourceHandouts/PrevalenceAndCorrelatesofEatingDisorders.pdf.

15. Sonja A. Swanson, Scott J. Crow, Daniel Le Grange, Joel Swendsen, and Kathleen R. Merikangas, "Prevalence and Correlates of Eating Disorders in Adolescents: Results from the National Comorbidity Survey Replication Adolescent Supplement," *Archives of General Psychiatry* (presently, *JAMA Psychiatry*) 68, no. 7 (July 2011): 714–723. doi:10.1001/ archgenpsychiatry.2011.22.

16. Centers for Disease Control and Prevention, "Youth Risk Behavior Surveillance—United States, 2011," *Morbidity and Mortality Weekly Report* 61, no. 4 (June 8, 2012): 39. Available at www.cdc.gov/mmwr/pdf/ss/ss6104.pdf.

17. Renfrew Center Foundation for Eating Disorders, *Eating Disorders 101 Guide: A Summary of Issues, Statistics and Resources*, September 2002 (revised October 2003), 3.

18. Renfrew Center Foundation, *Eating Disorders 101 Guide*, 4.

19. Renfrew Center Foundation, *Eating Disorders 101 Guide*, 3.

20. Sara Selis, "Binge Eating Disorder: Surprisingly Common, Seriously Under-treated," *Psychiatric Times*, April 3, 2007. Available at www.psychiatrictimes.com/articles/binge-eating -disorder-surprisingly-common-seriously-under-treated.

21. Kelly L. Klump, Cynthia M. Bulik, Walter H. Kaye, Janet Treasure, and Edward Tyson, "Academy for Eating Disorders Position Paper: Eating Disorders Are Serious Mental Illnesses," *International Journal of Eating Disorders* 42, no. 2 (July 2009): 99. doi: 10.1002/ eat.20589.

22. Lisa Hilton, "What's Wrong with Skinny?" *Daily Beast*, Entertainment & Fashion, February 8, 2010, www.thedailybeast.com/articles/2010/02/08/are-models-too-thin.html (accessed March 2013).

23. Peter Walker, "Inquiry Urges Health Checks for Models," *Guardian*, UK News, September 14, 2007, www.guardian.co.uk/uk/2007/sep/14/health.fashion (accessed March 2013).

24. Antonio Preti, Ambra Usai, Paola Miotto, Donatella Rita Petretto, Carmelo Masala, "Eating Disorders among Professional Fashion Models," *Psychiatry Research* 159, no. 1 (May 30, 2008): 86–94. doi: 10.1016/j.psychres.2005.07.040.

25. The Model Alliance, "Industry Analysis," modelalliance.org/industry-analysis (accessed April 8, 2013).

26. Roberts, *America the Beautiful*.

27. Roberts, *America the Beautiful*.

28. Kathleen McGuire, "Food Obsessed?" *Dance* magazine, October 2010, www.dancemagazine .com/issues/October-2010/Food-Obsessed (accessed March 2013).

29. Bess Kargman, *First Position*, First Position Films, 2011, www.balletdocumentary.com.

30. Kargman, *First Position*.

31. Kargman, *First Position*.

32. McGuire, "Food Obsessed?"

33. Rebecca Ringham, Kelly Klump, Walter Kaye, David Stone, Steven Libman, Susan Stowe, and Marsha Marcus, "Eating Disorder Symptomatology among Ballet Dancers," *International Journal of Eating Disorders* 39, no. 6 (September 2006): 503. doi: 10.1002/eat.20299.

34. Alice Schluger, "Disordered Eating Attitudes and Behaviors in Female College Dance Students: Comparison of Modern Dance and Ballet Dance Majors," *North American Journal of Psychology* 12, no. 1 (March 2010): 117.

35. Leah M. Kalm and Richard D. Semba, "They Starved So That Others Be Better Fed: Remembering Ancel Keys and the Minnesota Experiment," *Journal of Nutrition* 135, no. 6 (June 1, 2005): 1347. PMID:15930436.

36. Yolanda Diz-Chaves, "Ghrelin, Appetite Regulation, and Food Reward: Interaction with Chronic Stress," *International Journal of Peptides* 2011 (2011), Article ID 898450. doi: 10.1155/2011/898450.

37. Kent C. Berridge, Chao-Yi Ho, Jocelyn M. Richard, and Alexandra G. DiFeliceantonio. "The Tempted Brain Eats: Pleasure and Desire Circuits in Obesity and Eating Disorders," *Brain Research* 1350 (September 2, 2010): 43–64. doi: 10.1016/j.brainres.2010.04.003.

38. Pietro Cottone, Valentina Sabino, Marisa Roberto, Michal Bajo, Lara Pockros, Jennifer B. Frihauf, et al. "CRF System Recruitment Mediates Dark Side of Compulsive Eating," *Proceedings of the National Academy of Sciences of the United States of America* 106, no. 47 (November 24, 2009): 20016–20020. doi: 10.1073/pnas. 0908789106.

39. Devin Powell, "Overeaters and Drug Abusers Share Addictive Brain Chemistry," LiveScience, November 9, 2009, www.livescience.com/7959-overeaters-drug-abusers-share-addictive-brain-chemistry.html (accessed August 2012).

40. Carolyn Costin, MA, MEd, MFT, personal communication, September 30, 2013.

41. Justin Hunt, *Absent: A Justin Hunt Documentary*, Time & Tide Productions, 2010, www.absentmovie.com.

42. Maria Kang, "'Max Muscle Saved My Life,'" *Max Sports & Fitness*, March 2010, 42, digitaleditiononline.com/publication/?i=32129 (accessed March 2013).

43. Hunt, *Absent*.

---

a. "Addicted to Pizza," *Freaky Eaters*, season 1, episode 3, September 12, 2010, Shed Media US for TLC—a Discovery Company, www.tlc.com/tv-shows/tv-shows/other-shows/videos/freaky-eaters-addicted-to-pizza.htm.

b. "Addicted to Pizza."

c. Ryan Brown, "A Thin Spread," *Chronicle* (Duke University), February 9, 2011, www.dukechronicle.com/article/thin-spread (accessed February 2013).

d. Ruth (the author), July 10, 2013.

e. Kelly M., personal communication, July 10, 2013.

f. Cynthia Bulik, "Eating Disorder Behaviors and Weight Concerns Are Common in Women Over 50" (study summary), as reported to the National Eating Disorders Association, "Women Over 50," 2012, www.nationaleatingdisorders.org/women-over-50 (accessed February 2013).

g. "Eating Disorder Behaviors and Weight Concerns Are Common in Women over 50," *UNC Health Care and UNC School of Medicine: Newsroom*, June 21, 2012, news.unchealthcare.org/

news/2012/june/eating-disorder-behaviors-and-weight-concerns-are-common-in-women -over-50 (accessed February 2013).

h. Michael Inbar, "Plus-Size Model 'Shocked' at Being Made to Look Thinner," *Today: Style*, July 22, 2010, www.today.com/id/38358777/ns/today-today_style/t/plus-size-model -shocked-being-made-look-thinner (accessed April 2013).

i. Inbar, "Plus Model 'Shocked.'"

j. Susan Diesenhouse, "DANCE: In a Darwinian World of Weight Control," *New York Times* (archives), October 12, 1997, 2, www.nytimes.com/1997/10/12/arts/dance-in-a-darwinian -world-of-weight-control.html (accessed March 2013).

k. Bill Hewitt, "Last Dance," *People* (archives) 48, no. 4, July 28, 1997, www.people.com/ people/article/0,,20122756,00.html (accessed March 2013).

l. Ken Baker, "Heidi Guenther's Short, Tragic Life . . . and Death," *San Francisco Chronicle*, April 4, 1999, 3, www.sfgate.com/magazine/article/Heidi-Guenther-s-short-tragic-life-and -death-3490764.php#page-3 (accessed March 2013).

m. Colin Fernandez, "English National Ballet Chief Orders Dancers to Put on Weight after Audience Complaints That Stars Are Too Thin," *Mail Online*, News, April 15, 2012, www .dailymail.co.uk/news/article-2130067/New-English-National-Ballet-chief-tells-dancers -weight-vows-stamp-anorexia.html (accessed March 2013).

n. Sharma Apt Russell, *Hunger: An Unnatural History* (New York: Basic Books, 2005), 101.

o. Russell, *Hunger*, 105.

p. Richard Sine, "Competitive Eating: How Safe Is It?" WebMD, August 22, 2007, 1, www.webmd .com/food-recipes/features/competitive-eating-how-safe-is-it (accessed February 2013).

q. "Sonya 'the Black Widow' Thomas—Information and Eating Contest Results," EatFeats— Competitive Eating News, Database & Calendar, eatfeats.com/category/women/sonya- thomas (accessed February 26, 2013).

r. "Frequently Asked Questions," Insatiable Sonya: Competitive Eating's Black Widow (per- sonal website), sonyatheblackwidow.com/id2.html (accessed February 26, 2013).

s. Sine, "Competitive Eating," 2.

t. Tracey D. Wade, Anna Keski-Rahkonen, and James Hudson, "Epidemiology of Eating Disorders," in *Textbook in Psychiatric Epidemiology*, 3rd ed., ed. M. Tsuang and M. Tohen, chapter 20 (New York: Wiley, 2011), 343, as noted in NEDA, "What Are Eating Disorders?" (handout), 2012. Available at www.nationaleatingdisorders.org/sites/default/files/Resource- Handouts/GeneralStatistics.pdf.

Chapter 7

1. American Psychiatric Association (APA) Practice Guidelines, "Treatment of Patients with Eating Disorders, Third Edition, Part B," *American Journal of Psychiatry* 163 (supple- ment) (May 2006; AHRQ panel reviewed and revalidated, 2011). doi: 10.1176/appi .books.9780890423363.138660.

2. Frédérique R.E. Smink, Daphne van Hoeken, and Hans W. Hoek, "Epidemiology of Eating Disorders: Incidence, Prevalence and Mortality Rates," *Current Psychiatry Reports* 14, no. 4 (May 2012): 406. doi: 10.1007/s11920-012-0282-y.

3. Manal Ismail, "New Hope for UAE Sufferers of Eating Disorders," *National*, October 20, 2012, www.thenational.ae/news/uae-news/health/new-hope-for-uae-sufferers-of-eating -disorders (accessed March 2013).

4. APA Practice Guidelines, "Treatment of Patients with Eating Disorders."

5. Tony McNicol, "Japan Diet Risks on Rise: Problems with Eating Disorders Slip under the Radar," *Japan Times*, Community, August 3, 2004, www.japantimes.co.jp/community/2004/08/03/community/japan-diet-risks-on-rise.

6. Mariko Makino, Koji Tsuboi, and Lorraine Dennerstein, "Prevalence of Eating Disorders: A Comparison of Western and Non-Western Countries," *Medscape General Medicine* 6, no. 3 (September 2004): 49. PMID: 15520673.

7. Renfrew Center Foundation for Eating Disorders, *Eating Disorders 101 Guide: A Summary of Issues, Statistics and Resources*, September 2002 (revised October 2003), 4.

8. World Health Organization, "Number of Deaths: WORLD by Cause," Global Health Observatory Data Repository, 2012, apps.who.int/gho/data/node.main.CODWORLD (accessed March 2013).

9. NationMaster.com, "Mortality Statistics—Eating Disorders by Country (WHOSIS)," compiled January 2004, www.NationMaster.com (accessed March 2013).

10. Walter Kaye, "Mortality and Eating Disorders" (handout), National Eating Disorders Association (NEDA), 2012. Available at www.nationaleatingdisorders.org/sites/default/files/ResourceHandouts/MortalityandEatingDisorders.pdf.

11. Darryl Roberts, *America the Beautiful: Is America Obsessed with Beauty?* a film by Darryl Roberts and Sensory Overload Entertainment, 2007, www.americathebeautifuldoc.com.

12. Shan Guisinger, "Dangers of Dieting a Body Adapted to Famine" (special article for F.E.A.S.T.), March 2012, feast-ed.org/Resources/ArticlesforFEAST/DangersofDietingaBodyAdaptedtoFamine.aspx (accessed April 2013).

13. Jeffrey G. Johnson, Patricia Cohen, Stephanie Kasen, and Judith S. Brook, "Eating Disorders during Adolescence and the Risk for Physical and Mental Disorders during Early Adulthood," *Archives of General Psychiatry* (presently, *JAMA Psychiatry*) 59, no. 6 (June 2002): 545. doi: 10.1001/archpsyc.59.6.545.

14. Todd Tucker, *The Great Starvation Experiment: Ancel Keys and the Men Who Starved for Science* (Minneapolis: University of Minnesota Press, 2007), 214.

15. Janet L. Treasure, Elizabeth R. Wack, and Marion E. Roberts, "Models as a High-Risk Group: The Health Implications of a Size Zero Culture," *British Journal of Psychiatry* 192, no. 4 (April 2008): 243–244. doi: 10.1192/bjp.bp.107.044164.

16. Stephanie Covington Armstrong, "Digesting the Truth," NEDA—Stories of Hope, www.nationaleatingdisorders.org/stories-of-hope/digesting-truth-stephanie-covington-armstrong (accessed December 2012).

17. Cynthia L. Ogden, Margaret D. Carroll, Brian K. Kit, and Katherine M. Flegal, "Prevalence of Obesity in the United States, 2009–2010," NCHS Data Brief, No 82 (Hyattsville, Md.: National Center for Health Statistics, January 2012), 3. Available at www.cdc.gov/nchs/data/databriefs/db82.htm.

18. Darryl Roberts, *America the Beautiful 2: The Thin Commandments*, Harley Boy Entertainment, 2010, www.americathebeautifuldoc.com.

19. Ragen Chastain, "Who Is This Chick?" *Dances with Fat: Life, Liberty, and the Pursuit of Happiness Are Not Size Dependent* (blog), danceswithfat.wordpress.com (accessed April 2013).

20. Roberts, *America the Beautiful 2*.

21. Lynn S. Grefe, personal communication, April 23, 2013.

22. Communications Staff, "Full Mental Health Parity Is Now Law," APA Practice Central, November 6, 2008, www.apapracticecentral.org/news/2008/parity-law.aspx (accessed April 2013).

23. National Women's Law Health Center, "Eating Disorder Parity," hrc.nwlc.org/policy -indicators/eating-disorder-parity (accessed April 2013).

24. Eating Disorders Coalition for Research Policy and Action, "Influencing Policy: The FREED Act & Other Bills," 2013, www.eatingdisorderscoalition.org/influency-policy.htm (accessed September 2013).

25. NEDA, "National Eating Disorders Association Joins Off Our Chests in Battle to Launch Media and Public Health Act" (press release), January 31, 2012, www.nationaleatingdisorders .org/press-room/press-releases/2012-press-releases/national-eating-disorders-association -joins-our-chests-battle-launch-media-and-public-health-act (accessed April 2013).

26. Alia Beard Rau, "Arizona Bill Takes Aim at Airbrushed Women in Ads," *Arizona Republic*, February 14, 2012, www.azcentral.com/news/politics/articles/2012/02/14/20120214arizona- bill-takes-aim-airbrushed-women-ads.html (accessed April 2013).

27. Meghan Casserly, "Vogue's New Beauty Standard: No Underage Models or Eating Disor- ders," *Forbes*, May 5, 2012, www.forbes.com/sites/meghancasserly/2012/05/03/vogue-sets -new-beauty-magazine-standard-no-underage-models-or-eating-disorders/ (accessed April 2013).

a. McNicol, "Japan Diet Risks on Rise."

b. Judy Avrin and Danna Markson, *Someday Melissa* movie trailer, Someday Melissa, Inc., in association with Good for You Productions, 2011. Posted at www.nytimes.com/video/ style/1247467660335/someday-melissa-trailer.html (accessed June 30, 2013).

c. Arvin and Markson, *Someday Melissa*.

d. Robin Pogrebin, "A Mother's Loss, a Daughter's Story," *New York Times*, April 21, 2010, www.nytimes.com/2010/04/22/fashion/22Melissa.html (accessed March 2013).

e. Pogrebin, "A Mother's Loss."

f. Meredith Galante, "After Losing Teen Daughter to Bulimia, Totowa Mom Honors Her through Documentary," *Star-Ledger* (New Jersey), May 3, 2011.

g. Avrin and Markson, *Someday Melissa*.

h. Pogrebin, "A Mother's Loss."

i. Heidi Dalzell, "Wannarexia: A Dangerous Fad," *Examiner.com*, October 22, 2010, www .examiner.com/article/wannarexia-a-dangerous-fad (accessed March 2013).

j. Jeanie Lerche Davis, "Orthorexia: Good Diets Gone Bad," WebMD, November 17, 2000, www.webmd.com/mental-health/anorexia-nervosa/news/20001117/orthorexia-good-diets -gone-bad (accessed June 2012).

k. Lisa A. Flam, "When Eating Too Healthy Becomes Harmful," *Today: Health*, August 25, 2011, www.today.com/id/44264861/ns/today-today_health/t/when-eating-too-healthy -becomes-harmful/ (accessed July 2012).

l. Erik Strand, "Orthorexia: Too Healthy?" *Psychology Today*, September 1, 2004, www .psychologytoday.com/articles/200412/orthorexia-too-healthy (accessed September 2013).

m. Jane R. Hirschmann and Carol H. Munter, *Overcoming Overeating: How to Break the Diet/ Binge Cycle and Live a Healthier, More Satisfying Life* (Philadelphia: Da Capo Press, 2008), 1. www.overcomingovereating.com.

n. Eating Disorder Center of Denver, "'Drunkorexia' on the Rise in College-Aged Women," October 1, 2009, www.edcdenver.com/news-1/drunkorexia-on-the-rise-in-college-aged -women (accessed April 2013).

o. National Public Radio (NPR), "Shawn Colvin: 'Diamond in the Rough,'" *Diane Rehm Show*, WAMU 88.5 American University Radio, June 7, 2012. Transcript available at thedianerehm show.org/shows/2012-06-07/shawn-colvin-diamond-rough/transcript.

p. Rob Stein, "Obesity Epidemic May Have Peaked in U.S," *All Things Considered*, NPR Shots, January 17, 2012. Available at www.npr.org/ blogs/health/2012/01/17/145237480obesity-epidemic-may-have-peaked-in-u-s.

q. Roberts, *America the Beautiful 2*.

r. Perez Hilton, "New York Times Review Says Ballerina Is Too Fat!" *FitPerez* (blog), November 30, 2010, perezhilton.com/fitperez/2010-11-30-new-york-times-reviewer-says-ballerina-is-too-fat (accessed April 2013).

s. Maura Kelly, "Should 'Fatties' Get a Room? (Even on TV?)" *A Year of Living Flirtaciously* (*Marie Claire* dating blog), October 25, 2010, www.marieclaire.com/sex-love/dating-blog/overweight-couples-on-television (accessed April 2013).

t. Kelly, "Should 'Fatties' Get a Room?" (update).

u. "'Fatties' Blog Post Sets Off Online Uproar" (video clip), *Today: Health*, October 28, 2010, www.today.com/id/39868583/ns/today-today_health/t/fatties-blog-post-sets-online-uproar (accessed April 2013).

Chapter 8

1. Darryl Roberts, *America the Beautiful 2: The Thin Commandments*, Harley Boy Entertainment, 2010, www.americathebeautifuldoc.com.

2. Ginny Graves, "Health Controversy: Can You Be Fat and Healthy?" *Glamour*, Health & Diet, February 2012, www.glamour.com/health-fitness/2012/02/health-controversy-can-you-be-fat-and-healthy (accessed May 2013).

3. G. C. Patton, R. Selzer, C. Doffey, J. B. Carlin, and R. Wolfe, "Onset of Adolescent Eating Disorders: Population-Based Cohort Study over 3 Years," *British Medical Journal* 318, no. 7186 (March 1999): 765. doi: 10.1136/bmj.318.7186.765.

4. Heather Shaw, Eric Stice, and Carolyn Black Becker, "Preventing Eating Disorders," *Child and Adolescent Psychiatric Clinics of North America* 18, no. 1 (January 2009): 199. doi: 10.1016/j.chc.2008.07.012.

5. Lauren Cox, "Pro-Ana Websites Send Convoluted and Deadly Messages, Study Finds," *ABC News*, Health, June 17, 2010, abcnews.go.com/Health/MindMoodNews/pro-anorexia-websites-encourage-eating-disorders-send-mixed/story?id=10944783 (accessed May 2013).

6. Rachel Dretzin and John Maggio, *Frontline: Growing Up Online*, a FRONTLINE co-production with Ark Media, LLC, for WBGH/Boston Educational Foundation, 2007. Transcript available at www.pbs.org/wgbh/pages/frontline/kidsonline.

7. Dretzin and Maggio, *Frontline*.

8. Jenny L. Wilson, Rebecka Peebles, Kristina K. Hardy, and Iris F. Litt, "Surfing for Thinness: A Pilot Study of Pro–Eating Disorder Web Site Usage in Adolescents with Eating Disorders," *Pediatrics* 118, no. 6 (December 1, 2006): e1635. doi: 10.1542/peds.2006-1133.

9. Julie Weingarden Dubin, "Eating Disorders Amp Up with Technology," *SheKnows*, Parenting, February 22, 2013, www.sheknows.com/parenting/articles/948837/eating-disorders-amp-up-with-technology (accessed May 2013).

10. Drew A. Anderson, Jennifer D. Lundgren, Jennifer R. Shapiro, and Carrie A. Paulosky, "Assessment of Eating Disorders: Review and Recommendations for Clinical Use," *Behavioral Modification* 28, no. 6 (November 2004): 763–782. doi: 10.1177/0145445503259851.

11. Sara Selis, "Binge Eating Disorder: Surprisingly Common, Seriously Under-treated," *Psychiatric Times*, April 3, 2007. Available at www.psychiatrictimes.com/articles/binge-eating-disorder-surprisingly-common-seriously-under-treated.

12. National Eating Disorders Association (NEDA), "National Partnership between NEDA & SMH Brings Free Online Eating Disorder Screenings to the Public" (press release), February 19, 2013, www.nationaleatingdisorders.org/national-partnership-between-neda-smh-brings -free-online-eating-disorder-screenings-public (accessed May 2013).

13. Katherine Cruise, personal communication, October 3, 2013.

14. Michael P. Levine, PhD, personal communication, August 25, 2013.

15. Lynn S. Grefe, personal communication, March 23, 2013.

16. Dianne Neumark-Sztainer, Michael P. Levine, Susan J Paxton, Linda Smolak, Niva Piran, and Eleanor H. Wertheim, "Prevention of Body Dissatisfaction and Disordered Eating: What Next?" *Eating Disorders: The Journal of Treatment and Prevention* 14, no. 4 (September 2006): 278. doi: 10.1080/10640260600796184.

17. American Psychiatric Association Practice Guidelines, "Treatment of Patients with Eating Disorders, Third Edition, Part B," *American Journal of Psychiatry* 163 (supplement) (May 2006; AHRQ panel reviewed and revalidated, 2011). doi: 10.1176/appi.books .9780890423363.138660.

a. Lori Fradkin, "Diablo Cody Thinks Lena Dunham Is 'Our New Woody Allen,'" *HuffPost Women*, January 30, 2013, www.huffingtonpost.com/ 2013/01/30/diablo-cody-athena-film -festival-women_n_2569811.html (accessed May 2013).

b. Nanci Hellmich, "Athletes' Hunger to Win Fuels Eating Disorders," *USA Today*, Health and Behavior, February 5, 2006, usatoday30.usatoday.com/news/health/2006-02-05-women -health-cover_x.htm (accessed May 2013).

c. American College of Sports Medicine, "The Female Athlete Triad" (brochure), 2011. Available at www.acsm.org/docs/brochures/the-female-athlete-triad.pdf.

d. NEDA, "How to Help a Friend with Eating and Body Image Issues" (print brochure), 2012. Reprinted with permission from the National Eating Disorders Association. For more information visit www.nationaleatingdisorders.org or call NEDA's Helpline: 1-800-931-2237.

e. "Starved," *Wikipedia*, page last modified December 17, 2012, en.wikipedia.org/wiki/Starved (accessed October 2012).

f. Robert Lloyd, "'Starved' for Substance," *Los Angeles Times*, Entertainment, August 3, 2005, articles.latimes.com/2005/aug/03/entertainment/et-starved3 (accessed October 2012).

g. Margaret Wheeler Johnson, "Tracey Gold's 'Starving Secrets': Could On-Camera Recovery Work?" *HuffPost Women*, December 2, 2011, www.huffingtonpost.com/margaret-wheeler -johnson/tracy-gold-starving-secrets_b_1084528.html (accessed October 2012).

h. Daisy Dumas, "Anorexia Reality Show Starving Secrets Slammed by Eating Disorders Group for 'Putting Ill People on Television,'" *Mail Online*, Femail, December 5, 2011, www .dailymail.co.uk/femail/article-2070299/Anorexia-reality-Starving-Secrets-slammed-eating -disorders-group-putting-ill-people-television.html (accessed October 2012).

i. The Brits are as extreme about makeover TV as we are. In November 2012, the BBC Three channel spent a week's broadcasting looking into seven documentary segments that examined teenage body concerns—from plastic surgery to compulsive exercise to teen beauty pageants for the slender and super plus-sized.

j. "Portia de Rossi: My Life" (video clip), Cynthia McFadden interview with Portia de Rossi, *ABC News Nightline*, November 4, 2010, abcnews.go.com/Nightline/video/portia-de-rossi -life-12062192 (accessed March 2013).

k. John F. Morgan, Fiona Reid, and J. Hubert Lacey, "The SCOFF Questionnaire: A New Screening Tool for Eating Disorders," *Western Journal of Medicine* 172, no. 3 (March 2000): 164.

Chapter 9

1. National Eating Disorders Association (NEDA), Parent, Family and Friends Network, "Medical Management: The Medical Complications" (webinar), conducted by Joel Jahraus, MD, May 7, 2013.

2. Judy Avrin and Danna Markson, *Someday Melissa: The Story of an Eating Disorder, Loss and Hope*, Someday Melissa, Inc., in association with Good for You Productions, 2011, www.somedaymelissa.org.

3. Harriet Brown, *Brave Girl Eating: A Family's Struggle with Anorexia* (New York: William Morrow, 2010), 74.

4. Susan Donaldson James, "Anorexia Can Strike and Kill as Early as Kindergarten," *ABC News*, Health, February 25, 2012, 2, abcnews.go.com/Health/anorexia-nervosa-strike-kill-early-kindergarten/story?id=18581747 (accessed June 2013).

5. Jenny Graham, "Interventions: Another Option on the Road to Recovery," *Making Connections*, Winter 2012, 7. Available at www.nationaleatingdisorders.org/sites/default/files/MakingConnections/Winter2012.pdf.

6. Carefrontations, "What Does It Take to Put Together an Intervention?" (video clip), *LivingSoberToday*, May 24, 2013, www.youtube.com/watch?v=IpM43NnhFGI.

7. Graham, "Interventions," 7.

8. Northbound Treatment Services, "How to Find a Premier Drug Treatment & the Best Dual Diagnosis Center" (video clip), *LivingSoberToday*, March 1, 2013. www.youtube.com/user/LivingSoberToday.

9. Carolyn Costin, *The Eating Disorder Sourcebook: A Comprehensive Guide to the Causes, Treatments, and Prevention of Eating Disorders*, 3rd ed. (New York: McGraw-Hill, 2007), 99.

10. NEDA, "Medical Management."

11. Ruth (the author), June 17, 2013.

12. James, "Anorexia Can Strike and Kill as Early as Kindergarten," 2.

13. Mike Polan, "Hope for Parents," NEDA—Stories of Hope, 2013, www.nationaleatingdisorders.org/stories-of-hope/hope-parents-mike-polan (accessed June 2013).

14. Rebecca Murphy, Suzanne Straebler, Zafra Cooper, and Christopher G. Fairburn, "Cognitive Behavioral Therapy for Eating Disorders," *Psychiatric Clinics of North America* 33, no. 3 (September 2010): 611. doi: 10.1016/j.psc.2010.04.004.

15. Daniel Le Grange and Ivan Eisler, "Family Interventions in Adolescent Anorexia Nervosa," *Child and Adolescent Psychiatric Clinics of North America* 18, no. 1 (January 2009): 167. doi: 10.1016/j.chc.2008.07.004.

16. James Lock, Daniel Le Grange, W. Stewart Agras, Ann Moye, Susan W. Bryson, and Booil Jo, "Randomized Clinical Trial Comparing Family-Based Treatment with Adolescent-Focused Individual Therapy for Adolescents with Anorexia Nervosa," *Archives of General Psychiatry* (presently, *JAMA Psychiatry*) 67, no. 10 (October 2010): 1025. doi: 10.1001/archgenpsychiatry.2010.128.

17. Joel Yager, Michael J. Devlin, Katherine A. Halmi, David B. Herzog, James E. Mitchell, Pauline Powers, and Kathryn J. Zerbe, "Guideline Watch (August 2012): Practice Guideline for the Treatment of Patients with Eating Disorders, 3rd Edition," PsychiatryOnline, 2012. Available at psychiatryonline.org/content.aspx?bookid=28&sectionid=39113853.

18. Adrienne Juarascio, Jena Shaw, Evan Forman, C. Alix Timko, James Herbert, Meghan Butryn, Douglas Bunnell, Alyssa Matteucci, and Michael Lowe, "Acceptance and Commitment

Therapy as a Novel Treatment for Eating Disorders: An Initial Test of Efficacy and Mediation," *Behavior Modification* 37, no. 4 (July 2013): 459. doi: 10.1177/0145445513478633.

19. Harriet Brown, "Looking for Evidence That Therapy Works," *Well* (*New York Times* blog), March 25, 2013, well.blogs.nytimes.com/2013/03/25/looking-for-evidence-that-therapy -works (accessed June 2013).

20. National Public Radio (NPR), "New Treatments for Eating Disorders," *Diane Rehm Show*, WAMU 88.5 American University Radio, August 26, 2010, thedianerehmshow.org/shows/ 2010-08-26/new-treatments-eating-disorders.

21. NPR, "New Treatments for Eating Disorders."

22. Kourtney Wachter Gordon, personal communication, September 8, 2013.

23. Sophie Moura, "Starvation Nation: Inside a Groundbreaking Eating Disorder Facility," *Marie Claire*, June 20, 2011, www.marieclaire.com/health-fitness/news/eating-disorder-facility (accessed June 2013).

24. Ovidio Bermudez, featured quote, About Us, Eating Recovery Center, www.eatingrecovery center.com/about-us/eating-recovery-center-leadership/medical-and-clinical-leadership (accessed July 1, 2013).

25. B. Timothy Walsh, "Eating Disorders in Adolescents: Strategies for the Primary Care Provider—Focus on Anorexia Nervosa and *DSM-5*" (webinar). TeenScreen National Center for Mental Health Checkups at Columbia University, January 12, 2012.

26. Yager et al., "Guideline Watch."

27. American Academy of Child and Adolescent Psychiatry, "Psychiatric Medication for Children and Adolescents Part II—Types of Medications," *Facts for Families*, no. 29 (May 2012). Available at www.aacap.org/App_Themes/AACAP/docs/facts_for_families/29_psychiatric _medication_for_children_and_adolescents_part_two.pdf.

28. James M. Greenblatt, *Answers to Anorexia: A Breakthrough Nutritional Treatment That Is Saving Lives* (North Branch, Minn.: Sunrise River Press, 2010), 18.

29. Greenblatt, *Answers to Anorexia*, 241.

30. Greenblatt, *Answers to Anorexia*, 18, 241.

31. Greenblatt, *Answers to Anorexia*, 109.

32. American Psychiatric Association Practice Guidelines, "Treatment of Patients with Eating Disorders, Third Edition, Part A," *American Journal of Psychiatry* 163 (supplement) (May 2006; AHRQ panel reviewed and re-validated, 2011). doi: 10.1176/appi.books .9780890423363.138660.

a. Sonja A. Swanson, Scott J. Crow, Daniel Le Grange, Joel Swendsen, and Kathleen R. Merikangas, "Prevalence And Correlates of Eating Disorders in Adolescents: Results from the National Comorbidity Survey Replication, Adolescent Supplement," *Archives of General Psychiatry* (presently, *JAMA Psychiatry*) 68, no. 7 (July 2011): 722. doi:10.1001/archgenpsychiatry.2011.22.

b. Olivia Katrandjian, "Portia de Rossi: 'I Would Starve Myself Daily,'" *ABC News*, Entertainment (w/ GMA video clip), November 3, 2010, abcnews.go.com/Entertainment/portia-de-rossi-reveals-depths-eating-disorders-book/story?id=12033594 (accessed June 2013).

c. Katrandjian, "Portia de Rossi."

d. Julie Jordan, "Portia de Rossi: 'I Don't Want to Have Any More Secrets,'" *People*, November 3, 2010, www.people.com/people/article/0,,20438754,00.html (accessed June 2013).

e. Robert Schlossberg and Deborah Klotz, "Your Dentist, Your Friend," *Making Connections*, Spring 2012, 12. Available at www.nationaleatingdisorders.org/sites/default/files/Making-Connections/Spring2012.pdf.

f. NEDA, "Medical Management."
g. Roni Caryn Rabin, "Protocol to Treat Anorexia Is Faulted," *New York Times*, Health Research, January 2, 2012, www.nytimes.com/2012/01/03/health/research/anorexic-patients-can-be-fed-more-aggressively-study-says.html (accessed June 2013).
h. Rabin, "Protocol to Treat Anorexia Is Faulted."
i. Peter Joseph, *Zeitgeist: Moving Forward*, Gentle Machine Productions, 2011, www.zeitgeistmovingforward.com.
j. John Heminway, *Stress: Portrait of a Killer*, a co-production of National Geographic Television and Stanford University, 2008, killerstress.stanford.edu.
k. Kathryn Balch, "When Pregnancy and Eating Disorders Mix," *ABC News*, Women's Health, March 22, 2011, abcnews.go.com/Health/WomensHealth/pregorexia-pregnancy-eating-disorders-mix/story?id=13143285 (accessed June 2013).
l. Jennifer Tolman, "Eating Disorders: An Integrated Treatment Approach," 21st Annual Women's Health Care Symposium, September 16, 2011, www.peacehealth.org/Documents/Womens%20Health%202011%20Tolman.pdf (accessed June 2013).
m. Balch, "When Pregnancy and Eating Disorders Mix."
n. Ruth (the author), June 30, 2013.
o. National Alliance on Mental Illness, "Eating Disorders Fact Sheet," updated January 2013. Available at www.nami.org/factsheets/eatingdisorders_factsheet.pdf.
p. Jon Hamilton, "Ketamine Relieves Depression by Restoring Brain Connections," *All Things Considered*, NPR Shots, October 4, 2012. Transcript available at www.npr.org/blogs/health/2012/10/04/162299564/ketamine-relieves-depression-by-restoring-brain-connections.
q. Crystal C. Douglas, Jeannine C. Lawrence, Nikki C. Bush, Robert A. Oster, Barbara A. Gower, and Betty E. Darnell, "Ability of the Harris-Benedict Formula to Predict Energy Requirements Differs with Weight History and Ethnicity," *Nutrition Research* 27, no. 4 (April 2007): 194–199. doi: 10.1016/j.nutres.2007.01.016.
r. Timberline Knolls Residential Treatment Center, "Past Resident & Family Testimonials," www.timberlineknolls.com/why/testimonials (accessed July 9, 2013).
s. "Visiting Timberline Knolls" (video clip), *Demi Lovato: Stay Strong*, premiered March 6, 2012, on MTV Networks, www.demilovato.org/archives/5547 (accessed July 10, 2013).
t. "Demi Performs 'Skyscraper'" (video clip), *Demi Lovato: Stay Strong*.

Chapter 10

1. F.E.A.S.T. (Families Empowered and Supporting Treatment of Eating Disorders), "You Would Never Know She Had Been Ill," Parent Stories, 2012, feast-ed.org/Members/Parent Stories.aspx (accessed July 2013).
2. Theodora Aggeles, "Pinellas Teen Organizes Tampa Walk for Eating Disorders Awareness," *Tampa Bay* (formerly *St. Petersburg*) *Times*, November 26, 2010, www.tampabay.com/news/humaninterest/pinellas-teen-organizes-tampa-walk-for-eating-disorders-awareness/1136648 (accessed February 2013).
3. Chris Kuhn, "Bailey Monarch, Overcoming . . . One Step at a Time," *Skirt! Tampa Bay*, January 23, 2011.
4. F.E.A.S.T., "You Would Never Know She Had Been Ill."
5. F.E.A.S.T., "You Would Never Know She Had Been Ill."
6. Ruth (the author), August 1, 2013.

7. Carolyn Costin, "Carolyn Costin's New Book, *8 Keys to Recovery from an Eating Disorder*—Extended Version" (video clip), YouTube, March 6, 2012, www.youtube.com/watch?v=lFfBHEhQsh8.

8. Roger C., "The Origins of the 12 Steps," AA Agnostica, September 16, 2012, aaagnostica.org/2012/09/16/the-origins-of-the-12-steps (accessed July 2013).

9. American Psychiatric Association (APA) Practice Guidelines, "Treatment of Patients with Eating Disorders, Third Edition, Parts A & B," *American Journal of Psychiatry* 163 (supplement) (May 2006; AHRQ Panel reviewed and re-validated, 2011). doi: 10.1176/appi.books.9780890423363.138660.

10. Kelly M., personal communication, September 18, 2013.

11. National Public Radio (NPR), "New Treatments for Eating Disorders," *Diane Rehm Show*, WAMU 88.5 American University Radio, August 26, 2010. Transcript at thedianerehmshow.org/shows/2010-08-26/new-treatments-eating-disorders.

12. James Lock, Daniel Le Grange, W. Stewart Agras, Ann Moye, Susan W. Bryson, and Jo Booil, "Randomized Clinical Trial Comparing Family-Based Treatment with Adolescent-Focused Individual Therapy for Adolescents with Anorexia Nervosa," *Archives of General Psychiatry* (presently, *JAMA Psychiatry*) 67, no. 10 (October 2010): 1025–1032. doi:10.1001/archgenpsychiatry.2010.128; Daniel Le Grange, Ross D. Crosby, Paul J. Rathouz, and Bennett L. Leventhal, "A Randomized Controlled Comparison of Family-Based Treatment and Supportive Psychotherapy for Adolescent Bulimia Nervosa," *Archives of General Psychiatry* 64, no. 9 (September 2007): 1049–1056. doi:10.1001/archpsyc.64.9.1049.

13. Christina R., personal communication, June 6, 2013.

14. Kara N. Denny, Katie Loth, Marla E. Eisenberg, and Dianne Neumark-Sztainer, "Intuitive Eating in Young Adults: Who Is Doing It, and How Is It Related to Disordered Eating Behaviors?" *Appetite* 60, no. 1 (January 1, 2013): 13. doi: 10.1016/j.appet.2012.09.029.

15. Evelyn Tribole, "Intuitive Eating in the Treatment of Eating Disorders: The Journey of Attunement," *Perspectives*, Winter 2010, 12. Available at www.evelyntribole.com/resources/eating-disorders.

16. Jean L. Kristeller and Ruth Q. Wolever, "Mindfulness-Based Eating Awareness Training for Treating Binge Eating Disorder: The Conceptual Foundation," *Eating Disorders: The Journal of Treatment & Prevention* 19, no. 1 (January 2011): 49. doi: 10.1080/10640266.2011.533605.

17. Spryliving.com, "The Mindful Eating Marathon" (infographic), 26.2 Mindful Eating Tips! March 18, 2013, eatingmindfully.com/tools/26-2-mindful-eating-marathon-tips (accessed July 2013).

18. F.E.A.S.T., "Relapse," Eating Disorders Glossary, glossary.feast-ed.org/5-psychology-and-therapies/relapse (accessed August 12, 2013).

19. "Liza," personal communication, October 1986.

20. APA Practice Guidelines, "Treatment of Patients with Eating Disorders."

21. James I. Hudson, Eva Hiripi, Harrison G. Pope Jr., and Ronald C. Kessler, "The Prevalence and Correlates of Eating Disorders in the National Comorbidity Survey Replication," *Biological Psychiatry* 61, no. 3 (February 2007): 348–358. doi: 10.1016/j.biopsych.2006.03.040.

22. sztt, reader comment, March 11, 2011, to Renee Michael, "Health at Every Size?" *The 6th Floor: Eavesdropping on the Times Magazine* (blog), March 9, 2011, 6thfloor.blogs.nytimes.com/2011/03/09/health-at-every-size (accessed August 2013).

23. Margaret Marshall, "Embracing a Future of Giant Chocolate Chip Cookies" (audio clip), in "The Voices of Eating Disorders," *Well* (*New York Times* blog), by Tara Parker-Pope with

Karen Barrow, October 15, 2008, www.nytimes.com/interactive/2008/10/14/health/health guide/TE_EATINGDISORDERS_CLIPS.html (accessed August 2013).

24. Emily Hertz, "A Hard Climb Back to Health" (audio clip), in "The Voices of Eating Disorders" by Parker-Pope with Barrow.

25. Asha Brown, "There Is Always Hope!" National Eating Disorders Association (NEDA)—Stories of Hope, www.nationaleatingdisorders.org/node/915 (accessed August 2013).

26. "Rickywayne/Jessica (Texas)," *Heavy*, season 1, episode 2, January 24, 2011, A&E TV Networks, www.aetv.com/heavy/episode-guide.

27. Ericka Christina, "Learning How to Live Wholeheartedly," NEDA—Stories of Hope, www.nationaleatingdisorders.org/node/2762 (accessed August 2013).

28. L., "I Feel Like I'm Becoming the Person I Really Am," F.E.A.S.T.—Patient Letters, December 14, 2010, feast-ed.org/Members/PatientsSpeak/Patientspeak488.aspx (accessed August 2013).

29. Becky, "Becky's Recovery," The Joy Project, July 5, 2011, joyproject.org/580/beckys-recovery (accessed August 2013).

30. "Hannah," "Who Am I—a Recovery Essay," F.E.A.S.T—Patient Letters, August 31, 2011, feast-ed.org/Members/PatientsSpeak/patientWhoamIarecoveryessay.aspx (accessed August 2013).

31. Justin Shamoun, "Who Says You Have to Be Defined by Your Eating Disorder?" NEDA—Stories of Hope, www.nationaleatingdisorders.org/node/3195 (accessed August 2013).

32. Holly Alastra, "The Power of Forgiveness," Eating Disorders Resource Catalogue—Recovery, www.edcatalogue.com/stories-recovery/ (accessed August 2013).

---

a. Johanna S. Kandel, *Life Beyond Your Eating Disorder: Reclaim Yourself, Regain Your Health, Recover for Good* (Toronto, Ontario, Canada: Harlequin, 2010), 16.

b. Rick Nauert, "Estrogen Therapy Can Help Girls with Anorexia," PsychCentral, News, June 19, 2013, psychcentral.com/news/2013/06/19/estrogen-therapy-can-help-girls-with-anorexia/56242.html (accessed July 2013).

c. Zach Johnson, "Demi Lovato: I Finally Feel Like a Role Model," *US Weekly*, September 23, 2013, www.usmagazine.com/celebrity-news/news/demi-lovato-i-finally-feel-like-a-role-model-2011239 (accessed July 2013).

d. Raechal Leone Shewfelt, "Demi Lovato: I Still Struggle with Cutting, Bulimia," *Yahoo! Celebrity*, OMG Crush, March 7, 2012, celebrity.yahoo.com/blogs/crush/demi-lovato-still-struggle-cutting-eating-disorders-222223700.html (accessed May 2013).

e. "Demi Lovato, SAMHSA to Highlight New Strategies Proven to Help Young Adults with Mental Health and Substance Use Challenges" (press release), *Reuters Newswire*, April 29, 2013, www.reuters.com/article/2013/04/29/samhsa-lovato-idUSnPNDC02890+1e0+PRN20130429 (accessed May 2013).

f. Michael Cartwright with Ken Abraham, *Believable Hope: Five Essential Elements to Beat Any Addiction* (Deerfield Beach, Fla.: Health Communications, 2012), 80.

g. Cheryl Kerrigan, *Telling Ed No! and Other Practical Tools to Conquer Your Eating Disorder and Find Freedom* (Carlsbad, Calif.: Gürze Books, 2011), 182.

h. Carolyn Jennings, "Hunger Speaks," NEDA—Stories of Hope, www.nationaleatingdisorders.org/stories-of-hope/hunger-speaks-carolyn-jennings.

i. Carolyn Jennings, "Writing Can't Help My Recovery (or Can It?)," *Writing for Recovery Blog Series: A Guide to Journaling and Self-Discovery*, National Eating Disorders Association, May 31, 2013, www.nationaleatingdisorders.org/writing-cant-help-my-recovery-or-can-it.

j.   Carolyn Jennings, personal communication, September 3, 2013.

k.   Health at Every Size®, home page, www.haescommunity.org.

l.   Linda Bacon and Lucy Aphramor, "Weight Science: Evaluating the Evidence for a Paradigm Shift," *Nutrition Journal* 10, no. 9 (January 24, 2011), 1. doi:10.1186/1475-2891-10-9.

m.   EE, reader comment, March 10, 2011, to Renee Michael, "Health at Every Size?" *The 6th Floor: Eavesdropping on the Times Magazine* (blog), March 9, 2011, 6thfloor.blogs.nytimes .com/2011/03/09/health-at-every-size (accessed August 2013).

n.   Ginny Graves, "Health Controversy: Can You Be Fat and Healthy?" *Glamour*, Health & Diet, February 2012, www.glamour.com/health-fitness/2012/02/health-controversy-can-you-be -fat-and-healthy (May 2013).

o.   Kerrigan, *Telling Ed No!* , 106.

p.   Ruth (the author), August 21, 2013.

q.   *Seane Corn, Yoga from the Heart, Live at the San Francisco Conference* (exercise DVD, 132 minutes), Great Instructors Series from *Yoga Journal,* a production of *Yoga Journal* and Active Interest Media, 2007.

r.   CASAColumbia, *Food for Thought: Substance Abuse and Eating Disorders* (New York: National Center on Addiction and Substance Abuse at Columbia University), ii.

s.   Carolyn Cochran, Robert Malcolm, and Timothy Brewerton, "The Role of Weight Control as a Motivation for Cocaine Abuse," *Addictive Behaviors* 23, no. 2 (March–April 1998): 201. dx.doi.org/10.1016/S0306-4603(97)00046-4.

t.   Elizabeth Day, "Growing Up with My Sister, Amy Winehouse," *Observer* (the online magazine of the *Guardian*), June 22, 2013, www.theguardian.com/music/2013/jun/23/amy -winehouse-growing-up-sister (accessed August 2013).

u.   Janis Whitlock, "What Is Self-Injury?" (fact sheet), Cornell Research Program on Self-Injurious Behavior in Adolescents and Young Adults, 2010, 1. Available at www.selfinjury .bctr.cornell.edu/documents/what-is-self-injury.pdf.

v.   Rebecka Peebles, Jenny L. Wilson, and James D. Lock, "Self-Injury in Adolescents with Eating Disorders: Correlates and Provider Bias," *Journal of Adolescent Health* 48, no. 3 (March 2011): 310. doi: 10.1016/j.jadohealth.2010.06.017.

w.   Mary, "Mary," in *Thin*, by Lauren Greenfield (San Francisco: Chronicle Books with Melcher Media, 2006), 104.

Epilogue

1.   L., "I Feel Like I'm Becoming the Person I Really Am," F.E.A.S.T. (Families Empowered and Supporting Treatment of Eating Disorders)—Patient Letters, December 14, 2010, December 14, 2010, feast-ed.org/Members/PatientsSpeak/Patientspeak488.aspx (accessed August 2013).

2.   Carolyn Costin, *100 Questions about Eating Disorders* (Burlington, Mass.: Jones and Bartlett, 2007), 164.

3.   Theodora Aggeles, "Pinellas Teen Organizes Tampa Walk for Eating Disorders Awareness," *Tampa Bay* (formerly *St. Petersburg*) *Times*, November 26, 2010, www.tampabay.com/news/ humaninterest/pinellas-teen-organizes-tampa-walk-for-eating-disorders-awareness/1136648 (accessed February 2013).

4.   Anna North, "Are Parents the Real Cure for Eating Disorders?" *Jezebel*, August 16, 2010, jezebel.com/5613978/are-parents-the-real-cure-for-eating-disorders (accessed July 2013).

5. Portia de Rossi, *Unbearable Lightness: A Story of Loss and Gain* (New York: Atria, 2010), 287.

6. Jenni Schaefer, "Who Am I without Ed?" (video clip), Jenni Schaefer—Resources, 2013, www.jennischaefer.com/resources/#videos (accessed August 2013).

---

a. In October 2013, the Cohns transferred ownership of the Gürze Eating Disorders Resource Catalogue to Kathryn and Michael Cortese. Gürze-Salucore now takes care of compiling the catalogue and operating its website. Lindsay and Leigh are enjoying a well-deserved semi-retirement, but remain active in the communities they created. Learn more at www.gurzebooks.com/about.html.

Index

About the Author

Jessica Ruth Greene lives a lucky writer's life near the west central Florida coast, where she practices yoga, pitches in at her community radio station, and feeds whoever happens to drop by for dinner. You can contact her at jessicaruth .writes@yahoo.com.